Introduction to Concept Mapping in Nursing

in Nursing

CRITICAL THINKING IN ACTION

THE PEDAGOGY

Introduction to Concept Mapping in Nursing drives comprehension through various strategies that meet the learning needs of students, while also generating enthusiasm about the topic. This interactive approach addresses different learning styles, making this the ideal text to ensure mastery of key concepts. The pedagogical aids that appear in most chapters include the following:

Key Terms

Found in a list at the beginning of each chapter, these terms will create an expanded vocabulary. Students can use the text's online resources to see these terms in an interactive glossary and use flashcards to nail the definitions. Use the access code at the front of your book to access these additional resources.

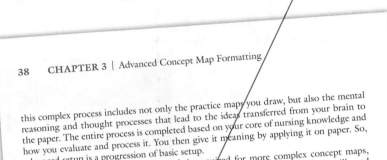

this complex process includes not only the practice maps you draw, but also the mental reasoning and thought processes that lead to the ideas transferred from your brain to the paper. The entire process is completed based on your core of nursing knowledge and how you evaluate and process it. You then give it meaning by applying it on paper. So, advanced setup is a progression of basic setup.

Because a more advanced approach is required for more complex concept maps, these maps are usually more expansive and complex. Your thought processes will need to be more advanced and refined as well. This chapter will lead you on a deeper path of questioning so that you can arrive at a destination of meaningful learning. This is critical thinking in action, and the results you see are what you put into expanding and honing it.

Key Terms and Definitions

- **Advanced concept map setup:** an extension of basic concept map setup where shape and color differentiation are utilized to refine the map for translation and readability
- **Concept map key:** a coded guide to color and shape included on the map to aid in interpretation
- **Uniformity** (as it applies to concept maps): selective use of shapes and colors with the advanced setup of a concept map
- **Concept map clarity:** the ability to interpret and follow the path of a concept map
- **Practice reflection:** the continuous and ongoing action of evaluating nursing knowledge and its application to refine and expand

Advanced Concept Map Setup

For use within nursing education, concept maps can become extremely detailed and large. If advanced formatting techniques are not employed, map information becomes crowded, difficult to interpret or read, and not very meaningful. Living concept maps focusing on nursing actions can become very expansive and contain a host of related concepts. A lack of utilized strategies to define, refine, and clarify all of them leads to a chaotic appearing map that is difficult to read, let alone learn from. Completing concept maps is not done to demonstrate solely what we know, but to help us to reflect on our knowledge base and the critical thinking abilities we are using to apply it. **Practice reflection** is the necessary act of evaluating and reevaluating what we know and how effectively we know it. **Advanced concept map setup** requires that reflective process for creating thorough and complete concept maps and allows us to assess and evaluate that knowledge simultaneously.

Because our goal for employing concept maps in nursing education is to promote and achieve strong critical thinking skills, we need to ensure that this is the purpose they serve. Creation, setup, and reflection of a completed concept map reinforce knowledge, critical thinking, and the analytical process of learning for application. The components of advanced setup are highlighted as follows.

Objectives

These objectives provide instructors and students with a snapshot of the key information they will encounter in each chapter. They serve as a checklist to help guide and focus study. Objectives can also be found within the text's online resources.

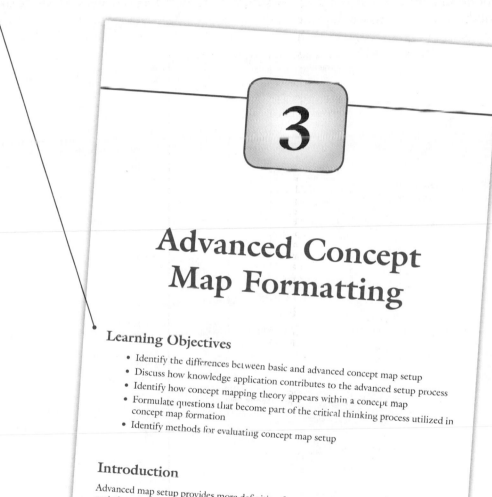

3

Advanced Concept Map Formatting

Learning Objectives

- Identify the differences between basic and advanced concept map setup
- Discuss how knowledge application contributes to the advanced setup process
- Identify how concept mapping theory appears within a concept map
- Formulate questions that become part of the critical thinking process utilized in concept map formation
- Identify methods for evaluating concept map setup

Introduction

Advanced map setup provides more definition for concept maps. It is essential for differentiation of concepts in a complex, living map. This process is very similar to the approach an artist takes when creating a painting. First come the thoughts and ideas of the painting's subject. Whether in thought or on paper, the artist begins to sketch a basic idea, followed by a simple rendering. Once that is achieved, in-depth consideration is given to dimensions, colors, and placement. Artistic expression is used to refine and tease out the specifics needed to perfect the final finished product.

When you create a map, you are that artist. Basic map setup is the rendering you create to "sketch" the path you want your map to take. It is important to realize that

Critical Thinking Activities

Students can work on these critical thinking assignments individually or in a group while reading through the text. Students can delve deeper into concepts by completing these exercises online.

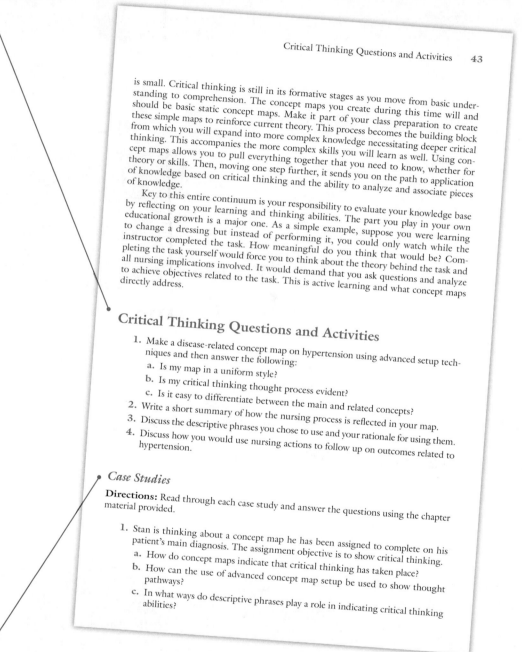

is small. Critical thinking is still in its formative stages as you move from basic understanding to comprehension. The concept maps you create during this time will and should be basic static concept maps. Make it part of your class preparation to create these simple maps to reinforce current theory. This process becomes the building block from which you will expand into more complex knowledge necessitating deeper critical thinking. This accompanies the more complex skills you will learn as well. Using concept maps allows you to pull everything together that you need to know, whether for theory or skills. Then, moving one step further, it sends you on the path to application of knowledge based on critical thinking and the ability to analyze and associate pieces of knowledge.

Key to this entire continuum is your responsibility to evaluate your knowledge base by reflecting on your learning and thinking abilities. The part you play in your own educational growth is a major one. As a simple example, suppose you were learning to change a dressing but instead of performing it, you could only watch while the instructor completed the task. How meaningful do you think that would be? Completing the task yourself would force you to think about the theory behind the task and all nursing implications involved. It would demand that you ask questions and analyze to achieve objectives related to the task. This is active learning and what concept maps directly address.

Critical Thinking Questions and Activities

1. Make a disease-related concept map on hypertension using advanced setup techniques and then answer the following:
   a. Is my map in a uniform style?
   b. Is my critical thinking thought process evident?
   c. Is it easy to differentiate between the main and related concepts?
2. Write a short summary of how the nursing process is reflected in your map.
3. Discuss the descriptive phrases you chose to use and your rationale for using them.
4. Discuss how you would use nursing actions to follow up on outcomes related to hypertension.

Case Studies

Directions: Read through each case study and answer the questions using the chapter material provided.

1. Stan is thinking about a concept map he has been assigned to complete on his patient's main diagnosis. The assignment objective is to show critical thinking.
   a. How do concept maps indicate that critical thinking has taken place?
   b. How can the use of advanced concept map setup be used to show thought pathways?
   c. In what ways do descriptive phrases play a role in indicating critical thinking abilities?

Case Studies

Case studies allow students to read and analyze real-life situations and apply what they have learned. They can be completed and submitted online.

Redeem the access code at the front of your book at www.jblearning.com. If you do not have an access code, one can be purchased at the site.

Introduction to Concept Mapping in Nursing

CRITICAL THINKING IN ACTION

Patricia Schmehl, MSN, RN
Faculty
Reading Area Community College
Reading, Pennsylvania

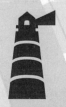

JONES & BARTLETT
LEARNING

World Headquarters
Jones & Bartlett Learning
5 Wall Street
Burlington, MA 01803
978-443-5000
info@jblearning.com
www.jblearning.com

Jones & Bartlett Learning books and products are available through most bookstores and online booksellers.
To contact Jones & Bartlett Learning directly, call 800-832-0034, fax 978-443-8000, or visit our website, www.jblearning.com.

Substantial discounts on bulk quantities of Jones & Bartlett Learning publications are available to corporations, professional associations, and other qualified organizations. For details and specific discount information, contact the special sales department at Jones & Bartlett Learning via the above contact information or send an email to specialsales@jblearning.com.

Production Credits

Executive Publisher: Kevin Sullivan
Acquisitions Editor: Amanda Harvey
Editorial Assistant: Rebecca Myrick
Production Editor: Amanda Clerkin
V.P., Manufacturing and Inventory Control: Therese Connell
Composition: Publishers' Design and Production Services, Inc.
Cover Design: Kristin E. Parker
Cover Image: © Petr Vaclavek/ShutterStock, Inc.
Printing and Binding: Edwards Brothers Malloy
Cover Printing: Edwards Brothers Malloy

To order this product, use ISBN: 978-1-4496-9879-9

Library of Congress Cataloging-in-Publication Data
Schmehl, Patricia.
  Introduction to concept mapping in nursing: critical thinking in action / Patricia Schmehl.
    p. ; cm.
  Includes bibliographical references and index.
  ISBN 978-1-4496-7900-2 (alk. paper)
  I. Title.
  [DNLM: 1. Education, Nursing—methods. 2. Concept Formation. 3. Learning. 4. Models, Nursing.
5. Nursing Theory. 6. Teaching—methods. WY 18]
  610.73—dc23
                                                    2012025794

6048

Printed in the United States of America
17 16 15 14 13   10 9 8 7 6 5 4 3 2 1

Contents

Introduction

A Note to Educators and Students

As a nurse educator I have discovered that a major goal of entry level nursing programs is to prepare nursing students who are confident and secure in the base knowledge and skills necessary to allow them to "hit the ground running" as new graduates. This presents the nursing educational community with a great challenge in that our student population is more nontraditional and diverse than ever before. Cultural and language diversity is a concern as well. We have to ask ourselves how we can provide the curricula and educational environment that will meet our students' needs, as well as the aforementioned goals.

Two of the most important concepts at the core of this process are critical thinking and the ability to apply theory to practice. These two concepts are interdependent and must be cultivated as each student travels the path from novice to the advanced beginner, prepared to begin independent practice. Successful practice and the assurance of quality standards of care in nursing practice cannot exist without the development of both, and our educational efforts must be strongly focused here.

Nursing faculty must also be cognizant of learning styles and the key role they play, not just in theory presentation, but also in a student's ability to move past simple learning to full comprehension and application. Creative strategies blended with approaches catering to each learning style are integral to this process. Effective teaching in this way fosters critical thinking with the result of enhanced knowledge application. Each concept blends with and touches on the other, yielding optimal educational outcomes. Concept mapping itself is part of this entire process.

As a nursing student, use of concept mapping theory is a key component in achieving performance goals as a graduate nurse. The reason for this is that it assists in building the base of knowledge so crucial to maintaining practice standards, as well as building the critical thinking skills to then apply that knowledge. In short, the use of concept mapping theory provides students with an opportunity to take learned theory and use it clinically. Cultivating nursing knowledge is all about building knowledge. Perhaps even as important, it is also about how that knowledge is used. Every piece of nursing theory has a place in application at the bedside. Concept mapping allows you to evaluate how sound that base of knowledge is and how effectively it is being applied. In this way it assists students in goal setting and self-evaluative practice reflection so essential to growth. A student's use of concept mapping in both learning and studying will yield positive results in critical thinking enhancement and knowledge application. The practice opens up wondrous possibilities of methods for relating and establishing relationships among concepts and helps students make sense of what "thinking like a nurse" is all about. In essence, it gives meaning to the role and actions of the nurse.

The purpose of this book is to lead faculty and students on a journey to optimal learning outcomes through the use of concept mapping in nursing education. Along the way, critical thinking and knowledge application skills will progress, be integrated into the maps, and allow for an assessment of both skills by faculty as well as students. This applies to classroom as well as clinical knowledge. You will begin to follow a student's progress as each map charts his or her thought processes related to critical thinking and knowledge application.

An important part of this journey is for students to reflect on their own progress, along with faculty feedback. Reflection is an essential part of critical thinking, enabling a student to be honest in self-appraisal. Each and every student plays an important role in his or her own success.

Concept mapping will meet the educational needs of all students, regardless of backgrounds or learning styles or the educational goals of faculty. As you will also see, the ways in which this process can be utilized are endless and limited only to your imagination. And so, let the journey begin. Follow me.

1

Understanding Concept Mapping

Learning Objectives

- Define concept mapping theory
- Identify the components of concept mapping theory
- Demonstrate how each component can be integrated into nursing education
- Explore how learning styles affect critical thinking
- Demonstrate and discuss how relationship analysis and critical thinking are integral to theory application
- Explain how learning styles and brain processing contribute to learning success
- Discuss the implications and impact of utilizing concept mapping to improve knowledge application
- Reflect on how past utilization of concept mapping has led to its application within nursing education
- Discuss and consider future implications and application of concept mapping in nursing

Introduction

The purpose of this first chapter is to introduce you to what concept mapping is. Every student's knowledge and perception of concept mapping is a little different. Within this chapter you will find answers to the questions you may have and be able to explore concept mapping theory and how it leads to meaningful learning and contributes to a completed concept map. A stepwise process that views the overall theory in addition to the separate segments will open your eyes to a whole other method of integrating meaning into all nursing knowledge. This information will redefine how you study, learn, and apply nursing knowledge. Whether you are a beginner, first-year student, or further along in the educational process, your critical thinking abilities will expand as you integrate this theory into your education. You will learn that asking questions that lead to more questions is not an exercise in frustration, but a sign of critical thinking growth. As your critical thinking skills deepen and grow, the answers will come, your confidence will grow, and you will feel a sense of satisfaction.

All nursing knowledge is based on a continuum from simple to complex. As you progress from the starting point and continue to the end point of graduation, more is demanded from you in terms of the knowledge base you must cultivate as well as the amount and type of knowledge you must apply in caring for patients. You will come to realize how concepts such as learning domains and learning styles strongly affect learning outcomes. As you read through this chapter, your goal should be to reflect on what you are learning and how you can implement that new knowledge to enhance your nursing education.

Although this book is directed at you, the nursing students, there are some sections in this first chapter that may address educational approaches. This allows you to see your education from a faculty perspective as well.

Before going further, we need to explore some of the terminology that will help explain some of the key concepts or thought processes used in the creation of and reflected within a completed map. Understanding those thought processes serves as the foundation of understanding actual map construction. These terms reflect the educational focus of a concept map and mapping theory.

Key Terms and Definitions

- **Critical thinking:** an in-depth thought process utilizing multiple information resources to question, make associations, and analyze data to form conclusions and consider actions and outcomes
- **Relationship analysis:** the process of comparing and contrasting concepts to make associations; interpreting similarities and differences between and among concepts, which allows for comprehensive learning
- **Theory-to-practice application:** the action of establishing a knowledge base and enabling utilization of that knowledge to enact practice decisions; providing rationales for decision making in practice
- **Learning styles:** methods through which one is able to effectively comprehend theory for meaningful learning from input related to aural, verbal, written, or visual information

- **Brain processing:** the brain's ability to accept, categorize, create associations, process, and give meaning and understanding to knowledge input
- **Learning domains:** categories of learning skills, behaviors, and outcomes a student must master within the continuum of learning, from simple to complex, comprising the cognitive, affective, and psychomotor spheres

Critical Thinking

Concept mapping, as it is used in nursing, serves as a pathway to the intersection of critical thinking and theory-to-practice application. To become a successful critical thinker in nursing, one has to be able to apply that thinking to nursing care. It is not enough to know about the pathophysiology of a disease process as stated in a textbook, or the steps followed through when performing a skill. As nurses we have to open up our minds and ask the "why" and "what else" questions that allow us to form a patient problem list, which then becomes the basis for our nursing actions. Yet, effective critical thinking is necessary for effective application, so both of those concepts are interrelated and very much interdependent, and serve as the basis of acceptable practice standards. A completed concept map provides a direct, real-time view of a nurse's thought processes. It allows both the educator and the learner to assess critical thinking abilities and the degree to which theory is being applied to practice. This is the basis of concept map theory.

Critical thinking has many definitions, and no single formal version has been accepted. It is generally defined as a higher level thinking that questions associations, the concepts of cause and effect, and judgment. It is often referred to as thinking about thinking. I like to describe critical thinking as a domino-like effect of a student's thought processes where one question stimulates a multitude of others. As this process continues, the questioning may diverge onto a variety of pathways where reasoning, judgment, and prior knowledge all play a part in considering solutions and answers to the questions. The questions are crucial to determine appropriate nursing actions. This process is actually the start of application, but the student may have difficulty recognizing that.

Although critical thinking is emphasized and integrated into nursing education from the very beginning of any nursing program, the largest growth of it usually occurs in higher educational levels when a student has cultivated a large base knowledge inventory and can now think about applying that to new knowledge in the classroom, as well as within the clinical setting.

In nursing education, the development and growth of critical thinking is necessary because it allows you, the student, to begin asking questions and making associations. Challenging yourself to question and make associations early on not only puts you on a quest for more knowledge but also allows you to gain confidence as your abilities deepen. Deeper critical thinking leads to improved decision making. Although this process begins in the classroom and the nursing lab, it quickly transitions to the clinical area and helps to lay the foundation of theory-to-practice application. Encouraging the process allows students to take an active role in their own learning.

One example of this would be when you question the difference between the textbook presentation of a disease process versus how it actually presents in a patient. For most students this is the first tentative step into the world of critical thinking. A book or lecture presents concrete facts in black and white (no pun intended). This is the disease process, this is the list of symptoms and how we address them, and so on. You listen and contemplate, take notes, and study the data presented. Some questions may surface, but until the information can be applied you may be uncertain as to what specific questions to ask. Putting that information together while assessing an actual patient is more than a little intimidating until you have the opportunity to examine, ponder, compare, and contrast. One of the main goals of nursing education must be to foster this process often and in as many ways as possible.

I have found that students realize the need for critical thinking, and have often heard the phrase, but really do not have a full understanding of what it means or how to integrate it into their goals for success. Each nursing program has a responsibility to not only define the term, but to define it for students within the context of each program and course. After all, critical thinking expectations assist in defining competencies, and students need to have full understanding of them if they hope to achieve them. Please do not assume that everyone has a full, comprehensive understanding of what critical thinking is and how it is to be applied. Most nursing student populations need an introduction to the concept, with repeated references and examples throughout the course of their nursing education to be able to fully grasp not only the meaning but also how to use critical thinking in application. A gradual approach is essential, because as the student gains knowledge and reaches the point of readiness for deeper application, questions become more involved, more frequent, and require much more consideration of scope and outcomes. During this phase it is very easy for a student to become overwhelmed. Questions are flowing in many directions, much as ripples in a pond after a stone's throw, and students may not know quite how to handle all of the questions, much less the answers. At this point, realization is dawning regarding responsibilities, independent thinking, and scope of practice. While this is what the faculty wants to see, these realizations can be more than a little overwhelming for students.

Another consideration in a gradual reinforcement of critical thinking theory and skill sets related to it is that part of the process involves student progression through the various **learning domains**. These domains increase in difficulty from simple knowledge to application and analysis. Each domain demands more knowledge—knowledge that takes on new meaning when combined with that which was previously learned. It also leads to more questioning and in-depth analysis of information, requiring the development of problem-solving skills concurrently with critical thinking skills. Within those categories are contained the various behaviors affecting learning. The three areas are: cognitive, affective, and psychomotor.

The cognitive sphere equates to knowledge and how it is used. Knowledge gradually progresses from simple memorization to the ability to analyze and apply what is learned. Critical thinking and relationship analysis may not be evident at lower levels on the continuum but should appear when comprehension occurs and continue to grow and expand along with increasing knowledge.

The affective sphere takes into consideration attitudes as part of the learning process and a student's reaction to learning. This may range from simple learning response to the ability to organize information.

Finally, the psychomotor sphere relates to skills in the educational process and how they are used and applied. To better understand this, visualize two paths running side by side. (See **Figure 1-1**.) One path is the continuum of learning domain progression, while the other is the progression of critical thinking abilities. Beginning nursing education is focused on general knowledge and memorization. Critical thinking at this point is focused on learning medical terminology, simple skills, and considerations of what nursing means. It is highly likely that during this phase, students are comparing their nursing education to past educational experiences, realizing the intensity and hard work needed to reach their goals. It is a time of first exposure to nursing theories and the foundation that will lead to comprehension. This phase would occur during the early portion of their first year of learning. Later on in that year, students will begin to amass more knowledge and begin to be able to consider associations. At this point, these associations would be along the lines of comparing proper steps in completing a procedure with omitted or incorrect steps; they are discovering what they do and do not know about how everything fits together. And so it goes as students travel the path from basic knowledge to application.

It is important to mention here that this process applies to nursing courses in any program type. The pathway described begins with the start of nursing education. Prior to that time, the presence and level of preexisting critical thinking abilities are highly individualized and dependent upon many factors and influences. For many students in either 4-year or community colleges, it is presumed that critical thinking as it applies to higher education is promoted and fostered early on. Thus, it would seem that a student should have some perception of and insight into these skills, but as we have discussed, that is not often the case. While I believe nursing is ahead of the game in this respect, nurse educators cannot lose sight of the fact that not every student comes into a nursing program with advanced critical thinking skills.

From all of this, I think it is easy to see several things. First, critical thinking does not occur in isolation and definitely includes the types of thought processes that lead to further investigation of associations and comparisons. Secondly, critical thinking as a part of nursing actions is a fact of nursing life, and its foundations are laid in nursing education. The way in which both students and faculty lay that foundation determines future successful practice. In fact, it is one of the cornerstones of all nursing practice. Finally, gradual integration serves as the most reliable method for meaningful application of critical thinking.

Figure 1-1 Learning domain and critical thinking ability progression.

Introduction/ Exposure	Beginning Comprehension	Advanced Comprehension/ Review	Application
Basic learning & memorization	Limited associations & comparisons/ questioning	Increased questioning, awareness of nursing actions	Critical thinking integration into all skills/actions
Critical Thinking Ability Progression		Integrated relationship analysis	Scope of practice awareness

Relationship Analysis

Relationship analysis may be a separate process within critical thinking, but as mentioned earlier, it is also an extension of critical thinking itself. The term refers to being able to see not only how concepts are associated, but also how they affect each other—questioning associations, outcomes, and actions. If this all sounds familiar, it is because it is closely aligned with what we know as the nursing process. It is also a necessary thought process that must be present for critical thinking to occur. For instance, we could read a paragraph on some type of pathophysiology. If we failed to link its meaning to nursing practice, what critical thinking could occur? Facts taken in isolation do not stimulate or allow for critical thinking. Relationship analysis translates into action—action in thought, reasoning, and judgment related to comparing and contrasting information. Basic relationship analysis occurs when, as a student begins the clinical experience, questions arise comparing theory on disease pathophysiology with the actual manifestations of it in a patient. The clinical experience is also the catalyst for comparing expectations with reality as far as skills and nursing actions are concerned. For example, taking a blood pressure appears to be a fairly simple and straightforward procedure. In the clinical setting, however, other considerations become important to completing the skill, such as cuff placement, prohibited use of an extremity, and equipment accuracy. So, the process is much deeper than simply comparing and contrasting. See **Figure 1-2** for a perspective on questions related to relationship analysis and how they meld with the critical thinking process. It is about examining all the related concepts, establishing associations, and categorizing. Beyond that, it is about taking that information and adding in meaningful learning that leads eventually to application. In many ways, this process of looking at relationships also involves troubleshooting, because the student learns a great deal about practice standards, therapeutic communication, safety, and scope of practice. The act of comparing also considers what is right about what they are doing and what is not. This may seem to be a different way of looking at this process but think about it: Critical thinking and all its components are integral to nursing practice. Because our practice translates into actions and those actions in turn define our practice, it all fits. Relationship analysis emphasizes the interdependence of information on actions and outcomes. This point is where the process begins to involve application.

The process is analogous to putting together a puzzle. Information is gathered, clustered, and separated into categories as needed until relationships appear. Learning that nothing is static in nursing is something I continually stress to students. While they may tire of hearing me say it, it is a statement that sums up concept mapping theory and is essential to the transition from learning to application. For instance, students learn early on in nursing theory that when a disease occurs in one body system, there are repercussions and manifestations in another. This is an early introduction to relationship analysis.

Another way in which relationship analysis is applied in nursing is when associations are made between a patient's diagnosis and abnormal laboratory or diagnostic test results. It is part of higher level thought processes and demonstrates a student's critical thinking abilities. I have seen that many students have difficulty making these associations, especially as they transition from the first year of nursing education to the second. It is not that students are unaware of these associations, but rather that they must condition themselves to think in a detailed way that allows for active thought processes involving relationship analysis. In any program, much more is expected from students in the second year, and rightly so. However, we have to remember that critical thinking growth, with

Figure 1-2 Analysis questions.

Topic	Analysis Questions
Assessment Finding	What meaning does this finding have as part of the patient's disease process?
	Is this finding a new one or "normal" for this patient?
	Does this finding necessitate any nursing actions at this time?
	Is there a difference between the textbook and what I am seeing?
	Does this finding indicate that my patient may be decompensating?
Skill	What factors must be considered to safely complete this skill?
	How should I proceed if something unexpected occurs?
	What nursing actions must occur after the skill is completed?
	Have I checked the physician's order prior to proceeding if necessary?
	What resources can be used to review this skill before proceeding?
Treatment	Why am I using these products to treat this wound?
	What documentation goes along with this type of treatment?
	What supplies are needed and where do I locate them?
	Have I educated my patient on how the treatment will be carried out?
	What follow-up care or action is necessary after completing the treatment?

relationship analysis as part of that, is honed gradually and incrementally. Identifying this process and introducing it early on in nursing education, as well as utilizing concept mapping to demonstrate it (both in lecture as well as clinically), allow for maximum achievement and competency.

It is also important to realize that this process applies to what students already know, compared to what they have yet to learn. While this may be obvious to educators, it is usually not so clear to students, especially those who are on the early pathway of nursing education. Often, students see what they have already learned as "old" material. You must not miss the important point that all nursing education already learned serves as building blocks and the foundation for future application. In any type of nursing program, there is a certain time lapse before this idea is firmly integrated. In fact, it may not totally "click" until the second year. I have had students tell me that they "shelved" previously learned information because they were not "using it!" I think it is extremely important to emphasize from day one that all information is relevant, necessary, and will need to be recalled in the future.

In summary, this process may find its beginnings in classroom theory but quickly extends into clinical practice and occurs in an incremental fashion. First, a student learns how to compare normal and abnormal assessment findings. This is often the focus in the first 2 years of nursing education, regardless of the type of program. As the student continues on the path of learning, other concepts are layered in and the process becomes more complex. The student recognizes the implications that diagnostic testing, laboratory testing, and medication effects have on nursing action and patient outcomes. This is the time when the student begins to truly realize and appreciate the nursing role: recognizing the full responsibility, scope of practice, and knowledge base needed to practice at appropriate and acceptable standards. It is important for nursing faculty to realize that this analytical ability is directly tied to critical thinking abilities. Educational goals must be focused on an incremental approach throughout the program.

Concept maps have a strong focus on outcomes and actions and lend themselves to use throughout nursing education. This is just a sampling to emphasize how relationship analysis–related thought processes are manifested. You may be able to think of many more related to patient education as well as various other patient care considerations. The meaning behind these questions is that a student asking or demonstrating them has progressed to the point where actions, responsibility for those actions, and outcomes are now being considered. Essentially, they mean that the student is already applying knowledge and critical thinking but may not recognize it. I say that because it is clear that some of the questions are simple, while others are more complex.

Theory-to-Practice Application

Theory-to-practice application is the ability of students to take what they have learned in the classroom and give it meaning at the patient's bedside. Sure, they may know what a rale is, but do they know what it means when they hear it? Do they know why it is present? How does it fit in with the patient's diagnoses? These and other similar questions, as we have seen, are all part of critical thinking and relationship analysis. Thinking critically is the jumping off point to students' realizations that more information is needed and, subsequently, that this information has meaning within the nursing process; it determines what assessments mean, why certain medications are needed, how laboratory and diagnostic tests fit into the equation, and, ultimately, what outcomes are desired. The realization that more information is needed is a big step forward in a student's growth on that pathway to advanced beginner. It is the point at which "everything clicks," and the light bulb goes on. From the foundational knowledge laid with previous education stems the essential components related to achieving application—knowledge of necessary nursing actions and outcomes determined through evaluating, revising, and implementing the plan of care; identifying abnormal findings; and following up to complete the process.

The ultimate goal of theory application to actual patient care is putting both critical thinking and relationship analysis into motion as nursing actions when planning the patient's care—not just the established plan, but the continual plan of care that changes along with the patient's condition and needs. It is ever changing, depending upon patient responses to treatment, new problems appearing during care, and so forth. This would also include, as stated earlier, a patient's holistic safety and communication needs, coexistent with any advocacy needs. This is what I like to call "the whole package." Remember, though, that on a continuum of learning this process is active and needs to be encouraged and stimulated from the beginning of nursing education.

I have found that if I lecture on this and use the phrase *theory-to-practice application*, students may not be able to grasp its meaning. I need to give examples and explain in detail what I mean and how they will carry it out. In their eyes it does not translate into an action, but a thought process. We are talking about second-year students here. They may have adequate base knowledge, but little understanding of how to utilize all that has been learned. While it comprises both of those things, educators must place a strong emphasis on the *action* part. Let's look at an example to better illustrate this process.

Suppose a student is assigned to a patient with chronic obstructive pulmonary disease (COPD). While the student may have some understanding of the disease process, he or she needs an awareness of how to plan care for that person related to nursing actions, follow up, and outcomes. At this point, questions must be introduced to spark that thinking process. Let's look at how a question-and-answer session could be used:

Q: What factors should be considered besides knowing what COPD is and how its pathophysiology occurs?

A: Before going into the patient's room, think about what this patient will look like. What might be different with his coloring, posture, overall appearance? How would this compare to what your book tells you?

Q: What other information would you need to help you care for this patient and where can you find that information?

A: It would be important to be aware of the patient's oxygen saturation via pulse oximetry and that a probe is in fact in place taking continuous measurements. Another consideration would be how the patient tolerates activity. Some questions to ask would be whether or not he uses oxygen at home or just needs it in the hospital. Be aware of the flow rate, assess that it is correct, and be sure it remains on. The patient may be experiencing a related diagnosis, such as pneumonia, which will exacerbate the COPD, so knowledge of chest x-ray results would be important to determine severity and degree of patient compromise. Also, be aware of the oxygen orders. Many times orders are given to titrate the therapy according to the patient's pulse oximetry. You would then need to document this more frequently, as well as the patient's response to the titration.

Q: How is safety in care managed with a patient with this diagnosis?

A: Suppose you enter the room and the patient is attempting to get to the bathroom. He has taken his oxygen off and placed it on the bed. You note moderate dyspnea and dusky nail beds. This now changes your patient's fall risk score, and safety measures should be instituted. If you note confusion, you should place a bed alarm, document the situation, and be sure to follow up with frequent safety checks and subsequent documentation. The patient will need education regarding limited activity restrictions and have the call bell in place to call the nurse when he needs to get out of bed. A urinal positioned where he can reach it would also be appropriate. Reinforcement of that education is important and may be repeated as needed. A focused assessment of the respiratory system would also be in order to help determine why this status change occurred.

Exercises and examples such as this are a wonderful way to get the students thinking. They are also important in helping them to make connections and think on their feet. In many programs, clinical patient assignments cannot be made prior to the clinical day, so students cannot benefit from researching patient-related information. They may have only 20 minutes or so to think about the diagnosis and their plan of care. This can be very stressful for students but at the same time may contribute to a vigilance that assists with raising care standards as far as student scope of practice is concerned. Deep foundational knowledge provides them with the means to look at all factors needed to determine the best, most effective nursing actions, while considering outcomes.

Another tactic that is beneficial to use when presenting this information is to link actions and decision making to the clinical evaluation tool. This reinforces that requirements are not random, but important in achieving competencies. This will also help to reinforce holistic considerations such as cultural and psychosocial factors influencing nursing actions and care-related decisions. Other important areas that can be drawn into this process are that of patient education and how the past medical history impacts the present plan of care. Concept mapping assists in developing thought processes related to critical thinking, knowledge assessment, and relationship analysis in ways that foster application. It is extremely important to recognize and inform the students that they are already aware of many of these processes and may in fact be applying them on a basic level. I am a firm believer in introducing these concepts from the start of nursing education. A gradual integration is less overwhelming and instills the standard for all three processes we have been considering. Including concept mapping theory and basic, static maps early on facilitates these goals. This also helps with underscoring the important fact that nothing learned in nursing education is without value. None of it is old and without later use or application.

One thing I have learned as an educator is that students need constant and continual reinforcement of information. Theory or skill-related presentations may be clear, but students do not have the knowledge base of faculty and are considering a multitude of knowledge facts at any one time. It is very easy for them to become distracted and miss something. Concept maps are tools that can be used to reinforce information along with learning concepts. This is the ultimate goal in nursing education, and it must be aligned with program competencies and can never occur in isolation. Critical thinking and relationship analysis are the building blocks integral to this process. When presenting concept map theory, it is important to mention that all of this content is already being used by students.

A concept map is a physical creation of those thought processes and thus can be used as a gauge of reasoning, judgment, and critical thinking abilities. **Figure 1-3** shows the interrelationships of these terms and concepts. The statement I make most often to

Figure 1-3 **Critical thinking, associations, and comprehension.**

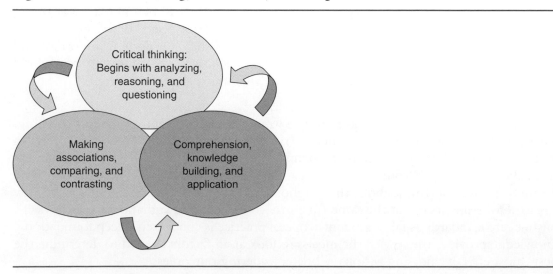

students is, "Nothing is static. What happens in one area of the body invariably affects the other." The same applies to the entire process just described. One thought leads to another, which leads to questions, which leads to actions, and so on.

In practice, this process is ongoing and occurs on a continuum of learning. With reflection and continued repetition, the student is able to progress in knowledge and the ability to apply it. An essential focus in attaining comprehension in learning is repetition and repeated exposure to a topic. Creating concept maps allows a student to see and utilize similar knowledge and application in a repeated pattern.

Figure 1-4 looks at this process in a different way. Figure 1-4a reiterates that, on a continuum of learning, application is the ultimate goal. Figure 1-4b briefly summarizes a student's progression to satisfactory attainment of applied nursing knowledge. It alludes to the progression of novice to advanced beginner and critical thinking thought processes evidenced. It can be applied to any type of registered nurse program of study. No matter the length of a program, the goals and competencies to be satisfied are very similar.

Figure 1-4 (a) The learning continuum; (b) Steps in learning.

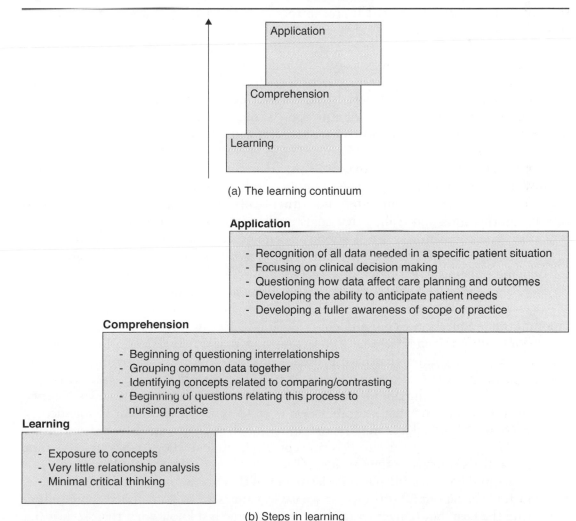

(a) The learning continuum

Application
- Recognition of all data needed in a specific patient situation
- Focusing on clinical decision making
- Questioning how data affect care planning and outcomes
- Developing the ability to anticipate patient needs
- Developing a fuller awareness of scope of practice

Comprehension
- Beginning of questioning interrelationships
- Grouping common data together
- Identifying concepts related to comparing/contrasting
- Beginning of questions relating this process to nursing practice

Learning
- Exposure to concepts
- Very little relationship analysis
- Minimal critical thinking

(b) Steps in learning

Learning Styles

Learning styles are methods through which we are able to learn and comprehend knowledge. Each style has an association with how our brains process incoming information. Without brain processing, we would be able to read a page of type, study a graph, or practice a skill, but never be able to organize, categorize, have memory of, or be able to apply that knowledge.

Much has been written and debated about learning styles. Some experts in education, as well as students, feel the whole concept to be myth rather than fact and that identifying learning styles may lead to labeling and compartmentalizing. In addition, there is no consistent agreement by experts on categories of learning styles, and a wide variety of titles have been assigned with overlapping information from different sources in some cases. I have also found that what can greatly affect these opinions is a student's or educator's perception or idea about what specific method is best regarding both studying and theory presentation to ensure comprehension in learning. Preconceived notions still exist that this method entails hours of reading prior to class, attending class and taking notes, then spending many more hours rereading and studying just from the book and the notes. This is an antiquated approach that does no justice to those who learn best through alternative methods.

Research will yield a variety of results, identified types, and characteristics. See **Figure 1-5** for a brief summary of learning styles. When you do research the various styles, please keep in mind that most of us use a combination of styles. It is also a good idea to research by characteristics rather than labels, because labels may be different in various resources and these terms are not the sole identification of our style of learning. It is much more important to recognize that those characteristics will identify behaviors that are more easily recognized than a one- or two-word label. The instant students see a certain set of behaviors within a style, they may exclaim, "that's me!" This is the jumping off point from which they may now start to look more deeply into how study, class preparation, and note-taking time is spent. They will either realize that they are on the right track or take another look and realize that adjustment is in order. So, it is not about pigeon-holing or labeling as much as it is about academic success within nursing education. I firmly believe that whatever the program, nursing faculty need to take responsibility for introducing learning style theory, even in a small way. It may be true that others know a bit more about it or have the methods and time to explain it more fully; however, we are the ones who can integrate it successfully into nursing curricula for the best results. We tailor all other education to our student populations, so why not this as well?

Having summarized all of that, the fact remains that we do all learn differently and there are research studies that have proven a link between use of learning styles and enhancement in critical thinking abilities; pairing the correct learning style with each student's brain processing abilities equals academic success. Through my own observations, most students find that a combination of styles is actually the best fit for success. In order to provide equal learning opportunities for all students, faculty needs to ensure that each student has exposure to this concept. Each student, then, needs to make time for opportunities to explore the various styles.

I always find it interesting when I ask students if they are aware of their learning style. I usually find that about 50–60% forget what a learning style is, a small percentage admit to hearing the term but remember nothing else, and the rest know what their style is but have never used it to study! The fact is that most, if not all college campuses, introduce

Figure 1-5 Learning styles.

Visual/Seeing	Although a student may comprehend some concepts from reading, the process is greatly enhanced when photos, graphs, and animations are used.
Auditory/Listening	If this is the dominant learning method, taping notes as well as employing other auditory methods, such as an audio book, are keys to enhance learning.
Verbal/Writing	The printed and written word dominates this style so that learners benefit from reading, rereading, and note taking.
Kinesthetic	This is pure "hands on" learning where sensory interaction is necessary to comprehension and application.

this topic early on in college life, yet many students are not using this valuable resource. I have addressed learning styles in my lectures, as a presentation in a remedial nursing course, and within concept mapping presentations and have witnessed student success in enhancement of critical thinking abilities and thus improvement in clinical and academic performance. I issue a challenge to all nurse educators to become more familiar with learning styles, promote student awareness of them, and integrate them into your curricula. Our goal in nursing education is to attain competency in knowledge application, which defines our scope of practice. It is obvious we cannot reach this goal realistically unless we tailor our educational methods to our future nurses. If a student cannot progress from learning to comprehension, then true application is impossible.

Another point to be aware of with learning styles is that using them is not confined to class preparation time. In addition to aiding comprehension and the process of incoming information, learning styles speak to environmental and social factors in learning, as well as study skills. A learning style must be integrated into all parts of learning to be valuable. Note-taking templates may need to be altered to reflect material organization the way a student "sees" it. This may be different from outline formats as well as presentation formats, but it is what will actually be meaningful to the student. Many students do not realize that learning styles also impact studying. Each style has a component of environmental considerations. These include factors related to effective studying such as choosing a quiet environment versus studying in a group. Some students may benefit from background noise while others need extreme quiet. Those students with a tendency toward oral or audio learning styles may find it helpful to read aloud while studying or reviewing taped lectures. In addition, in auditory learning styles comprehension is affected by the tone of emphasis a speaker uses as well as nonverbal communication. When studying, factors such as background noise and the presence of others play key roles in whether effective studying actually occurs. An example I have used is as follows:

> Have you ever read a chapter while studying, only to find yourself reviewing certain portions over and over? Did it seem as though you really weren't retaining anything? More than likely, this occurred because the verbal style of learning is not your dominant style and spinning your wheels using it wasted time and didn't benefit you in the least. Of course, a well rounded knowledge base must be intact before anyone can truly apply a specific style to learning for optimum outcomes. It is very helpful for students to have a

working knowledge of their particular learning style prior to attempting complex, living maps.

In addressing studying, it is also beneficial to emphasize that effective study time is essential for developing a knowledge base within which critical thinking and relationship analysis can occur. One exercise I have used in the past is to have students make a monthly calendar. For each week, three main categories are logged according to hourly increments and color coding. The three main areas are:

1. *Personal time:* This might entail anything from getting a massage or knitting a blanket to having a mammogram.
2. *Family time:* This category may include activities such as taking children to a movie, planning family meals, or spending time with a sibling.
3. *School time:* This area highlights study time allotted related to nursing education.

A student should see a pattern showing that the majority of their time is spent studying. Information gleaned from this activity is valuable as it opens students' eyes to how little they may actually be studying. The color assigned to school time should be seen frequently and take precedence. Adequate time plus effective time equals meaningful study time. Some ground rules for this exercise include that a student must be honest about the data and be willing to use the data as a goal-setting tool for improvement. For instance, sitting with an open book on your lap while watching TV does *not* add up to either effective or adequate study time! Neither does trying to study while eating or making your child's lunch.

I cannot emphasize enough that knowing one's style and employing it in *all* areas of learning are necessary if progression to application can occur. Such multifactorial processes really make effective learning quite a challenge at times, especially when each student learns and processes just a bit differently than the others in a large classroom group, but these multifactorial educational processes are necessary to ensure that all students' needs are met. Although extremely important in theory knowledge, these methods are also integral to skills learning as well.

Learning styles are applied to concept mapping in one way through map formatting. A student will format a map according to how material is processed and organized. In another way, an in-depth knowledge of a learning style allows a student to more easily identify concepts as well as how to organize, cluster, and analyze how all of the pieces fit together. This is in itself an example of comparison/contrast.

Learning Styles and Brain Processing

As we have seen, learning styles are directly related to **brain processing**. A student's map formatting is partially determined through brain processing. While most literature identifies that we definitely use our entire brain for learning and reasoning, one side is usually dominant and determines how we best learn. As you research this topic in more depth, please be aware that this research is ongoing and often updated. The majority of newer research into brain function has shown evidence that both sides of our brains work in harmony to process incoming information from a variety of sources and senses. The bottom line is that brain processing, however it is defined, is very much a key component in each person's learning style and ability to take in and give meaning to learning. Additionally, a student will learn more regarding how creativity plays a role in education along with insight into how they follow directions.

Knowledge of this process becomes very important when maximizing the potential of concept mapping in nursing education because it will tell us how each student categorizes the information provided, which determines how relationship analysis is carried out. This information is also a predictor of how a concept map is set up for optimal learning. For example, when learning about body system pathophysiology, some students look at the main problem (or the whole), before identifying and separating the process into segments for comparison and relationship analysis. Other students may need to identify each segment of the problem and its relationship to the whole before being fully able to consider and understand the pathophysiology. In other words, understanding brain processing aids both faculty and students in the understanding of learning styles, which opens a window directly into our capacity to pass beyond learning to achieve the ultimate goal of applying knowledge. The entire miracle of learning styles and how our brains process input gives great insight into how learning, and subsequently, comprehension and application are allowed to occur. Once again, their labels are not as important as the behavioral characteristics they define. What is far more important is that students' awareness of how their brains work leads to reflection and introspection. An opportunity is also provided for them to take a more active role in successful and meaningful learning. This should serve to generate more knowledge, leading to increased self-confidence. For instance, if a student is performing suboptimally, either clinically or academically, a part of the problem may be stemming from ineffective studying. A student who consistently attempts to learn and study using a style not congruent with their processing is going to spend a great deal more time studying but getting nowhere. While this will not solve every student's learning difficulties, it is definitely worth addressing. Time involved in research may also be a factor, but it is time well spent.

The brain as a whole is able to accept and store information. It is also able to make its own data associations, draw on past experiences, and cluster and/or separate data into categories. Until incoming information is stored, it cannot be truly processed. Both long- and short-term memory are a part of this process. If we were able to look inside our brains and visualize thought processing, it would no doubt appear as a very complex concept map with far-reaching and ever-expanding associations. If you really think about this, the meaning of it all does become clearer. Let's suppose that you are viewing a photograph. Your mind instantly associates the camera that captured the scene, and many memories surrounding it are triggered. Other associations would include emotions, actions, and feelings about the photograph and its subject. How amazing is that? What the mind does with information and how it works is exactly what a concept map is able to demonstrate! Students learn a most valuable lesson about how they think and can actually see it evidenced on paper. What better learning and teaching tool could we possibly have? Insight into learning is a major component of successful education. Concept mapping allows for the mental multitasking essential to brain processing, critical thinking, and application. All of these things are interconnected.

From a nursing perspective, imagine that students are learning about nursing actions associated with the postoperative patient. Once they know that stasis is a major catalyst for postoperative complications, their minds can now create a link between nursing actions that would prevent stasis. Creating nursing actions in the plan of care for mobility, anti-embolism stockings, and sequential compression devices would address stasis of blood; incentive spirometry along with coughing and deep breathing would be necessary for preventing stasis of secretions; and finally, mobility and fluid intake would assist with prevention of urinary stasis. Thinking this plan of care through is necessary, but putting it down as a concept map not only reinforces the ideas but also allows students to visualize their choices and where they may have missed a step. It is a reflection of practice and previously learned information all rolled into one. It is sometimes helpful for students to be able to picture a patient in their minds—either someone they have provided care to or a friend or family member. Along with reflection, this assists with solidifying the information relative to nursing actions and allows for application.

This is how learning styles and effective studying are connected with brain processing and aligned with concept map theory. This fact also demonstrates why simple learning and memorization are inadequate for achieving the ability to apply theory. A student needs to move forward and be able to comprehend, make associations, and develop in-depth critical thinking skills prior to applying.

Now, if we isolate how the left sides of our brains take in information, we could see that if this side dominates, the learner prefers written information for information processing.

Learning through the written and spoken word is orderly, sequential, and logical to these individuals. When analyzing data, they will look at each smaller segment of data affecting the whole before being able to consider or understand the larger process. A more detailed example is this: Suppose a student is going to be learning about renal failure. A dominant left brain processor would read the chapter thoroughly, take notes in an outline form, and focus on the symptoms and abnormal assessment findings before considering and analyzing the type of failure or the specific causes. This is a reality-based approach. When considering nursing actions and problem solving for this patient, these students would consider each problem and how to address each one in turn. Data would be somewhat isolated at first so that this learner could derive meaning from each individual piece. Completing each step allows future consideration of the whole and how all of it fits into the pathophysiology of renal failure. See **Figure 1-6**.

In contrast, right-sided brain processors utilize a more random approach to learning and need specific directions and introductions for concepts to be completely understood. Emotions, sensory input, and short-term memory are dominant methods used in this style of learning. A particular concern with this type of learner is the ability to link data and draw conclusions. These learners may feel that they need multiple attempts when learning for comprehension and become easily frustrated. A hands-on style combined with visual components is best as they process and attempt to understand the main problem, first, to obtain an overview, before smaller segments can have meaning. For this student to best understand renal failure, seeing animations or other visual demonstrations provide for comprehensive learning. They would benefit first from understanding what renal failure is and then what results from it. Outlines and reading will not lead to any meaningful and productive learning. They may have trouble learning as quickly as the left brain processor. See **Figure 1-7**.

Learning styles and brain processing work hand in hand, playing a major role in advanced learning. Another way this becomes valuable is in application of nursing actions. Learning styles and brain processing play a role in critically analyzing relationships necessary in clinical decision making and care planning. Everything we have been discussing

Figure 1-6 **Theory application.**

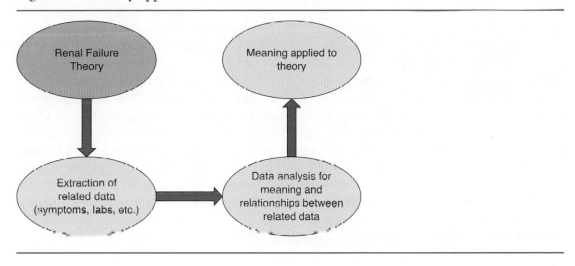

thus far becomes a major part of nursing education, whether academically or clinically. All of this information is essential to achievement of appropriate practice standards. The nursing process embodies all of this as an essential knowledge base that is necessary for assessment of data culled from the physical examination and holistic considerations to plan, implement, and evaluate care.

At this point you may be asking how all students can benefit from the use of concept mapping, given all the variations in learning styles and brain processing. While this will be addressed in more detail in subsequent chapters, I think it is appropriate to consider it here. Keep in mind that each map is a direct transmission of thought processes to paper. That in itself is helpful as it contributes to learning success.

To address all learning styles and brain processing preferences among various student populations, we need to incorporate beneficial types of resources. This is not to say that they be made available, but included as an integral part of presentation and review. As nurse educators, we need to be creative in integrating these resources into lecture outlines,

Figure 1-7 **Brain processing and application.**

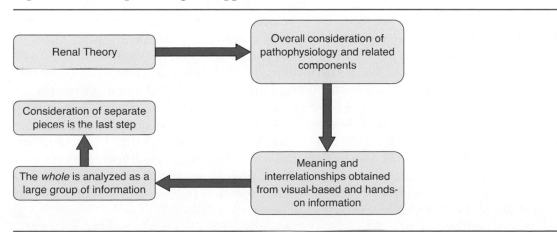

course outlines, and informational resource repositories. School libraries are especially necessary collaborators assisting with obtaining, cataloging, and reserving these materials. The nursing computer lab can be utilized for software-based programs, other forms of stored programs, and web-based resources. Within today's online learning options, such as ANGEL and Blackboard, files and folders containing links to audio, video, and other various learning resources can be posted for students to access off campus, anytime and anywhere. In that same theme, handheld electronic devices are now the rage. They allow a student to download an ebook or other electronic resource, even self-created documents, useful in either classroom learning or clinical situations. While cost may be a factor, the portability of voluminous data is easier than ever and its value cannot be ignored. How many students do you know who would rather lug several heavy books to the clinical site instead of a small, comparatively weightless electronic device?

All of the information discussed in this chapter will directly influence concept map setup. As stated earlier on, all concepts in concept mapping and nursing educational theories are directly interrelated.

A Bit of History

While the use of concept mapping in nursing education is relatively new, its use in other educational arenas has been going on since the 1970s. Initially developed and utilized in the field of science, in time various educational specialties adopted the method for use involving both team and individual work. The eventual and continued development of concept mapping then morphed into a variety of formats appealing to sectors outside education, including business and even the National Aeronautics and Space Administration (NASA). Simply formatted maps were commonplace and used mostly for educating. Eventually, many more formatting types were developed, leading to expanded uses such as problem solving, thought provocation, creativity, and considering possible outcomes based on decision making. As time passed, limited, static maps morphed into more complex, even grandiose living maps used by students and educators in almost every field of education. What began as a simple tool used solely for education by educators has exploded into a movement embracing concept maps in all areas of education from kindergarten through advanced academic settings and beyond. There are as many styles and layouts of concept maps as there are ways to employ their use. Data input for the maps contains everything from numbers, to mini outlines, to pictures and graphs.

Along with this boom has been the development of concept mapping software. For those computer-savvy students, this software is appealing because it is easy for them to understand and speaks to visual learning styles and creativity. Many students find it easier to generate a computer-based map rather than a hand-drawn one. I always advocate free resources included with textbooks, including providing web-based access. Programs are available for purchase, but some can be quite expensive. Why pay when free resources exist? Another reason I say this is because students need time to develop the type of map formatting that is congruent with individual learning styles and suits their learning needs. This process may take a bit of time initially and is best done with pencil and paper. As time progresses and students are comfortable with the process, a transition to computer-based map generation is certainly an option. One such option is the use of office software. An example of this is Microsoft Word.

The nursing profession has used concept mapping for educational purposes since about 2006. Although the list of resources is small, that list grows every year. Just a few years ago Internet searches for the use concept mapping yielded mostly nonnursing references. Today, a search will indicate that programs throughout the country are integrating use of these teaching/learning tools into curricula. Stimulating creativity and critical thinking, concept maps are able to merge knowledge with care planning and outcomes and to encourage questioning that gives rise to more effective and complete critical thinking. From my standpoint, they also assist faculty in evaluating that critical thinking process so important to preparing new graduates for practice. They allow students to evaluate the depth of critical thinking ability and key into areas of strength, building self-confidence while also allowing them to see where they need to work harder. When used in certain ways, concept maps can make a stronger statement about scope of practice and nursing action accountability than any admonishing statement ever could. Maps can be used by educators within lectures, as simple tools for skills learning, and by students for everything from note taking to studying to presentations. They are also beneficial tools in individual or group assignments.

What of the Future?

Because you have decided to purchase this book, it is obvious that you want to learn more about concept mapping and the implications of its use in nursing education. My hope is that your quest for knowledge in this area continues. You may be inspired to create your own uses and integration of the process into your practice. Go for it! The true beauty of the process is the myriad uses and creativity it inspires. Continue to learn and then share that knowledge with others. Collaborative efforts do not exist solely for bedside nursing in patient care, but also in nursing classroom and clinical education settings. Creativity is necessary in all forms of nursing education, and concept mapping theory feeds that need. Whether a map is simple or complex, plain or colorful, a multitude of benefits are provided. I envision future directions and trends for the use of concept mapping in nursing education to include:

- Formal research that demonstrates positive outcomes with use of concept maps in nursing education
- Expanded use of concept mapping in all forms and at all levels of nursing education
- Rapid growth in resources related to concept mapping
- Integration of concept mapping use within healthcare settings
- Continued correlation with skills and theory in nursing textbooks
- Incorporation of maps into patient-based teaching plans
- Nursing programs employing concept map materials as required resources
- Use of concept mapping rubric data to assess learning, specifically critical thinking outcomes

The nursing landscape is changing rapidly. There are more opportunities for nurses than ever before in a wide variety of roles and settings. Technology integration within those roles and settings will continue to expand and grow. While computer-based care strategies have their benefits and do provide rapid access to useful information, they do not and cannot replace the need for a strong base of nursing knowledge where critical thinking and all its facets comprise the cornerstone of care standards. Nursing care standards must always meet the bar that evidence-based research sets. The Quality and Safety Education for Nurses (QSEN) project, along with the Institute of Medicine (IOM), has established initiatives to improve quality and safety in nursing. Funded by the Robert Wood Johnson Foundation, this initiative includes faculty development promotion and student preparatory strategies to achieve those goals through setting the following competency objectives:

- Patient-centered care
- Teamwork and collaboration
- Evidence-based practice
- Quality improvement
- Safety
- Informatics

As a stakeholder in your chosen profession, personal nursing education goals must reflect these competencies for consistent, quality improvement in care. Knowledge equals safety, assurance of quality care standards, and nursing profession empowerment.

The future use of concept mapping within nursing practice begins now with a single step. That step is the journey you have just begun: to learn about concept mapping theory and then create your own concept maps. It will not take long for you to envision and enact other ways to use the maps for more effective learning. As with anything else, you can never realize all of the possibilities until you try. This is your chance to utilize creativity—to individualize the maps for a multitude of learning objectives. Concept maps are magical tools having the ability to be tailored and shaped into a variety of formats as individualized as the student who creates them.

Summary

Learning about concept mapping theory is the first step on your pathway to further develop a knowledge base with the ultimate goal of applying what you have learned. You have learned that the main components of concept mapping theory are important because they:

- Assist with the development and growth of critical thinking skills
- Demonstrate how to use critical thinking to view differences and similarities among and between data to analyze relationships
- Allow you to consider and set goals for using learned knowledge in practice related to nursing actions and outcomes

These components will be visible within the maps you will create because they contribute to the demonstration of each concept. It is important for you to recognize that all learning is based on this theory, whether you use concept maps or not. The maps are a necessary part of cultivating the skills and critical thinking abilities for successful application. Through them you will be able to see how you critically think—the steps your mind takes to process and apply education. Think of this as a wonderful tool with multiple uses and a strong contributor to your success in nursing.

Critical Thinking Questions and Activities

1. In your own words, explain what is meant by the term *critical thinking*. Research the definition and compare it with your explanation.

2. How is relationship analysis related to critical thinking?

3. Provide an example of how relationship analysis is used in determining a nursing action.

4. How does eventual theory application stem from critical thinking and relationship analysis?

5. Take a moment to think about how you learn. The last time you studied, what method made it easier for you to start to comprehend it—for example, written, aural, or visual?

6. Reflect on ways you learn currently. How will what you have read change this process?

Case Studies

Directions: Read through each case study and answer the questions using the chapter material provided.

1. Jane is a first-year nursing student who will be performing a Foley catheter insertion for the first time. Although she learned during the skills lab to place the insertion kit on the bed, her patient is confused and not able to consistently follow directions. Jane has decided to use the bedside table because she has a better chance to maintain sterility of the kit and safely perform this procedure.

   a. How does Jane's decision making demonstrate critical thinking?

   b. What other considerations are necessary prior to proceeding?

   c. What types of processes are entering into Jane's decision making and nursing actions?

   d. What resources and prior knowledge has Jane used to assess the situation and plan the skill completion?

2. Dan is in his second semester as a nursing student and feels as though he is not doing as well academically as he could be. Family obligations take his time away from school, and the time he does spend studying feels futile. Although he reads, he cannot seem to remember what he read and then spends time re-reading until he becomes so frustrated he has to stop. Dan has set aside 5 hours weekly to study but does not feel he has fully comprehended what he read.

   a. What should Dan's first step be in evaluating his problem?

   b. What are some valuable resources Dan could use?

    c. What other activities might be used to help Dan?

    d. What are some goals Dan can set to be successful?

3. Sandy is a second-year student who is studying pulmonary pathophysiology. Although this topic was presented during her first year, more of it will be applied during her clinical experiences this year. In addition, Sandy knows that exam questions will be at a higher level requiring application. She is feeling nervous about how to proceed and maintain her success from last year.

    a. In what ways can Sandy evaluate her knowledge so that she can see that she has comprehended it and can now apply it?

    b. How can critical thinking assist this process?

    c. How are nursing actions parts of knowledge application?

> **WWW** For a full suite of assignments and additional learning activities, use the access code located in the front of your book to visit this exclusive website: **http://go.jblearning.com/schmehl**. If you do not have an access code, you can obtain one at the site.

References

Benner, P. (1984). From novice to expert: Excellence and power in clinical nursing practice. *American Journal of Nursing, 84*(12), 1480.

Caputi, L. (2011). Critical thinking skills and strategies. Retrieved from http://www.lindacaputi.com/userfiles/Thinking_Skills_Explained(1).pdf.

Caputi, L., & Blach, D. (2008). Teaching nursing using concept mapping. Glen Ellyn, IL: College of DuPage Press.

Johnson, L., & Lamb, A. (2000–2011). Critical and creative thinking—Bloom's Taxonomy. Retrieved from http://eduscapes.com/tap/topic69.htm.

King, M., & Shell, R. (2002). Teaching and evaluating critical thinking with concept maps. *Nurse Educator, 27*(5), 214–216.

Schuster, P. M. (2002). Concept mapping: A critical-thinking approach to care planning. Philadelphia, PA: F.A. Davis.

Simpson, E., & Courtney, M. (2002). Critical thinking in nursing education: Literature review. *International Journal of Nursing Practice, 8*(2), 89–98.

Taylor, L. A., & Littleton-Kearney, M. (2011). Concept mapping: A distinctive educational approach to foster critical thinking. *Nurse Educator, 36*(2), 84–88.

2

Map Components and Basic Formatting

Learning Objectives

- Identify the components of a concept map framework
- Describe how descriptive phrases are used to signify nursing actions
- Compare and contrast static concept maps from living concept maps
- Discuss the similarities and difference among and between primary and secondary related concepts
- Discuss how formatting of a concept map demonstrates relationship analysis
- Review how concept mapping theory influences formatting

Introduction

Learning about concept mapping theory was our first step toward creating a concept map. Just as nursing education occurs on a continuum involving building blocks of knowledge, so too does concept mapping education. A knowledge base of information on the theory behind the maps is necessary prior to moving forward. Because that has already been completed, we need to look at what basic components comprise the physical layout or formatting of a concept map. This process then becomes a pathway to understanding what information is needed to fill in and complete the map, as well as to see how the entire process stems from concept mapping theory.

During this journey you will come to know a great deal about how you think: how you perceive, take in, and process all information. Based on previous educational experiences, whether nursing based or not, you may already feel you are in tune with this process. Your perceptions may be that, using a barometer of test grades, you have accomplished and attained personal goals for learning, processing, and studying. However, applied thought processes in nursing education require much more in-depth thinking and analysis than other types of education you have had. Critical thinking abilities must be cultivated, nurtured, and increased exponentially as your education progresses. Critical thinking in nursing equates to applying knowledge constantly. Every nursing action involves reasoning and comparison and contrast through relationship analysis, and critical thinking is at the center of that process. Concept mapping will be an integral process to nurturing and developing these skills. Each map will be a visual example of how you think and reason to make decisions and carry out actions. At times this process may feel frustrating because you may not be used to thinking so deeply and with such in-depth analysis. As time passes it will become second nature, but you must be patient with yourself. As a nursing novice there is much yet to be explored, experienced, and learned. Reflection will be important to compare where you have been to where you are going. Remember, it is a journey. Setting goals as you proceed will provide measurable milestones in regard to critical thinking abilities and relationship analysis. Let's begin by learning more about each map component and methods through which we can compose and format the maps.

Key Terms and Definitions

- **Concept map:** a diagrammatic teaching and learning tool demonstrating relationship analysis between a main concept and its related concepts; it promotes critical thinking skills
- **Descriptive phrases:** phrases used within a concept map to explain interrelationships between and among concepts as well as to denote an action between concepts
- **Main concept:** the focal point of a concept map from which all ideas and relationships stem
- **Related concept:** any data, information, or idea that has a relationship with the main concept
- **Primary related concepts:** data, information, and ideas that have direct interdependent relationships with the main concept
- **Secondary related concepts:** data, information, and ideas that have indirect but interdependent relationships with the main concept
- **Static concept maps:** concept maps demonstrating simple interrelationships and concepts for simple application related to knowledge and comprehension
- **Living concept maps:** Concept maps demonstrating multiple, complex interrelationships and actions for in-depth, complex application related to analysis

What Is a Concept Map?

Before we can consider the components of a concept map, we need to consider what a map actually is. A **concept map** is a *diagram* of ideas/concepts and how each interrelates. A main idea or concept is the central focus. Then, in order for relationship analysis to take place, a subgroup of related ideas/concepts is added. This is a key point of concept map theory: Map construction must definitely indicate a main idea/concept, related ideas/concepts, and not only how both relate and interconnect with each other, but also how the related ideas themselves interconnect. All components are needed for meaningful learning.

Point A, or the starting point, is the main focus or topic. Point B signifies the endpoint of how the map identifies interrelationships between the main topic and all of the related ones. For example, let's suppose we are considering how a patient will respond to a dose of furosemide (Lasix). The drug dose is our main focus. Related concepts would include side effects, actions, and purpose of using this drug for this patient, among other factors. If we mapped this out, what would be demonstrated between points A and B would be how we linked those relationships. In other words, point A is where we begin by identifying the map's main focus and all things that relate to that focus. Point B is the end result of the associations we have made. The path between A and B is the analytical process. Your focus will be directed toward this area as you consider, compare, and analyze information, ideas, and relationships. It is also where the hard work related to thinking will take place. When you begin this process, some relationships will be very simple, straightforward, and easy to analyze. As you progress and your educational knowledge base builds, many more factors must be taken into consideration to realize what relationships exist; then completely identify them to make all of the possible associations. One way in which concept maps assist with this critical thinking growth process is that constructing maps requires you to research information. This serves several purposes. It forces you to clarify and review and remember, which is another step in fully comprehending that information for application. The time you put into creating concept maps is valuable for knowledge and critical thinking growth. Hard work pays off with big rewards. As your knowledge level and ability to apply grows, so will your confidence. This is because increased thought processing gives meaning to nursing actions and assists with decision making, prioritization, and organization.

As an integral part of the critical thinking process, this diagram stimulates ongoing questions in a domino-like effect. As more questions form, more analytical perspectives occur, resulting in more questions, and so on. Questions spring from looking at point A and asking what things affect, are related to, and are affected by point A. See **Figure 2-1** for a pictorial representation of this process. The multitude of questions floating through your mind may cause initial frustration, but you will quickly realize that questioning is an essential part of the analytical process that comprises critical thinking. Questions stimulate you to look at relationships, see connections, and make decisions related to actions. Without those precious questions there can never be any answers. We need answers to relate concepts and see associations.

Figure 2-1 **The critical thinking process.**

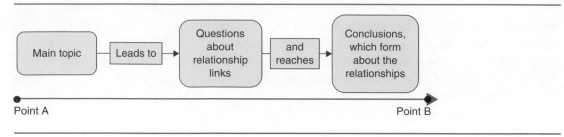

In concept maps relating to nursing theory, point A becomes a patient problem or focus area. Point B translates into nursing actions and outcomes. Remember that to get from point A to point B we need critical thinking skills that allow for identification of concepts and ideas, as well as the ability to demonstrate the links and connectedness between the identified ideas and concepts. A well-founded knowledge base contributes to the critical thinking skills leading to analysis and eventual application. Because students may have difficulty employing these types of thought processes, it is important for faculty to utilize, integrate, and reinforce this in all student interaction.

As a student, you may be able to see that a disease or abnormal assessment finding is a problem to focus on, but at the same time have varying degrees of difficulty in identifying an abnormal laboratory test as an area of concern. You may also have difficulty seeing the link between broad categories and abstract concerns as problems that need to be considered as part of the nursing care plan and necessitating actions. These are examples of both the simple and complex interrelationships we have been discussing. It is essential to remember that any patient problem or area of concern requires a nursing action of some kind, and various levels of thinking and reasoning abilities are necessary to reach conclusions. Concept maps will be a valuable tool for identifying these concepts and incorporating them into nursing care.

Let's take another look at some examples related to this. Suppose your patient is alert and oriented but speaks no English. You might be thinking that the simple way to address this problem is to call for an interpreter. If we put this situation into what was discussed in the previous paragraph, point A would be the language barrier. Point B would then become successful communication. But communication is not the only concern or focus of it. You need to ask yourself such questions as:

- What is this patient's perception of health care?
- Is there complete understanding of the treatment plan?
- What cultural concerns impact the nursing process and any formulated nursing actions?

Most decisions we arrive at have resulted from multiple questions and analytical processes. Very few nursing actions result from a single thought or piece of data. Everything is connected.

Another example of this is safety. Students are aware that safe care is to be provided in all instances and settings but may have difficulty isolating specific contributors to safe care practices or their roles in preventing an untoward event. Part of this may have to do with how a student sees the nursing student role and scope of practice. A crucial piece of thinking critically is the ability to project and visualize how you would proceed if you were the primary care nurse. You need to have a recognition and awareness of the fact that potential problems are in your scope of practice responsibilities and part of critical thinking thought processes. I often stress to students that although a student's scope of practice may have limitations, he or she is still responsible for these things and a collaborator of the care team. At the very least, making the co-assigned registered nurse (RN) aware of a potential problem is part of the solution, whether you are able to carry out the steps of an action or not.

Another broad category to be mindful of is patient education. It is important for students to know that patient education takes a variety of forms—from informal conversations to formal sit-down sessions—and includes everything from medications, to treatments, to clarifying physician statements, to diagnostic testing and discharge instructions. If point A in this instance is the topic to be taught and point B is the assessment of that education, the analysis that occurs between those two points is extremely important. It cannot solely focus on the educational method used. To be successful and have the ability to be assessed, we would need to first assess the patient's learning style and preferences in learning—how each patient best learns for comprehension.

I mention all of this because we have spoken a great deal about specifics, isolating individual problems and areas of focus for specific nursing actions. This plays a necessary part not only in the nursing process, but in establishing the plan, implementing it, and following up on it as well. This process defines our nursing actions, considering each one in turn, as part of the whole care continuum. If you really think about it, when care is provided to a client, is all the care lumped together, given at one time in the same way? Of course not. Specific, carefully planned nursing actions are employed to identify and address each patient problem. It stands to reason then that problems must be seen individually and acted on one by one. But, the broader categories also have strong implications for practice. In an age when there are so many collaborators in every care setting, there may be some role confusion among students and questions as to who takes care of and regulates what aspect of care. I have seen this come out in concept maps and have reinforced the fact that although there are collaborators, the nurse is responsible for overseeing all care. The information entered into a map has its origins in actions that are identified through analysis of many relative factors.

It is important to note here that although the concept map takes the shape of a diagram, the tool can be and is compatible with *any* learning style. It is not solely a tool for visual learners. This fact will become more evident as we move along. Also, no matter what that style is, the individual parts as well as the whole must be considered in the plan of care and the concept map, just as they are within the nursing process. How this is achieved is slightly different for each student, as we have seen. Our role as nursing educators is to help students find methods enabling them to see isolated and narrow foci of knowledge as well as the wider and broader components of knowledge, both of which can and must be applied in nursing care.

A **static concept map** is one that contains ideas and information that change little over time. They are also more fact based and somewhat concrete. For instance, a simple skill such as taking a temperature varies little except for the route by which it is obtained and perhaps the device used. Static maps are great for studying simple concepts and note taking. Another way to explain it is that these maps are simpler in that they contain fewer concepts, fewer relationships to be analyzed, and thus fewer steps to travel from point A to point B. Because they are smaller and simpler, it is easier to see relationship links in these maps. They are wonderful for teaching specific steps used in performing a skill.

In contrast, **living concept maps** feature more involved and complex interrelationships, generate more in-depth questions, and necessitate ongoing analysis. Contents of these maps continually evolve, expand, and require revision. You would create a living map when demonstrating nursing actions for a client with multisystem pathophysiology. Much more critical thinking and knowledge are a necessity because each step in the analytical process is taken out farther to reach an endpoint. The list of related concepts is larger, and this means that the number of interrelationships is larger as well. Next, we will learn about map setup and contents.

Basic Map Components

In order to create the type of diagram that allows for relationship analysis, the following components are needed. (Each component is explored in finer detail as we progress through the chapter.)

Shapes

Shapes not only help contain information (concepts and related ideas); they also assist with categorization and structuring of a concept map, as well as sequencing and flow of information. Any size or color and any shape can be useful. Each shape can hold one word, a small sentence, or even a list. In addition, pictures, graphs, and charts may also be used. The ability to adapt the maps in this way not only provides for multiple learning opportunities, but also application to all learning styles. In some situations, font, size, and color of text may be adjusted to emphasize or focus on a key concept within the shape. It does not matter what shape is chosen. Here are some commonly used shapes.

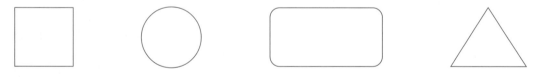

Lines and Arrows

As shapes contain component information, so lines and arrows are used to show connections, links, and interrelationships between ideas. A simple line connecting two shapes, for instance, generates questions immediately. How are the components connected? How does each relate to the other and reflect back to the main concept? All of this gives birth to critical thinking processes; stimulates learning, the beginnings of the comparison and contrast process; and finally, the beginnings of practice application. Alternative line styles may be used to show direct versus indirect relationships between concepts, a common link of categories within a map, dependent relationships, cause-and-effect relationships, and much more. Paired with a shape, curved arrows may indicate sequencing and/or an ongoing process. As a map expands in size and scope, lines become very important in being able to follow links and meanings associated with data groups. Demonstrating relationships always begins with connecting lines and arrows.

Descriptive Phrases

Descriptive phrases, or connective phrases, are necessary to tell the story of inter-relationships within a map. Although the word "phrase" is used, a variety of formats are acceptable. Some situations warrant a single word, while others may call for several words or a short sentence. Descriptive phrases are written or typed along or across the lines or arrows to further describe interrelationships and connectedness between and among the main concept and related concepts. They should always be action based. These phrases are helpful in promoting independent thoughts that lead to more independent action and self-confidence. They also play a major role in creating and establishing associations not just between concepts but in nursing actions as an extension of applied knowledge.

Within nursing concept maps, descriptive phrases can be tailored to the main focus of the map. For example, if the map's purpose is to identify nursing actions, action verbs reflecting them should be utilized. Similar sets of phrases can be created to reflect the main goal of the map.

What phrase you choose is limited only to your imagination. Some common descriptive phrases include:

- Results in
- Stems from
- Is associated with
- Caused by
- Leads to
- Is manifested by
- Affects
- Monitor for
- Follow up
- Assess
- Educate
- Actions needed
- Signifies
- May result in
- Is related to
- Signifies a need for
- Indicates
- Prevents
- Promotes
- Requires
- In response to
- Follow up with
- Necessitates collaboration with
- Implies
- May lead to

You will be able to add to the list as you begin to create your own concept maps. Often, recalling a patient you cared for will help in this process. For example, if you cared for a patient with diabetes and her finger stick glucose was 250, what did you do about that? Most likely you assessed her for any hyperglycemic effects and then informed your co-assigned RN. If you were completing a map of your nursing actions for this patient, you could use the descriptive phrase "immediately assessed for" to show that action.

Maybe you are trying to show a link between an elevated creatinine level and acute renal failure. You can use the phrase "is related to" to demonstrate that you see that particular link. So, the action demonstrated with descriptive phrases occurs in two ways: first, as an action the student has taken in response to a patient problem or concern; and second, as a verbal expression demonstrating a critical thinking link between concepts. *Maps are all about action—action of thought, connection, performance, application, planning, and follow up.* Actions directly reflect on a student's critical thinking abilities.

Actions resulting from thoughts refer back to critical thinking and the reasoning and deductive processes you use to reach conclusions about the actions you will carry out. In this way, the descriptive phrases you choose serve as a bridge between your knowledge base and which information within that repository you select to make decisions regarding actions. This process includes viewing data and clustering similar facts and data together while isolating and separating dissimilar data. This is also the phase of decision making where we put relationship analysis into action. Asking questions is a helpful step in reaching the proper conclusions. Let's refer back to the first example described earlier. The following question set would be helpful in reaching a conclusion that results in nursing actions appropriate to the situation.

1. Is this result abnormal?
2. What symptoms or assessment changes can accompany this value?
3. What nursing actions are utilized to address this?
4. What are the priority actions?
5. What medications, treatments, or other interventions are required to prevent deterioration?
6. What actions must be completed now and which must occur later?
7. What actions could prevent this from happening again?

These questions reflect concept mapping theory and will not only help to reinforce it but will also assist you in improving your critical thinking abilities. Using these questions consistently in clinical situations and case studies will soon make them a habit. Keep a laminated copy in your pocket and be sure to refer to it often.

A Main Concept and Related Concepts

The **main concept** is the map's focus and information starting point. **Related concepts** are those things that extend from and relate back to the main concept. The rest of the map will stem from ideas related to the main concept. These concepts are used to fill in the shapes. Then, as stated earlier, any lines and descriptive phrases utilized tell the rest of the story. When we move from simple, skill-focused static maps to the multi-focused and more complex living maps, the main topic becomes a *patient problem* and the related concepts become *related problems*.

Examples of patient problems include:

- A nursing diagnosis
- An abnormal laboratory result
- A behavior
- An abnormal assessment finding
- An adverse event

The related concepts would become extensions of the related problems such as:

- A secondary diagnosis occurring as a result of the original diagnosis (such as dizziness resulting from gastrointestinal bleeding)
- Effects seen secondary to the abnormal laboratory finding\(manifestations resulting from hypokalemia)
- Manifestation of a behavior (flat affect and refusal of treatment secondary to depression)
- A multisystem effect related to an abnormal finding (chest pain occurring with altered states of oxygenation)
- An extension of an adverse event (a patient loses consciousness after experiencing severe hypotension)

Related concepts can take the form of a single word, a short statement, or a question. They may be determined by both actual as well as anticipated problems.

As we build on this information, it easy to see how valuable concept maps are. The information provided in this section also demonstrates how a well-rounded knowledge base is essential, along with strong critical thinking skills, to reach the conclusions necessary to demonstrate clinical competency. For instance, if key information is missing for a stated patient problem and/or the student does not take actions out far enough, fails to consider outcomes, or omits key steps, it is most likely that the student has not developed adequate critical thinking skills. I would caution though that the concept map should always be paired with clinical performance. There are instances where a student has thorough knowledge of the patient and demonstrates (either verbally or through actions) adequate critical thinking and clinical judgment skills but may omit those steps in a concept map. This might be the case when a student is still developing skills and has not had many opportunities for application on the clinical site. It can also occur if a student is utilizing map formatting incongruent with personal learning style. So now you may be asking, "Well, which one is it?" To be able to fully evaluate a student, you have to know that student. That is the answer. You must be familiar with how students perform, critically think, problem solve, and apply knowledge. This is usually more difficult for faculty with large clinical groups where there never seems to be enough time to directly observe all students in the group or a situation where faculty have not had time in a new semester to glean this information. Unless all students are new, as is the case with an incoming freshman class, it is helpful for faculty on various levels to compare notes and gain an awareness of student performance. For upper level faculty, looking back at evaluation forms and the previous grading may indicate those students at risk who will need additional assistance developing knowledge and skills. Many students are not able to truly integrate all previously learned information until sometime during the second year of nursing education.

So, creative concept map construction provides us with either a static, unchanging document useful in learning simple concepts or a living document that can be revised as needed for optimal learning. The possibilities are truly endless. A concept map can be as simple or detailed as possible dependent upon the focus and purpose. A basic construction format is shown in **Figure 2-2**.

As you can see, the basic formatting pictured shows an arrow linking a main concept to two other concepts. This would be evident even if the descriptive phrases were not present. The double-pointed arrows indicate an interdependent relationship between both subconcepts and the main one. You could also infer that because the boxes containing the subconcepts are touching, they also interrelate with each other. The double-pointed arrow has been added to emphasize this. To alter the format, different shapes may be used to signify the main concept and the related concepts.

Looking at this example, it can be said that reading a concept map is similar to reading symbols, interpreting code, following a road map, or using a type of sign language. For some students, it may feel as if they are learning a new language. In reality, concept mapping is nothing more than a different way to express and interpret knowledge. Students may not realize that they are already doing these things. Mapping them out feels new and different. What impacts this are the various ways students are able to take in, process, and give meaning to what is learned.

Integrating concept map theory early on and aligning the simplicity or complexity of maps with your individual learning and critical thinking abilities is the most productive approach. Using concept mapping theory terminology in various educational settings reinforces this process. Students can then learn to think in that mode of always looking at relationships between data and actions. Bringing that process consistently into all education, whether to skills practice, the classroom, or the clinical setting will result in enhanced critical thinking. It would be continually reinforced and students would most likely make an easier transition to that higher level that nurse-like thinking educators want them to attain. I feel strongly that nursing programs are already doing this. What I am saying is not brand new, however, I do feel that we may need to integrate concept

Figure 2-2 **Basic concept map construction.**

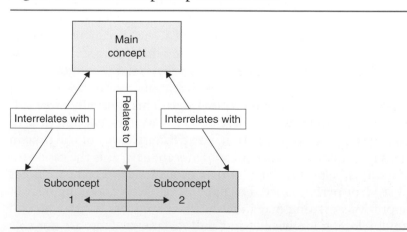

mapping theory more fully into curricula and introduce it on day one so that this type of thought process becomes ingrained and graduates will be better able to track their critical thinking and knowledge application abilities. We need these data to move forward with the most effective ways possible of preparing our nursing graduates.

Summary

This chapter has been one of the building blocks in taking concept mapping theory and integrating it into our nursing practice via application. The concept mapping theory sets the stage so to speak for the key players starring in the map. It is a necessary step in providing meaning to the information we add into the map. It could be compared to preparing the scenery when preparing for a stage play. The scenery and background used help to shed light and meaning on what the play in its entirety or each individual scene is trying to convey.

The star players having major roles are the main and related concepts. The entire concept map revolves around and derives its meaning from those two components. Identifying the main concept results from an awareness of your patient—of all data, history, and facts pertinent to that patient and the list of problems or concerns that arise from that data. These become the foci necessitating nursing actions. Critical thinking and relationship analysis allow us to view a collection of information, analyze it, and draw conclusions. This mirrors the nursing process, which also plays a key role in the entire process. If you are having difficulty with comparing and contrasting, it may be helpful to think about this process in various ways. For instance, you could think of a patient problem or concern in terms of normal/abnormal, comparing patient findings to those in your text. Another method I find helpful would be action/result. You can ask yourself, "If I carry out this particular action, what is the result? How will that address the problem? Are other actions needed?" So you see, questions are at the heart of this entire theory and process of concept map creation as well as in the application of it.

A concept map is central in the care planning process and is a care plan itself. The plan focuses on patient problems, and strongly on problem-based nursing action. This is in contrast to recording only patient data and nursing diagnoses. Traditional care plans focus on a narrow part of the nursing process while concept maps look at the entire care continuum. It is important to recognize that while both are valuable, concept maps are the only tool that completely demonstrates your thought process related to decision making, clinical judgments, and nursing actions.

Critical Thinking Questions and Activities

1. Discuss nursing care situations that would be used in the creation of a static concept map.
2. Create a simple static concept map from an example you cited in activity 1, answering the following questions after its completion:
   - Identify and explain "point A."
   - Identify and explain "point B."
   - What factors did you analyze to go from point A to point B?

3. Identify the main and related concepts in the following scenario:

   • You are caring for a patient who has had an appendectomy. This is his second postoperative day and he is complaining of incisional pain, feeling warm, and feeling weak and nauseous. He is coughing frequently during your assessment, but his cough is weak and nonproductive. He tells you he knows he would feel better if he could "spit something up." He is receiving a large volume IV of Lactated Ringer's solution infusing at 100 milliliters per hour, and he has yet to get out of bed.

4. Discuss how critical thinking and relationship analysis were used to identify the main and related concepts in activity 3.

5. Create at least two new descriptive phrases.

Case Studies

Directions: Read through each case study and answer the questions using the chapter material provided.

1. Sheila has been assigned a patient who is to be discharged home today. Sheila is unprepared for this experience and is not sure exactly how to proceed. She has never done a discharge before except on a theoretical patient in the nursing lab. She does remember that the patient will need information on medications to take at home but not much else.

   a. What other information is needed in order to prepare for her patient's discharge?

   b. What is the "point A" for this procedure?

   c. What types of descriptive phrases can be used to define her nursing actions?

   d. What are the main concepts used in a concept map on patient discharge?

   e. What would the secondary concepts be?

2. Ted's instructor has asked him to construct a short problem list and possible nursing actions for them using the patient he cared for today. He will be presenting this in post-conference tomorrow. The following is Ted's list of his patient's information:

   ✓ D.F. is 78 years old and admitted from an assisted living facility

   ✓ Admitting diagnosis: post fall from tripping over his walker

   ✓ Fractured right hip

   ✓ Past medical history (PMH): anemia, hypertension, osteoarthritis, and hardness of hearing bilaterally

   ✓ Current situation: Buck's traction in place, NPO for surgery in the morning, large volume IV infusing at 75 milliliters per hour

   a. Make a list of the patient's problems.

   b. What nursing actions can be used to address the identified problems?

   c. What additional information is needed to complete the problem list for this patient?

   d. What are some nursing diagnoses for this patient? Create at least four.

3. A group of students is having a discussion about all the things concerning a patient situation that become part of the problem list.

    a. Summarize the types of patient information used to create a problem list.

    b. Why is this information a problem or concern?

    c. How can this information be used to create a concept map?

> **WWW** For a full suite of assignments and additional learning activities, use the access code located in the front of your book to visit this exclusive website: **http://go.jblearning.com/schmehl**. If you do not have an access code, you can obtain one at the site.

References

All, A. C., Huycke, L. I., & Fisher, M. J. (2003). Instructional tools for nursing education: Concept maps. *Nursing Education Perspectives, 24*(6), 311–317.

Harpaz, I., Balik C., & Ehrenfeld, M. (2004). Concept mapping: An educational strategy for advancing nursing education. *Nursing Forum, 39*(2), 27–36.

Novak, J. D., & Cañas, A. J. (2008). The theory underlying concept maps and how to construct and use them. Retrieved from http://tuyunta.com/papers/Concept%20Maps.pdf.

Tanner, C. A. (2006). Thinking like a nurse: A research-based model of clinical judgment in nursing. *Journal of Nursing Education*. Retrieved from http://jxzy.smu.edu.cn/jkpg/UploadFiles/file/TF_0692810354_thinking%20like%20a%20nurse.pdf.

3

Advanced Concept Map Formatting

Learning Objectives

- Identify the differences between basic and advanced concept map setup
- Discuss how knowledge application contributes to the advanced setup process
- Identify how concept mapping theory appears within a concept map
- Formulate questions that become part of the critical thinking process utilized in concept map formation
- Identify methods for evaluating concept map setup

Introduction

Advanced map setup provides more definition for concept maps. It is essential for differentiation of concepts in a complex, living map. This process is very similar to the approach an artist takes when creating a painting. First come the thoughts and ideas of the painting's subject. Whether in thought or on paper, the artist begins to sketch a basic idea, followed by a simple rendering. Once that is achieved, in-depth consideration is given to dimensions, colors, and placement. Artistic expression is used to refine and tease out the specifics needed to perfect the final finished product.

When you create a map, you are that artist. Basic map setup is the rendering you create to "sketch" the path you want your map to take. It is important to realize that this complex process includes not only the practice maps you draw, but also the mental reasoning and thought processes that lead to the ideas transferred from your brain to the paper. The entire process is completed based on your core of nursing knowledge and how you evaluate and process it. You then give it meaning by applying it on paper. So, advanced setup is a progression of basic setup.

Because a more advanced approach is required for more complex concept maps, these maps are usually more expansive and complex. Your thought processes will need to be more advanced and refined as well. This chapter will lead you on a deeper path of questioning so that you can arrive at a destination of meaningful learning. This is critical thinking in action, and the results you see are what you put into expanding and honing it.

Key Terms and Definitions

- **Advanced concept map setup:** an extension of basic concept map setup where shape and color differentiation are utilized to refine the map for translation and readability
- **Concept map key:** a coded guide to color and shape included on the map to aid in interpretation
- **Uniformity** (as it applies to concept maps): selective use of shapes and colors with the advanced setup of a concept map
- **Concept map clarity:** the ability to interpret and follow the path of a concept map
- **Practice reflection:** the continuous and ongoing action of evaluating nursing knowledge and its application to refine and expand

Advanced Concept Map Setup

For use within nursing education, concept maps can become extremely detailed and large. If advanced formatting techniques are not employed, map information becomes crowded, difficult to interpret or read, and not very meaningful. Living concept maps focusing on nursing actions can become very expansive and contain a host of related concepts. A lack of utilized strategies to define, refine, and clarify all of them leads to a chaotic appearing map that is difficult to read, let alone learn from. Completing concept maps is not done to demonstrate solely what we know, but to help us to reflect on our knowledge base and the critical thinking abilities we are using to apply it. **Practice reflection** is the necessary act of evaluating and reevaluating what we know and how effectively we know it. **Advanced concept map setup** requires that reflective process for creating thorough and complete concept maps and allows us to assess and evaluate that knowledge simultaneously.

Because our goal for employing concept maps in nursing education is to promote and achieve strong critical thinking skills, we need to ensure that this is the purpose they serve. Creation, setup, and reflection of a completed concept map reinforce knowledge, critical thinking, and the analytical process of learning for application. The components of advanced setup are highlighted as follows.

Shapes

Using size and color with *shapes* will help to identify categories and relationships. This can be achieved in several ways:

- Shapes can be clear but outlined with different colors for emphasis and focus.
- Use separate colors to differentiate between main concepts and subconcepts.
- Use a larger size or different shapes for various categories.
- Shapes may be overlapped or touching to signify a codependent relationship.
- Cluster shapes to show multiple relationships or associations by using smaller shapes to surround a larger one.
- Alternate text colors or fonts within shapes to separate ideas and concepts or to link them.
- Shapes can be used as symbols to illustrate a point or to emphasize. For example, a small triangle could be used as a caution sign:

Shapes assist with information organization and can indicate differentiation while highlighting relationships at the same time.

Lines

Styles and colors of *lines* are just as important as shapes in creating and tailoring information within concept maps. Bold, dark lines might be used to demonstrate a primary relationship between concepts, while dashed lines could signify secondary relationships. The color choice for a line can indicate an emphasis or relationship. Curved lines and arrows can demonstrate a stronger link between concepts where a sequential or cause-and-effect relationship is shown. Many lines will appear in living maps demonstrating multiple connections all over the paper. It is of utmost importance to make clean lines with a clear path. Along with lines, *arrows* of various colors and degree curve help define sequencing and interconnected links. Arrows are sometimes underused as creative and meaningful ways of demonstrating this. A simple pattern of straight arrows can branch off of a main concept to indicate expanding effects of it. Double-ended arrows are great for demonstrating dependent relationships. Colored, curved arrows are a very effective way to show causal and sequencing relationships.

A crucial concept to remember when using lines, shapes, and color in larger maps is that **uniformity** is a priority. Using a wide variety of inconsistent styles can make for a very confusing map and detract from what you truly want to demonstrate.

Descriptive Phrases

Also, use of a coded **key** will be very helpful with larger maps containing multiple concepts and relationships. Actually, a key should be required for optimal interpretation.

No matter how large or small your map is or the purpose for it, *always use descriptive phrases.* Viewing a map is the launching point for examining relationships and their interactions, but the phrases make us take another look and begin the question-and-answer process that forms the basis of critical thinking. A map can never have too many descriptors. Repeated use of descriptors adds exposure to learning, leads to questioning that ensures comprehension, and aids in the ability to apply what is learned. See **Figure 3-1** (descriptive phrases are contained within the clear boxes).

Often, these larger, more complex living maps contain small groupings or clusters of information, which are then linked to other clusters and groupings. The flow of information then becomes extremely important so that the "trail" can be followed. Associations made may affect multiple clustered groups and related concepts. **Clarity** and organization are essential to creating a meaningful map. Descriptive phrases need to be well chosen to assist with defining actions and the links between and among concepts.

Figure 3-2 shows additional descriptive phrases from a standpoint of patient problem-based application. As stated earlier, descriptive phrases are all about action. Although some can almost strictly indicate a nursing or performance action and others a heavier thought-based emphasis, many times both actions can appear in one phrase because application is taking place. Application of knowledge links critical thinking to applied action.

Through this chart, a link appears between nursing diagnoses and the concept mapping process. Because the nursing process embodies critical thinking and application and nursing diagnosis determination is integral to this, it is important to demonstrate this. Follow through is an important part in completing the circle from assessment to evaluation. The purpose of descriptive phrases is to assist us with considering and addressing outcomes within our actions. I am always emphasizing to students the need to *follow*

Figure 3-1 **Descriptive phrases.**

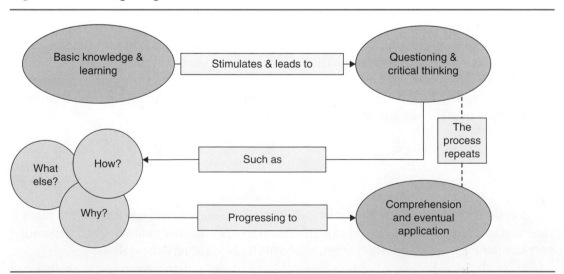

Figure 3-2 **Additional descriptive phrases.**

Phrase	Action Based	Thought Based	Concern/ Problem	Possible Use
Educated patient about	✔		Knowledge deficit	New medication ordered on discharge
Documented	✔		Evaluation of planning	Follow up of treatment effectiveness
Redressed per protocol	✔	✔	Impaired skin integrity	Carries out orders related to wound care Shows an awareness of protocols and follow through
Notified	✔	✔	Need for collaboration	Recognizes the need for collaborators to complete care, whether as part of the care team or other departments (lab, x-ray)
Relates to		✔	Disease process	Recognition of an abnormal lab value stemming from the pathophysiology
Is caused by		✔	Symptomatology	Linking of abnormal assessment finding with a specific disease process

up and follow through. I have repeated this often because until students become more comfortable with in-depth critical thinking and gathering all the facts they need for effective application, they sometimes falter when completing the nursing process through to evaluation so that outcomes can be considered. Some of this faltering is no doubt a confidence issue as well as uncertainty in acting somewhat independently. Freshmen are used to very structured learning where they are guided in large part out of necessity. As students move toward the completion of their nursing education, they will be expected to act more independently. Critical thinking, clinical judgment, and clinical reasoning abilities must all expand and deepen to meet those requirements.

Concept Map Key

Use of a coded **concept map key** will be very helpful with larger maps containing multiple concepts and relationships. A key is a requirement for optimal interpretation. This might be the last thing you add to your completed concept map. This will be extremely important for interpretation from several perspectives:

1. Your map will be easier to follow and interpret. A complex, living map is much easier to follow when the reader is guided by a coded key. Main concepts are easily identified, and it is much easier to clarify related concepts as well. Each

component, whether a line or shape, will have an assigned color, similar to a map legend, which definitively demonstrates how it is used.

2. Advanced setup techniques allow key features to pop off the paper and stand out. The key then helps to define their places in the critical thinking and association-forming processes.

3. This allows the instructor to assess your critical thinking abilities in terms of the nursing process and outcome achievement.

4. Reviewing your concept map using the key offers you an additional opportunity to reflect on your own thinking processes and assess your own competency. **Figure 3-3** is an example of a coded key.

The key you use can be expanded to include how clusters of information relate to each other and to some other important component. In the case of a nursing-based concept map, for example, one cluster may relate to an item in the patient's past medical history, as well as to the main problem. You will see other examples of this throughout the text. The main thing is to expand the key as needed to show each and every link you have provided.

Summary

We have now journeyed from basic concept mapping theory to basic and advanced setup components of a concept map. Setting up any concept map stems from your understanding of concept mapping theory. Integral to that process is your knowledge base. When you take those first tentative steps in nursing education, your knowledge base

Figure 3-3 **Example of coded key.**

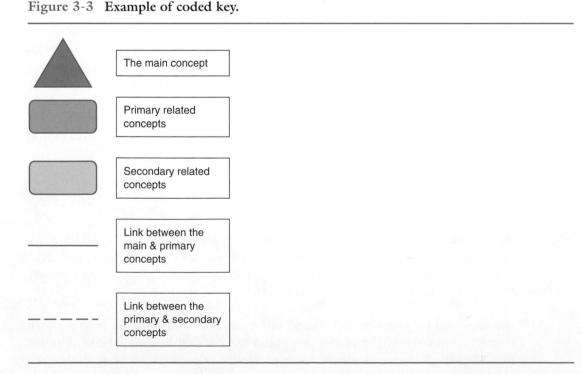

is small. Critical thinking is still in its formative stages as you move from basic understanding to comprehension. The concept maps you create during this time will and should be basic static concept maps. Make it part of your class preparation to create these simple maps to reinforce current theory. This process becomes the building block from which you will expand into more complex knowledge necessitating deeper critical thinking. This accompanies the more complex skills you will learn as well. Using concept maps allows you to pull everything together that you need to know, whether for theory or skills. Then, moving one step further, it sends you on the path to application of knowledge based on critical thinking and the ability to analyze and associate pieces of knowledge.

Key to this entire continuum is your responsibility to evaluate your knowledge base by reflecting on your learning and thinking abilities. The part you play in your own educational growth is a major one. As a simple example, suppose you were learning to change a dressing but instead of performing it, you could only watch while the instructor completed the task. How meaningful do you think that would be? Completing the task yourself would force you to think about the theory behind the task and all nursing implications involved. It would demand that you ask questions and analyze to achieve objectives related to the task. This is active learning and what concept maps directly address.

Critical Thinking Questions and Activities

1. Make a disease-related concept map on hypertension using advanced setup techniques and then answer the following:
   a. Is my map in a uniform style?
   b. Is my critical thinking thought process evident?
   c. Is it easy to differentiate between the main and related concepts?
2. Write a short summary of how the nursing process is reflected in your map.
3. Discuss the descriptive phrases you chose to use and your rationale for using them.
4. Discuss how you would use nursing actions to follow up on outcomes related to hypertension.

Case Studies

Directions: Read through each case study and answer the questions using the chapter material provided.

1. Stan is thinking about a concept map he has been assigned to complete on his patient's main diagnosis. The assignment objective is to show critical thinking.
   a. How do concept maps indicate that critical thinking has taken place?
   b. How can the use of advanced concept map setup be used to show thought pathways?
   c. In what ways do descriptive phrases play a role in indicating critical thinking abilities?

2. Andrea wants to construct a concept map for her clinical experience so that she can remember the four assessment methods.

   a. What type of concept map would this be?

   b. What is the difference between static and complex concept maps?

   c. How are nursing actions and outcomes determined using concept mapping theory?

3. Andy and Melissa are discussing and reviewing the nursing process. They want to better understand how to demonstrate its use within a concept map.

   a. Identify the steps of the nursing process.

   b. What types of patient information would fall into each step of the nursing process?

   c. What nursing actions come from each step?

   d. How does each action demonstrate application of nursing knowledge?

   e. How can a concept map be used to reinforce following up and following through on patient problems?

WWW.   For a full suite of assignments and additional learning activities, use the access code located in the front of your book to visit this exclusive website: **http://go.jblearning.com/schmehl**. If you do not have an access code, you can obtain one at the site.

References

Clayton, L. H. (2006). Concept mapping: An effective, active teaching-learning method. *Nursing Education Perspectives, 27*(4), 197–203.

Mueller, A., Johnston, M., Bligh, D., & Wilkinson, J. (2002). Joining mind mapping and care planning to enhance student critical thinking and achieve holistic nursing care. *International Journal of Nursing Knowledge, 13*(1), 24–27.

Schuster, P. (2000). Concept mapping: Reducing clinical care plan paperwork and increasing learning. *Nurse Educator, 25*(2), 76–81.

The Data-Gathering Process

Learning Objectives

- Explore the sources of information utilized in creating a nursing-based concept map
- Demonstrate how patient-based information in a concept map relates back to concept mapping theory
- Describe how nursing knowledge supports and defines nursing actions
- Define patient problems and create a patient problem list
- Analyze relationships within the problem list to differentiate between primary and secondary problems

Introduction

This chapter will be the next step on the path leading to construction of a completed concept map. Thus far you have learned about concept mapping theory, which laid the foundation for understanding thought processes and theoretical components related to concept mapping. That information leads you to question and reflect on what you know and how that knowledge is used in patient care. More reflective questions were generated when we explored the basic diagrammatical components of a concept map. Critical thinking is all about asking questions, reasoning to obtain the answers, asking more questions, and evaluating knowledge as this process continues. Now we move toward a more specific nursing focus to question what types of information should be included in a nursing-based concept map and why. What sources are necessary, how is that determined, and what specific information should be extracted related to the nursing actions used to complete a plan of care? Everything you have learned thus far is part of this entire reasoning process. A nursing-based concept map cannot be either fully understood or completed without a working knowledge of the specific patient data to be included as well as its origins. When a patient problem list is formulated, you will need to have knowledge of and be able to recognize every bit of information contributing to a patient problem or concern. This applies to both static and living concept maps. While this may seem to be quite a daunting task, do not panic. On some level you are already utilizing concept mapping theory in your learning. You are already comparing and contrasting facts and other data on some level. Concept mapping forces you to explore all of these things in more detail and to utilize them constantly. This is how you benefit and grow in knowledge, critical thinking, and self-confidence.

All but the most simple skill-related concept maps are related to nursing actions. A simple, static concept map may require the inclusion of less information than a more complex one, but the same information is still necessary. This chapter explores those valuable sources and how you can utilize them to extract the data necessary to formulate a concept mapping–based plan of care. Nursing actions are formulated based on patient problems. Those problems must be identified and extracted from various sources to then formulate a complete plan of care.

Key Terms and Definitions

- **Subjective data:** patient-related information obtained directly from patient statements
- **Objective data:** patient information the nurse obtains from patient assessments, behaviors, nonverbal cues
- **Related diagnostic data:** patient information utilized in formulating nursing diagnoses and planning care, originating from laboratory results, diagnostic testing, procedure outcomes, and treatment responses
- **Patient problems:** a listing of patient concerns contributing to the plan of care as derived from subjective, objective, and related diagnostic data
- **Active problems:** problems contributing to the current plan of care and that threaten homeostasis
- **Inactive problems:** problems not related or contributing to the current plan of care
- **Past medical history (PMH):** the patient's inclusive past medical history
- **Past surgical history (PSH):** the patient's inclusive past surgical history
- **History of present illness (HPI):** the circumstances surrounding the patient's hospital admission; the symptomatology and events leading the patient to seek medical care

Nursing Action Rationales

All nursing knowledge is designed for two very specific purposes: 1) to establish an extensive and sound knowledge base for critical thinking–based application of that knowledge, and 2) to guide nursing actions per evidence-based practice rationales and standard of care guidelines. As you have discovered, gaining the knowledge is only part of ultimately satisfying a goal of formulating nursing actions. Recognizing and determining interrelationships among the various theoretical teachings, comprehending how they fit into patient care decisions, and then translating them into nursing actions is the ultimate achievement goal. Every nursing action we perform originates from this starting point. *A specific rationale guides specific actions.* Rationales explain the purpose of and the reasoning for a particular action. No action should be performed without an awareness of the rationale behind it. No nursing action is random—each and every one has meaning based on research and accepted standards. Cultivating strong critical thinking skills will enable you to interpret and associate pieces of knowledge and learn how to use them in applying knowledge. This gives meaning to nursing actions. Knowledge really is power. Critical thinking allows examination of knowledge from many perspectives and angles: gathering like data, separating unlike data, and making comparisons and contrasts.

Overall, recommended nursing actions are based on nursing research, evidence of best practices based on that research and patient outcomes. This does not mean that recommended actions are generalized or one size fits all. If you think back to what you read about learning domains, the psychomotor and affective spheres are useful in individualizing and tailoring nursing actions to specific patient needs. These spheres allow us to see each patient as an individual with specific needs. This is holism in action. Because nursing actions are parts of the nursing process and *are* the plan of care, each action of the entire plan is patient need focused.

So, we know that rationales related to knowledge, nursing research evidence, and care standards *guide* nursing actions. But what *determines* or leads to a nursing action? In other words, why is a nursing action carried out? To what do the rationales apply and to what stimuli are they responding? Patient problems and concerns obtained from various sources are the stimuli for those nursing actions. Patient problems and concerns can be more broadly defined as any abnormal finding or patient need in response to alterations in physical and/or mental health requiring a nursing action. **Figure 4-1** summarizes these concepts.

This also includes those nursing actions resulting from physician orders. An abnormal finding may also refer to treatments and interventions such as tubes, lines, and dressings. You may gain a better understanding of this concept by comparing a healthy person requiring none of those things to a patient who does require these treatment measures and interventions to maintain homeostasis.

Patient Problems

Let's explore **patient problems** in more detail as they relate to nursing actions. Each patient has specific needs related to a main problem, which is a disease, illness, or syndrome. Those needs translate into specific problems or areas of concern, which then become stimuli for nursing actions. The nursing actions comprising the plan of care are in response to the main problem as well as the required treatment interventions. If you take

Figure 4-1 **Nursing action rationales.**

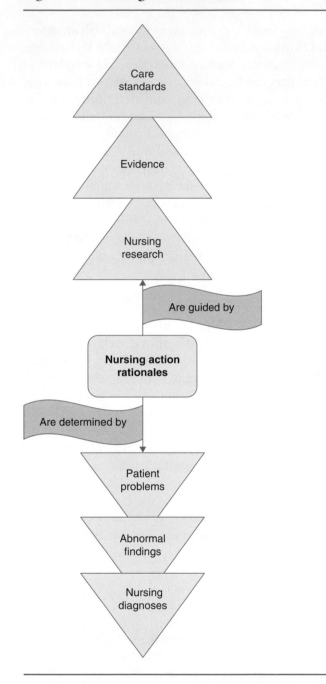

all of this from a standpoint of critical thinking and concept mapping theory, this means recognizing and examining all facts related to each specific patient's main problem plus all other related information involved in nursing actions within the plan of care. **Figure 4-2** will help to put this into perspective.

This chart is another form of the Kardex or plan of care. When you are on the clinical site looking at the Kardex (or whatever the plan of care is known as within a specific facility), all of the following things should appear there. This is the information you use

Figure 4-2   **Patient problems.**

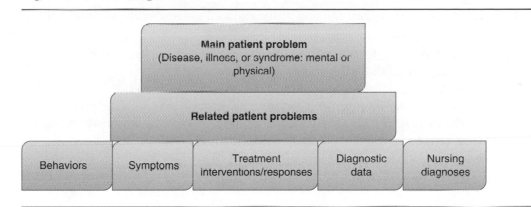

to plan and organize your care, via nursing actions, for the day. Let's look at each category for some more detailed examples.

Patient Behaviors and Symptoms

Behavioral assessment is a major component of the plan of care for many reasons. A patient problem list must always include behaviors because they are an extremely important component for assessing needs, responses, and outcomes. Nursing actions resulting from assessing behavior may occur in response to:

- Unexpected responses where safety concerns arise: confusion, violence, withdrawal, care refusal, increased fall risk
- Behavioral responses to education that assist with determining effectiveness and compliance
- Postural behaviors indicating possible distress: a hand over the heart when complaining of chest pain, postures indicating respiratory distress, inability to move independently
- Nonverbal cues not compatible with verbal cues
- Behaviors indicating adverse effects related to symptoms, deterioration, or treatments
- Behaviors and responses reflecting a patient's perception of health, illness, and medical care

Symptoms play a major role in defining illness and determining the origin of problems. The term *differential diagnosis* is used when the cause of symptoms is unclear and several origins are likely. The critical thinking process allows for comparisons and contrasts in this case to reach conclusions and is usually multidisciplinary. Nursing actions related to symptoms are used to:

- Describe what is occurring through documentation and reporting
- Focus on generalized and specific body system involvement

- Determine deterioration and the need for more interventions
- Determine and demonstrate nursing actions and follow up/follow through within the standards of care
- Monitor continuously for the resolution or exacerbation of symptoms as well as the appearance of additional symptoms

Monitoring *treatment interventions and responses* is part of the nursing process and another major area of origin in regard to nursing actions. Critical thinking questions related to nursing actions in this area include the following:

- To which part of the patient problem does this particular treatment or intervention apply?
- What is the expected response from this treatment as well as an unexpected one I might see?
- What nursing actions are necessary before, during, and after the intervention?
- If the treatment is a tube, dressing, or line, what is my responsibility for management of this treatment?

Treatments and interventions can run the gamut from observations to monitoring and management, recording and reporting data, and troubleshooting equipment. More detailed examples of treatments and interventions, along with their related nursing actions in this category can be found in **Figure 4-3**. As you can see in the figure, actions may take the form of assessments, administrations, observations, monitoring, and many other forms. Anything you do for a patient is a nursing action. Most of the actions discussed have been tangible and purpose driven. There are such things as intangible actions that may seem difficult to define such as emotional support, using alternative treatments to manage pain, or simply holding a patient's hand or using active listening to show advocacy and support.

Documentation, Reporting, and Communication

A major component of all actions is documentation. Documentation is the evidence that a nursing action has been carried out. It also explains why that particular action was necessary, how it was carried out, and how the original problem was treated and addressed. Documentation is a written description of the nursing process and justifies how standards of care have been met.

In addition to documentation, reporting is just as important. Communication is one of the most important and most utilized nursing actions. Reporting is a nursing action and a necessary communication skill in care-related standards and competencies. Patient satisfaction surveys focus on communication effectiveness as one component of evaluating completeness in care provided. **Figure 4-4** summarizes interdisciplinary, collaborative reporting as a necessary component in nursing actions.

Reporting patient concerns and data to the physician can take place during rounds or on the phone. Necessary items to report include patient responses to currently ordered treatments, patient concerns, laboratory values, diagnostic test results, vital signs, and changes in a patient's status.

Figure 4-3 **Treatments, interventions, and nursing actions.**

Treatment/Intervention	Nursing Action(s)
Medication	Safe, timely administration
	Observation for responses and side effects
IV fluid (large volume)	Monitor site for infection or infiltration
	Infuse fluid per orders
	Maintain site patency
Foley catheter	Measurement and documentation of accurate intake and output, ensuring patency, infection prevention
	Maintaining a leg band
NG tube insertion	Irrigation, medication administration
	Measuring and recording length of tube outside the body each shift
	Securing the tube and assessing skin integrity
Aerosol treatments	Collaboration with respiratory care
	Monitoring for effectiveness and need for additional treatment
Activity	Ensure appropriate safety measures are in place
	Adjust activity to patient symptoms/responses
Procedures	Educate patient
	Pre-procedure vital signs and preparation
	Post-procedure monitoring and tolerance
	Ensure standards and protocols are followed
Wound care	Observe and record data related to depth and stage
	Prevent pressure on wound site
	Redress and treat as ordered and in collaboration with wound care nurse

Reporting to nursing colleagues may involve communicating patient needs to nurses during the current shift or reporting factual information to the charge nurse/facilitator. It may also include giving or receiving shift-to-shift report. Nonnursing colleagues may or may not be directly involved in care but are nonetheless part of the communication process. For instance, nursing assistants (patient care technicians) will need to know about new orders that affect what care they give (a new order for fingerstick glucoses to be done, activity orders, etc.). The unit secretary may need to know that the patient has left the unit for a test or has been discharged. Knowledge of all team members and their specific roles will guide your communication reports to them.

Reporting to patients and their families is different from education-based communication. Patients need to be informed about who their care providers are, what the plan of care will be, and how changes in their condition affect that plan. The patient's family and/or support system must be included in this process. Patients have a right to know

Figure 4-4 Communication.

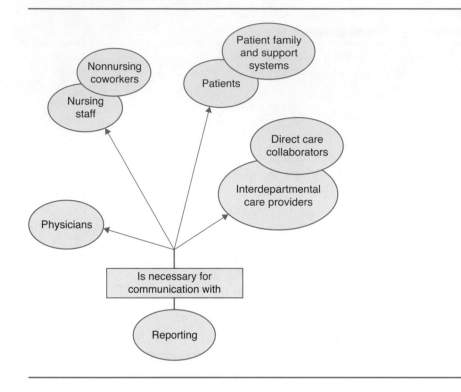

laboratory and test results. They also have a right to have an active part in any care decisions as well as to refuse proposed care and treatments. As a student, it may not fall within your scope of practice to be responsible for all of these things, but you still need to have an awareness of them. Ongoing communication with patients and their families is a part of advocacy and has been shown to prevent misunderstandings.

Direct care collaborators provide or authorize patient care. They are members of such disciplines as social services, respiratory care, physical therapy, intravenous (IV) therapy, laboratories, and case management. Other care providers having an indirect, more peripheral role in care include radiology technologists, computerized axial tomography (CAT) scan technicians, and pharmacists.

No matter who you are reporting to, it is extremely important to relay specific facts in a clear and concise manner. All nursing actions must be carried out with safety in mind, and communicative reporting is no different. Providing incorrect or incomplete information can result in patient care errors. In an effort to prevent errors and improve communications related to reporting, the nursing profession has assisted in developing and implementing a technique known as SBAR. This format is useful in reporting whether you are communicating with a physician, collaborator, or nursing colleague. In many institutions SBAR is now mandated for use in shift-to-shift reports as well as in physician reporting and in interdepartmental patient transfers. For example, it is used when a patient is sent for a diagnostic test or when a patient is transferred to another bed assignment. The technique is summarized as follows:

S: This signifies the *situation*. It includes patient identification and information related to a concern, event, or problem.

B: This section includes pertinent *background* information including current treatments, medications, vital signs, laboratory results, and patient status.

A: Information to be included in this section signifies *assessment* of what is currently occurring.

R: *Recommendations* related to advocacy and treatment strategies are to be included here.

Please keep in mind it does *not* replace a written report but directs and guides an oral one for better overall communication. Think about it. If a patient was blind, confused, or non-English speaking, how would a radiology technician performing an x-ray know that? It may be written on the chart but missed by the technician. The SBAR technique has been included in interdepartmental training. The technologist now knows to look for the form and have an awareness of important information pertaining to that patient, thus promoting safety and communication. Figures 4-5 and 4-6 provide more in depth examples of using the SBAR technique in two patient care–related situations: physician communication and patient transfer to the radiology department.

Diagnostic Data

Analyzing **related diagnostic data** is a necessary part of all patient care. As you increase your nursing knowledge and care for more patients, you must necessarily become more aware of diagnostic data and how they fit into the plan of care. Remember when I mentioned that phrase, "nothing is static?" Laboratory and diagnostic testing results fit that statement. A diagnostic test is ordered to assist in diagnosing disease. That sounds like a relatively simple statement, but it is not. A physician's order for a diagnostic test has many implications for nursing care. First, it helps us to understand cause and effect, which is used in the relationship analysis component of critical thinking. We learn to

Figure 4-5 SBAR example: Nurse to physician communication, based on a patient with shortness of breath.

S	List patient room number, age, admitting diagnosis, and PMH.
	State whether the physician you are calling is the attending or a consult and why the patient was first seen.
	State all information related to the complaint: in this case lung sounds, subjective and objective information, oxygen saturation, when it began, and what you did to address it thus far.
B	Provide information on other complaints related to this, related current events, other system assessments if applicable (e.g., tachycardia), recent chest x-ray results, ABGs, or other related laboratory tests.
A	Sum up your assessment of the problem and whether or not the patient is decompensating.
R	Suggest and ask for further orders.

Figure 4-6 SBAR example: Nurse to interdepartmental care provider, patient is being sent for a chest x-ray.

S	List patient name or nickname, allergies, age, room number, and the reason for the transport as well as why the test is being performed.
B	Provide information needed to safely complete the ordered test.
	Include information on language barriers, mental or sensory deficits, and any tubes or lines to be kept secure during the procedure.
	Another important piece of information is whether or not the patient is in any type of isolation.
A	Add that the patient is stable for transfer.
	Other important information would be to add whether the patient needs to have the head at a certain angle, be kept NPO, is prone to hypoglycemia, etc.
	A phone extension can be added if questions arise.
R	In this situation, the only recommendation would be to add comments to call with results or any other comments the ordering physician has specified.
	Some physicians prefer to view x-rays themselves and ask to be notified when the test is complete.

compare normal function or results to the abnormal or unexpected ones. It also helps us to better understand how the body functions, both in disease and wellness. Along with these concepts, we learn how tests are performed and how that affects patient education prior to the test as well as any monitoring that must be done afterward. Many diagnostic tests are invasive. The more instrumentation used and the more substances administered during the tests, the more nursing actions we need to perform after the test. Patient tolerance of any procedure is an important point to note in the assessment of outcomes and documentation.

Pre-procedure preparation may include an array of actions including simple patient education, medication administration, the completion of complex checklists, or placement of an IV line. Post-procedure nursing actions may range from having to only document patient tolerance to checking the status of an invasive procedure site to monitoring for adverse medication effects.

Another impact of diagnostic testing on nursing actions is their interpretation. If you are preparing a patient for diagnostic testing, part of your responsibility is to have knowledge of what the results mean. Results obtained will have three possible outcomes related to your nursing actions, based upon the complexity of the particular test:

1. No orders will change.
2. A few new orders will be received.
3. Many new orders will be received.

For example, let's say your patient has had a colonoscopy. When the patient returns, your nursing actions are partly to assess tolerance of both the procedure and any conscious sedation administered. In addition, you need to have knowledge of why the test was performed. If it was performed because of rectal bleeding, you will want to know what the findings are, if any biopsies were done, and if any active bleeding was seen. This will help you to anticipate any possible patient compromise and further orders. Possible orders to anticipate if there is active bleeding would be for a surgical evaluation and the typing and crossmatching of blood products. So, with every exposure your patients have to diagnostic testing, the more you are able to learn. As you continue to expand your knowledge level and critical thinking abilities you will see patterns emerge—common pairings between symptoms, diseases, and the diagnostic tests ordered. Of course, the condition of your patient prior to the test will also be a determining factor in this process.

You will also be able to see common patterns emerge in laboratory testing. However, because many of the same tests are ordered on almost every patient, this process takes a bit more thinking. Basically, to maximize learning in this area, you will need to make it a point to focus on specific testing as it relates to every disease or syndrome you study. I cannot emphasize enough that making connections through analysis, comparison, and association is what it takes to truly makes things stick. So the nursing implications in this case are to have an awareness of normal and abnormal levels of a test as well as the symptoms you will see when abnormal results are present. Abnormalities seen with laboratory tests fall into a continuum, ranging from severely decreased to severely increased (see **Figure 4-7**). Each type of test has a normal range. Within that range, no abnormal symptoms occur. However, symptoms can occur even if the level is either mildly decreased or mildly elevated. Nursing actions are necessary when an abnormal level leads to patient symptoms, especially when they are severe or pronounced. At the very least your actions are to recognize the abnormal level, have an awareness of possible symptoms, and monitor the patient. More severe imbalances necessitate making the coassigned nurse or physician aware and to be alert for further orders. If a laboratory test is abnormal, one question

Figure 4-7 Continuum of laboratory results.

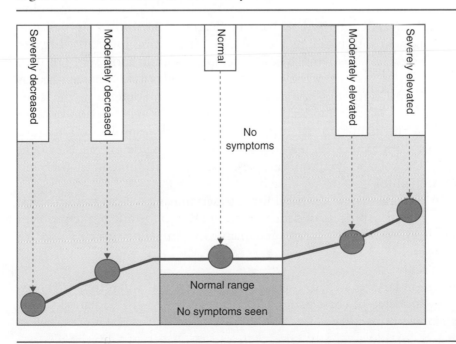

you will want to ask yourself is, "when is the next time the test is to be drawn?" If none is ordered, then one needs to be.

The difficult part in not only learning but applying this information is that for many types of laboratory tests, abnormalities can translate into very subtle symptoms. Also, for some tests the abnormal value occurs in tenths of a point. Although you may see it and feel it is insignificant, every tenth counts. Lack of symptoms may mean there are metabolic changes occurring at the very least. The huge concern with that is a patient's condition can suddenly change and not for the better. Therefore, the more you know about your patient the better. I am not just talking about facts, data, and numbers. Know your patient's baseline status, assessments, and behaviors, because these are all the factors utilized in critical thinking processes in creating the plan of care.

The other thing to remember is that while certain laboratory values are specific to organ systems (such as liver function tests), others may be altered in a wide variety of disease states, some which are occurring simultaneously. Electrolyte values are one example of this. Any abnormal value becomes a patient problem because it has the potential for leading to symptoms and a change in a patient's status.

Nursing Diagnoses

Nursing diagnoses are especially valuable for identifying patient problems that require specific nursing actions. As a part of the nursing process, formulating a nursing diagnosis is the second step. A patient or situation is assessed and from that assessment originate specific nursing diagnoses, constructed for that particular patient. Because each diagnosis specifies a patient problem or area of concern, each also requires a nursing action, or more likely several actions or a series of actions. The point of nursing diagnoses is not to satisfy a certain step within the nursing process, but to identify problems that need to be addressed and possibly resolved through nursing actions. Construction of nursing diagnoses easily demonstrates relationship analysis: the cause and effect of how a certain nursing diagnosis relates to a disease state or symptom. Isn't this what concept mapping theory and critical thinking are comprised of? Nursing diagnoses are another tool readily available to you that will help with building and refining critical thinking skills. **Figure 4-8** contains the nursing diagnosis template. This template should look very familiar. Formulating nursing diagnoses is part of the standard of care and is a skill that always has a place in patient care. Step 1 is to assess the patient or situation and determine the focus of concern. The next step is relationship analysis and critical thinking in action because you need to analyze how the main focus relates to the disease state or problem. The third step is to state how this main focus area, now the identified nursing diagnosis, is evident or manifested. Lastly, the specific symptoms are described. It is all linked together and all components are needed for it to make sense.

Let's look at a few nursing diagnoses. In addition to serving as a review, this information will be used to explain the process of data extraction used to formulate the problem list. The color coding utilized in the figure may help to isolate the segments used to formulate the diagnoses.

1. *Acute pain* secondary to a diagnosis of acute myocardial infarction (MI) <u>as manifested by</u> midsternal chest pain rated 8 on a scale of 1–10, radiation to left jaw, and shortness of breath.

Figure 4-8 Nursing diagnosis template.

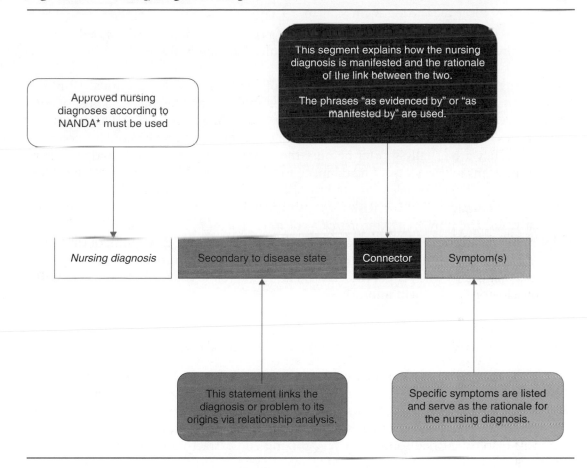

This diagnosis makes a statement relating the problem, which can also be thought of as a complaint, concern, or focus, to a disease state. Critical thinking and the ability to make associations must be used to link the specific complaint to its cause. While some diagnoses can clearly be linked and appear to be straightforward, others are not. To be able to fully recognize and associate links of information, you need that strong knowledge base we spoke of earlier as well as sound critical thinking abilities. The symptoms noted here are classic for myocardial pain and are acute.

2. *Altered oxygenation* related to chronic obstructive pulmonary disease (COPD) exacerbation as evidenced by capillary refill of greater than 3 seconds, pulse oximetry reading of 88%, and evidence of pneumonia on chest x-ray.

By formulating this nursing diagnosis, recognition is demonstrated regarding the link between pneumonia and an exacerbation of COPD. Abnormal focused assessment findings within the pulmonary system, as well as systemic effects, can be related to both processes. Comparison is made between the patient's baseline status, the findings related to the COPD, and how the presence of pneumonia has affected it.

3. *Impaired skin integrity* related to prolonged bed rest as evidenced by stage two sacral ulcer measuring 2 cm × 2 cm × 1 cm.

This nursing diagnosis demonstrates a connection made between bed rest and a break in skin integrity. Knowledge of ulcer staging is also evident.

Nursing diagnoses are a great tool for applying and improving critical thinking through analysis and association. From these seemingly simple statements, a host of connections are made where problems are identified and from which nursing actions spring.

These examples reflect real problems. Nursing diagnoses can also be used for potential problems. They are usually shorter because the problem has not yet occurred and there are no symptoms in every case. The template for those types of diagnoses looks like this: *Risk for (or at risk for)* problem related to specific illness or situation.

A brief example would be: Risk for sepsis related to current urinary tract infection. In most cases, the phrases *as manifested by* or *as evidenced by* are not necessary. If signs are present related to the risk, they can still be included. Remember to think of the entire process as making connections. The act of considering future problems is anticipating problems that change the plan of care. As you hone and refine your critical thinking skills, your anticipatory ability will improve.

Recognizing and Extracting Patient Problems

Now that we realize nursing actions come from patient problems, we need to think about the sources for those problems. In order to identify the patient problems or areas of concern, which then lead to nursing actions, we need to know where to find them. These problems will become the basis for our patient problem list and used to construct a concept map. Identified sources for recognizing and extracting those problems are:

- Subjective patient data
- Objective patient data
- The patient database
- The **HPI** (history of present illness)
- The **PMH** (past medical history)
- The **PSH** (past surgical history)
- Laboratory and diagnostic findings
- Psychosocial information
- Admitting diagnosis

Each of these sources is valuable for use in collecting and connecting all the necessary information needed for problem identification. Problem identification leads to the formulation of nursing diagnoses and ultimately the plan of care. As mentioned earlier, the sources also assist in creating the concept map problem list.

Subjective Data

Subjective data are information obtained directly from the patient in a verbal exchange and can be obtained by several methods. In a formal interview process such as completing the health history or database, specific questions can be asked. The point of completing those two documents is to find out all we possibly can about our patient. This process often uncovers problem areas that may not have been previously identified but that will impact the plan of care. Similar information can be obtained during structured educational sessions or during treatments. Another method is to utilize casual conversation during bathing or an assessment to elicit subjective information. Information obtained can range from additional physical assessment findings to psychiatric/psychosocial factors impacting care to information relating to how the patient learns. All of this information impacts how holism is applied in care: how the plan is tailored to the patient's specific needs.

Subjective data can also include verbal exchanges between other staff, the physician, and various collaborating disciplines. For example, if a patient was admitted through the emergency department (ED), the ED staff has made note of the subjective data they obtained. The physician would have seen the patient there and recorded notes and orders. Perhaps an aerosol treatment was administered. The respiratory therapist would record assessments, notes, and outcomes related to that.

Objective Data

Objective data originate from three sources and are comprised of your observations during interactions with the patient. The first source is the physical assessment. Whether focused or generalized, it allows you to form a baseline assessment of your patient's condition. It is also a great opportunity for knowledge recall as you compare normal textbook findings with those your patient exhibits. Every student–patient interaction is a "mini classroom" and a valuable learning experience. Learning while doing is a great way to apply knowledge and a very effective educational process.

Patient behaviors are another important component of objective data. Patient behaviors are compared with verbal statements for congruency. Many times verbal cues are a mismatch with nonverbal ones and provide insight into a patient's state of mind. State of mind can impact perception and understanding of illness as well as compliance.

The third source of objective data is the related diagnostics we have spoken of previously. These include laboratory and diagnostic test results. Applicable types of results include anything ordered for your patient. Set a goal to be aware of the results for each and every test your patient has had. Key examples are:

Laboratory Tests	Diagnostic Tests
Electrolytes	Echocardiogram
Complete blood count (CBC)	Nuclear scans
Liver function tests (LFTs)	CAT scans
BUN, creatinine	Arteriograms
Blood, urine, and sputum cultures	Colonoscopies
Wound cultures	Esophagogastroduodenoscopies (EGD)
24-hour urine results	Ultrasound
Biopsy samples	Cardiac catheterization
Body fluid sample results	Magnetic resonance imaging (MRI)

In order to use subjective and objective data, you will need to first recognize the problem. Some problems are very straightforward, while others may be more obscure. Constructing a plan of care for a concept map means being able to identify a piece of data as a problem. As stated earlier, a problem can also be defined as a patient need, an area of concern, or anything related to your patient that requires a nursing action. All information about the patient found on the chart is a combination of subjective and objective data. This includes the HPI as well as the PMH and PSH. To summarize, that means a problem can be:

- A mental symptom
- A physical symptom
- A line or tube
- Refusal of a medication or treatment
- An educational need
- An abnormal laboratory test
- A safety concern
- A need for collaborative care

It is evident that some problems are very easily identified while others are more difficult. This is why strong critical thinking skills are so important. Critical thinking skills allow you to recognize important problems and concerns related to your patient and then use them to create a plan of care or *action plan* geared to addressing them. Enhanced thought processes also allow for categorization of patient problems. Abnormalities gleaned from assessments only partly address all we need to consider. Isolating only physical symptoms would remove the holism component that is used to consider the psycho-social-spiritual aspects related to patient care, as well as the collaborative care aspects.

Data become problems and problems become the basis for nursing actions. Your theoretical knowledge base and critical thinking skills will assist you in recognizing that something related to your patient is a problem. Only then can you act on it. A helpful acronym is RE-ACT:

R   Recognize the problem and its impact on the plan of care.

E   Engage actively in investigation and analysis of the problem.

A

C   Act on it.

T

Being able to extract the necessary information to formulate a plan of care and a problem list for concept mapping requires three things: *recognition* of the problem; having complete knowledge of your patient, which includes knowing what information is important and *where to find it*; and the critical thinking and reasoning abilities necessary to *translate* those findings into problems and nursing actions. This requires the ability to research appropriate sources of information. Appropriate research sources have been listed earlier but can be summarized as:

1. The patient—via assessments and verbal interactions
2. The physician—via documented notes and verbal exchanges
3. Care collaborators—via documentation and verbal reporting
4. The chart—whether electronic or hard copy because much of the data needed is collected in one place

The Patient's Medical Record

If you have not yet had many opportunities to fully review a patient's medical record, now is the time. Knowing how and where to research information will allow more rapid identification of problems. Care of your patient must always include knowing all you can about your patient. This means organizing your time to allow for regular review of information. The process of patient problem identification is not meant to be once and done. It is a living, ongoing process just like the nursing process, which never ceases as long as the patient is under our care.

The first step is knowing where to look for important information. In some institutions, there may be several separate sources of the patient record. There may be hard copy charts mainly used for physician and collaborator use and a separate "bedside" chart used exclusively for nursing documentation. In other facilities, the hard copy or electronic records may contain all of these items. Take a look at **Figure 4-9**.

Figure 4-9 **Navigating the medical record.**

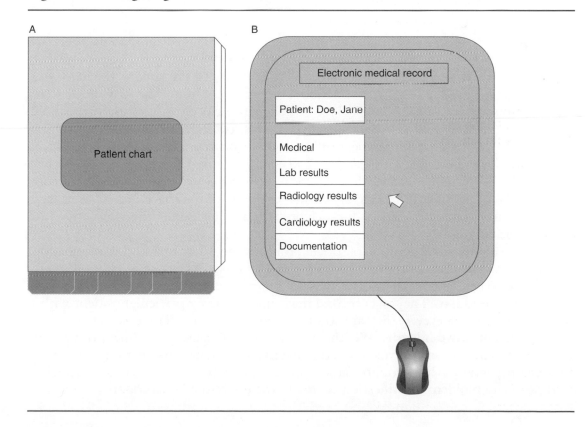

The hard copy chart (Figure 4-9a) shows organization of materials by tabs. Each labeled tab frequently contains the following information:

- *Admission information.* This information is generally derived from the admissions department and reflects personal patient information such as address, date of birth, marital status, next of kin, insurance, and billing information.
- *History and physical.* This tab contains the admission diagnosis, HPI, PMH, PSH, and the medical treatment plan.
- *Progress notes.* Progress notes provide a running multidisciplinary commentary on patient problems and care team responses. Usually physician based, each medical specialty is represented and documents the medical problem list and planned treatments. In many facilities, multiple disciplines are now documenting in this section so that true collaborative care is assured.
- *Consults.* This section contains physician consultation forms from when the first patient visit occurred.
- *Physician orders.* All orders are seen here.
- *Results.* Usually multiple tabs are used to divide laboratory, radiology, and cardiology results.
- *Miscellaneous.* Other tabs normally seen are those for other multidisciplinary charting. Some examples are IV therapy flow sheets, physical therapy, and respiratory therapy. The purpose of these sections may include charting treatments, tracking data, and having one concentrated area for following the timeline of collaborator-specific care.

Figure 4-9b depicts a computer screen for an electronic medical record. There are many different types of software. Most feature tabs on one side of the page similar to the tabs on a hard copy chart. While some of the tabs may be the same as the hard copy chart, others may group related information. For instance, a results tab may break down further into specific results. A medical records tab may break down into specific sections featuring the history and physical, operative reports, consultant reports, and progress notes. Becoming familiar with patient information through use of these various sources will ensure that you have the most current and comprehensive knowledge of your patient and assist with problem identification. All forms utilized, whether within the hard copy chart or electronic medical record, are permanent parts of the chart and stand as legal records of care. Mandatory actions for each problem and its resultant nursing actions are documentation.

We have discussed recognition of patient problems and where to find this information. Let's address data extraction from these sources a bit more. As far as the physical assessment is concerned, abnormal assessments signify problems because they are a deviation from normal findings. They may be "normal" findings for a particular patient with a particular disease; however, they are still not a normal finding. These objective assessments are often easy to identify. Whether you are using a focused assessment or generalized head-to-toe assessment, you will recall that the following assessment methods are to be used: inspection, percussion, palpation, and auscultation. **Figure 4-10** depicts data extraction and problem identification related to the use of these methods.

Figure 4-10 Problem extraction from the physical assessment.

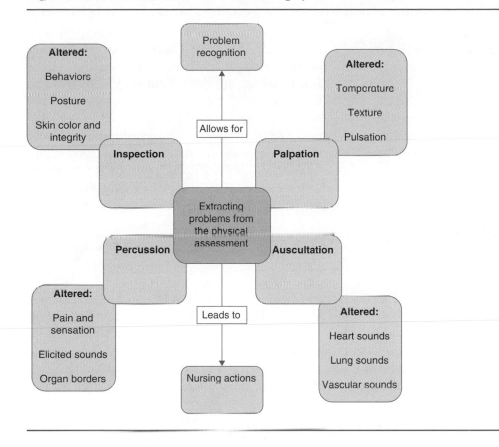

Suggested steps to use during the assessment process include: *Identify* the findings as a problem or concern, consider the problem to *formulate* a nursing diagnosis from it and analyze it by making associations and considering cause and effect, and then *decide* on appropriate nursing actions related to the problem. These steps are part of the RE-ACT acronym described earlier. The steps are broken down and a bit more specific. Using nursing diagnoses not only reinforces use of the nursing process but also assists with recognition and use of cause and effect—components of critical thinking used consistently in concept mapping. Once you begin thinking this way, it will quickly become a habit. The stronger your critical thinking skills are, the easier it becomes. In addition, once you have completed these steps, you will begin to visualize the necessary nursing actions. After a short period of time, linking problems with actions through the use of concept mapping will become second nature.

Objective data are then paired with subjective data to identify additional problems. Subjective data, whether in the form of verbal responses or behaviors, can become a problem or concern requiring an action; for example:

- The patient tells you she wants to leave because she has no insurance. This becomes a collaborative problem requiring an action to ensure compliance and future health concerns.

- Your patient denies pain but is grimacing and tachypneic. A nursing action is needed to determine why this mismatch between statements and behaviors is occurring.
- The patient states he takes all of his medications daily. One of those medications is warfarin (Coumadin) and the pro-time result is subtherapeutic. Nursing actions necessary for this problem would be re-educating the patient on Coumadin and determining his current level of knowledge.

Researching the medical record will yield results regarding subjective and objective data collected by other members along the care continuum that are ongoing problems requiring a current nursing action. For example, a patient exhibiting withdrawn behavior in the ED will not suddenly end that behavior on arrival to your unit. Using the medical record as a source yields a host of information from which patient problems can be extracted.

Admission Tab

Personal information related to living conditions, a support system, and insurance will assist you in formulating problems and actions related to holistic or psychosocial needs. For example, if the patient's address indicates residence in an extended care facility, this is an abnormal finding. It generates questions such as: Why has the patient been living in an extended care facility? What is the patient's baseline status? Often, this status means that either physical and mental limitations or both have been noted. This may guide actions related to education and safety.

Lack of a support system or death of a spouse may result in depression or other mental health problems requiring nursing actions such as monitoring, medications ordered to treat those disorders, and follow up with a physician as well.

Because insurance dictates treatment and treatment settings, knowledge of this status is necessary as collaborative care is essential to ensure the standard of care. Nursing actions focusing on collaboration with social services and case management will ensure access to appropriate care and services.

These types of nursing actions relate to psycho-social-spiritual needs. Alterations in this area may necessitate consulting other collaborators such as a psychiatric care team as well as pastoral care personnel. In this instance, nursing actions result from advocacy and go hand in hand with monitoring for treatment effectiveness and safety alterations.

The History and Physical Tab

This area is ripe with patient problems. The admission diagnosis and HPI provide information on what the patient's chief complaint was, as well as the events surrounding it, that led the patient to seek care. Let's suppose that a patient came to the ED for care for right wrist pain. An x-ray subsequently showed evidence of a fracture. This information allows you to extract problems such as pain, the need for preoperative education, and the possible alteration in neurovascular status in the right upper extremity. However, more meaning and further problems can be identified when considering the HPI. Suppose you find in report that the patient is 88 years old and fell. This should stir your critical thought processes and initiate questions such as:

1. Was this a simple mechanical fall?
2. Did a syncopal event or other event precipitate the fall?
3. Was there a loss of consciousness or a witness to the incident?
4. Was the patient injured in any other way?
5. Was the patient recently ill, dehydrated, or complaining of other symptoms?

Information found within the PMH may also yield important findings. Perhaps the patient has a history of falls. Maybe there is a history of hypotension, heart disease, dizziness, or other contributing symptoms that led to the fall. Some PMH is always relevant and will always be a part of the plan of care mandating nursing actions. Some examples of this are:

- *Anemia.* This can contribute to orthostatic hypotension secondary to further volume depletion in a surgical patient or altered states of oxygenation in a medical patient.
- *COPD.* Bed rest, pneumonia, anemia, and other diagnoses and problems may exacerbate COPD.
- *Diabetes.* Illness raises the body's stress levels and demand for glucose. Glucose control is difficult and leads to actions related to glucose management. Frequent blood glucose measurements and insulin coverage are mainstays of treatment. In addition, the patient must be monitored for hypoglycemia secondary to treatment as well as hyperglycemia from ineffective treatment response.

As stated earlier, nothing is static and everything connects and relates to everything else. The more you educate yourself on your patient, the more problems become evident. This also should mean the generation of more questions, deeper critical thinking, and more nursing actions. This entire process also allows for reflection on your current knowledge and skills along with what you have yet to learn and apply.

Progress Notes

Progress notes summarize patient problems. Reading these daily will assist in review of established problems and alert you to new problems. The plan of care must be assessed in an ongoing manner, every shift and every day. The plan of care needs to evolve along with the patient problems. This includes the formulation of nursing diagnoses and nursing actions. Reviewing this section also can promote discussion with the physician regarding patient needs and any progress or lack thereof. It is also a great way to learn about associations. The treatment plan is outlined within progress notes. From this you will see treatments associated with diagnoses, diseases, and problems. Common patterns will emerge and either validate what you have already learned or teach you something new.

Consultants

This section allows for identification of consultants along with planned treatments, prognoses, and associations. In addition, you will learn about accepted treatment guidelines and protocols. Another common pattern exists between diagnostic testing and complaints or problems. Many patient problems and their resultant nursing actions originate from this area.

Physician Orders

Physician orders connect with the treatment plan and diagnosis and serve as another learning experience. As you make associations between orders and the illnesses or complaints they stem from, you are reinforcing what you already know and adding to that base of knowledge to apply it. Problems created from physician orders usually relate to a need for a new order, alterations required for an existing order, and discontinuation of an order. **Figure 4-11** provides examples of each. Critical thought processes can be evidenced in each of the examples. Relationship analysis is also evident.

The Results Tab

Results are normally broken down and separated by specialty area. Each area is explained below, along with the potential problems.

Laboratory Results

Laboratory results include any specimen from any source that the laboratory receives for analysis. These include blood, tissues, body cavity fluid, synovial fluid, spinal fluid, urine, and biopsy specimens. Problems are formulated based on either abnormal results, symptoms related to the abnormal results, or both. Some examples are:

- A patient is experiencing symptomatic hyperkalemia.
- Spinal fluid analysis has given a positive result for bacterial meningitis.
- Synovial fluid aspirate has shown evidence of uric acid crystals.

All of these would be new problems requiring physician notification, anticipated orders for new treatments, and ongoing monitoring.

Figure 4-11 **Examples of problems with physician's orders.**

Problem Type	Examples
Need for a new order	*Your patient has a low hemoglobin result and a blood transfusion is needed (per the plan from the progress notes).*
	Action: You make the physician aware of the result and receive an order for one unit of packed red blood cells
Need for current order alterations	*A patient has been experiencing hypotension and has antihypertensive medications ordered.*
	Action: You advocate for either hold parameters or changing the dose or frequency.
Need for order discontinuation	*Your patient was NPO for an abdominal scan. The results are normal and the patient is hungry.*
	Action: You call and report the scan results to the physician and tell him the patient is requesting a diet. An appropriate diet order is received.

Radiology Results

Radiology results include those from several subdepartments within the larger radiology department: CAT scan, MRI, ultrasound, x-ray, arteriography, and interventional radiology. Most patient problems generated from this category relate to abnormal results. Abnormal results from this type of testing usually signify altered function and symptomatology. Common problems resulting in nursing actions from within this category would be related to status changes and symptoms secondary to:

- A mass or tumor
- Bleeding
- Pneumothorax
- Pneumonia
- Hemothorax
- Fracture
- Obstruction
- Perforation
- Complications from receiving contrast dye

In the case of arteriography and interventional radiology, patient problems arise from procedures that are invasive and during which medications for conscious sedation are administered. Problems requiring nursing actions may include bleeding, neurovascular status change, tube placement monitoring, and troubleshooting and sedation reactions. Interventional radiology is a discipline that is frequently used for procedures such as:

- Peripherally inserted central catheter (PICC) line placement
- Thoracentesis
- Chest tube placement
- Abscess drainage tube placement
- Urostomy tube placement

Because all of these are abnormal findings, problems requiring actions can include monitoring for patency and possible infection, maintaining dressings, noting and documenting drainage color and amount, and education on the purpose of the lines and how they fit into the treatment plan the physician has established.

Cardiology Results

Cardiology results are another large category. Tests in this category whose results can impact patient care include:

- Electrocardiograms (ECGs)
- Echocardiograms
- Stress testing
- Cardiac catheterization

- Tilt table testing
- Holter monitoring
- Telemetry monitoring

Problems and their associated nursing actions result from rate and rhythm changes, symptoms related to rate and rhythm changes, ECG changes occurring during chest pain, abnormal test findings requiring physician notification and subsequent testing, and adverse patient events related to deterioration from any of the aforementioned procedures or findings.

The Miscellaneous Tab

As mentioned earlier, many other collaborators may be assigned tabs for various reasons. Problems can be interdisciplinary and require nursing actions focusing on communication and documentation. For example, if your patient has had a PICC line placed and 3 days later the dressing is curling, then a redressing is required. Because many facilities stipulate that the IV therapy team perform this, your nursing action would be to notify them for the site to be redressed. Although they will respond and carry out this action, your responsibility is to oversee care. Thus, you would follow up by observing that this is accomplished in a timely manner. You would also document your findings related to the curled dressing, what you did to address it, and then chart that it was completed by the IV team.

Another example might be that your patient was ordered to have physical therapy. When the therapist arrived, the patient refused because of complaints of severe weakness. This response would prompt you to ask why the patient is so weak and perhaps evaluate his or her status again, along with orthostatic vital signs and hemoglobin level. In a post-surgical patient, blood loss anemia can lead to these symptoms. Although the physical therapist may document this event, you must also document and follow it up. In addition, you would notify the physician, because an order has not been carried out.

Gathering All the Information Collected to Formulate a Plan of Care

Data extraction from patient information is not only important within the nursing process but also in the formulation of the plan of care. It is a necessary component in determining nursing actions. It is important to remember that patient problems can be **active**, **inactive**, or collaborative.

In general, the problem list for a concept map needs to contain every problem identified from each available source. In most instances, the Kardex supplies the most current problems and the nursing actions are clear. Although this provides a partial listing of patient problems and the actions are a combination of medical and nursing focused care, the Kardex content originates from physician orders and therefore is medically based. While this is appropriate, it does not fully address the nursing aspect. The care provided to a patient is always to be holistic, and specific nursing problems and actions must be formulated to ensure this. It will help if you think of the term *patient problems* to signify any problem or concern that affects the patient not only physically, but also psycho-social-spiritually. This allows tailoring the plan of care to each specific patient. Combining concept mapping with this process means we can also view critical thinking and decision-making skills as the process is completed. Let's consider how to set up a problem list on a generalized basis. Research and planning must be done before you assume care of a patient.

From the material presented in this chapter, you should now have a clear idea of what data or information you will need to collect to formulate a problem list. Now we need to discuss how this can actually be carried out. **Figure 4-12** summarizes data types and the steps to obtain them. One of the first methods for obtaining information to use for the problem list is during your first exposure to the patient chart or Kardex. With the

Figure 4-12 **Data/information types.**

Information Type	Source	Research/Assess	Action Results From
Physical	Subjective Objective Medical & collaborative records	Medical record: • H&P • HPI • PMH • PSH • Documentation forms Patient interaction	Physical assessment Verbal exchange Research
Mental/ Emotional	Subjective Objective Medical & collaborative records	Admission report Shift-to-shift report Patient interaction Past interdepartmental staff notations	Physical assessment: • Behaviors • Nonverbal cues • Verbal cues Verbal exchange Research
Social/Spiritual	Subjective Objective Medical & collaborative records	Medical record: • Nursing database • Physician documentation • Interdepartmental documentation Verbal report from consultant or pastoral care personnel	Research Verbal exchange Physical assessment
Diagnostic	Medical record	Results tab or designated results area	Research Computer printout Verbal report

necessary information in mind along with a plan, this process becomes streamlined. It would be in your best interests to arrive at the clinical site early so that you have the time necessary to become familiar with your patient and can begin this process. During this time there are key questions you should be asking. These questions reinforce information research and how to link nursing actions with the patient information and data you collect:

1. What is the patient's admitting diagnosis and what problems or areas of concern can you identify from them?
2. How does the HPI contribute to the problem list?
3. What significant PMH will impact the plan of care and what actions will stem from it?
4. What medications have been ordered and what nursing actions can result from administering them?
5. What laboratory and diagnostic tests have been ordered and what are the results?

Plan of Care Format

Each facility has a specific plan of care format. You will need to become familiar with its format and layout to better navigate it. In general, information is organized in the following manner:

- A section near the top that includes patient identifiers, the admitting diagnosis, code status, isolation status if it applies, and allergies
- The physician orders affecting nursing actions containing the following:
  - Activity
  - Diet
  - Treatments: fingerstick glucose, wound care, oxygen therapy, respiratory treatments, and so on
  - IV therapy and access type: large volume solutions, total parenteral nutrition (TPN), any drips used in treatment such as heparin, and so on
- An area listing medical consults and care team collaborators
- A section listing the timing and frequency of laboratory and diagnostic tests

Some Kardexes may contain nursing diagnoses or specific patient information such as sensory deficits and fall risk. If not found on the Kardex, this information should be communicated during report so that vital information affecting nursing actions is not omitted. For instance, information that a patient is legally blind, severely hard of hearing, or mentally retarded is vitally necessary in formulating a plan of care because it affects every nursing action you take.

Some items of information not generally included on the Kardex are medications, laboratory or diagnostic test results, and treatment responses. Thus, the research you do will be necessary to collect all appropriate data.

The next way of obtaining additional information and perhaps even answering some of the questions you have asked yourself is during the shift-to-shift report. Staff nurses caring for patients will have in-depth knowledge of your patient. If the questions you have posed have not yet been answered, be sure to ask them at this time. Better knowledge of patients and their needs means a better ability to formulate problems, plan effective actions, and provide a quality standard of care.

Once these steps have been completed, quickly research anything you may have forgotten and begin to jot down problems. Remember, this does not have to be a detailed list just yet. Jotting down ideas of problems throughout the day will help you to think about your plan of care, as well as nursing actions, nursing judgment, and decision making related to nursing actions. Reinforcement and association analysis is the basis of concept mapping theory and this is putting it into action.

Figure 4-13 demonstrates the importance of interacting with staff and collaborators to answer questions and collect information. While much can be obtained from the medical record, essential pieces of information are always gleaned from verbal exchange and questioning as well. So, research refers to reviewing the chart in addition to interaction with all members of the healthcare team. Direct patient contact plus collaborative interaction plus research equals in-depth knowledge of patient problems and will lead to effective nursing actions. In the course of any nurse–patient interaction, multiple senses and methods are used to collect and analyze multiple sources of important information that then contribute to the problem list and resultant nursing actions.

Now let's create a sample list following the steps and methods outlined earlier. Suppose you arrive on the clinical site and your Kardex contains the following information (most Kardexes/plans of care are simple black and white, computer-generated forms).

Figure 4-13 Sample patient medical record.

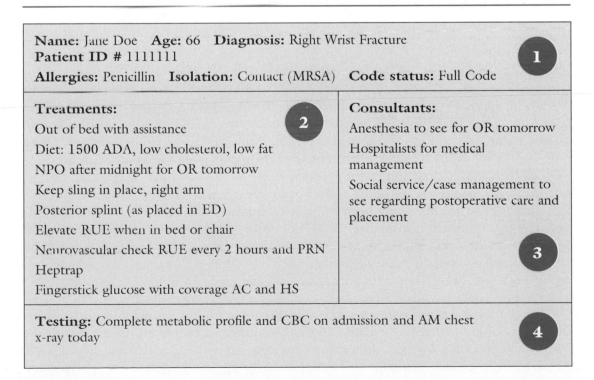

Name: Jane Doe   **Age:** 66   **Diagnosis:** Right Wrist Fracture
Patient ID # 1111111

1

Allergies: Penicillin   **Isolation:** Contact (MRSA)   **Code status:** Full Code

Treatments:

2

Out of bed with assistance

Diet: 1500 ADA, low cholesterol, low fat

NPO after midnight for OR tomorrow

Keep sling in place, right arm

Posterior splint (as placed in ED)

Elevate RUE when in bed or chair

Neurovascular check RUE every 2 hours and PRN

Heptrap

Fingerstick glucose with coverage AC and HS

Consultants:

Anesthesia to see for OR tomorrow

Hospitalists for medical management

Social service/case management to see regarding postoperative care and placement

3

Testing: Complete metabolic profile and CBC on admission and AM chest x-ray today

4

Section one identifies several problems and areas of concern:

- The patient has a wrist fracture and will have pain that needs to be assessed and managed.
- More information must be obtained regarding the stability of the fracture and any planned treatment.
- An allergy to penicillin is a problem and medications must be researched for any cross-sensitivity.
- The patient is ordered to have contact isolation for methicillin-resistant *Staphylococcus aureus* (MRSA). Questions to research would be whether the infection is active or inactive. Patients with past evidence of MRSA must be isolated until repeat cultures are negative. The patient and her family will need education regarding the isolation requirements and proper donning and disposal of garb.
- A status of full code signifies that you must be ready to respond in the event of a code blue.

Already, five problems or areas of concern have been identified. The next step would be to begin thinking of the resulting nursing actions.

Section two identifies problems related to treatments and safety concerns. An order for activity with assistance should prompt some questions:

1. Does the patient require some assistance because of something in the PMH or because her fracture site needs to be stabilized constantly or both?
2. The patient could have a high fall risk assessment because of past history of falls or secondary to pain medication. A fall would definitely contribute to complications.

The patient's diet order hints at both a diabetic and cardiac history. The fingerstick glucose order does as well. Further research is needed to satisfy questions regarding this. Appropriate resources are listed in Figure 4-12. NPO status signifies a need for patient education as well as alerting other staff and the dietary department that the patient receives no oral intake after midnight. The next several orders assist with identifying actual and potential problems related to the wrist fracture. These would be fracture displacement, pain, and possible neurovascular compromise. Actions related to these problems take priority. One problem related to any IV therapy is the potential for infection and maintaining patency of the access device.

Section #3 could be considered an area of concern. Nursing actions related to consultations are: Ensuring they have been completed and the patient is actually seen. If this is not actually witnessed, information would be found within the medical record as stated earlier. Another action would be to be present during the visit so that questions can be answered and any nursing care concerns can be relayed. A consult for placement should prompt investigation. A wrist fracture rarely results in a need for placement outside the home unless the patient is generally weak or has difficulty with self-care.

Laboratory and diagnostic testing require nursing actions because it must be ensured that the tests are actually completed and the results must be placed on the chart. So, while not a "problem" per se, they are areas of concern with mandated nursing actions. As part of this process, nursing knowledge must be applied to determine whether the results fall into a normal range or not and what symptoms accompany an abnormal level. Each facility determines which tests complete a basic metabolic profile. The nurse needs to have knowledge of this. Generally, this umbrella term includes the following tests:

- BUN
- Creatinine
- Electrolytes
- Glucose
- Calcium

The CBC will measure the hemoglobin, hematocrit, and mature and immature blood cell measurements.

As you can see, the Kardex review only scratches the surface where patient problems are concerned. The review generates questions and the need for research of the medical record. Those steps, in combination with critical thinking and relationship analysis, result in a patient problem list and the nursing actions accompanying them. Theoretical nursing knowledge must be sound for this to take place. Knowledge really is power!

Developing a Checklist for Patient Problems

With all of the sources available and data to be collected, it is prudent to utilize a checklist to identify patient problems. This then becomes the catalyst for nursing actions. It will allow you to categorize and picture the appropriate number of steps needed to complete an action. You will find a template in **Figure 4-14**. Please remember that any attachments originating from the patient's medical record must be used only by permission according to your school or clinical facility's policy. In most cases this means that no patient-related documents may be removed from the facility for outside use. Any patient-related document must have the patient's name removed per Health Insurance Portability and Accountability Act (HIPAA) privacy/confidentiality laws. In the problem list collection tool, only the patient's initials are used. This tool provides plenty of room to record data so that no information is needed beyond the clinical setting to complete a concept map.

This template will assist with improving critical thinking in several ways:

- It will allow you to evaluate your research abilities.
- It will promote relationship analysis through connecting concepts such as symptoms and diseases.
- You will develop a deeper understanding of how patient problems and concerns affect nursing actions.
- You will see improvements in patient care judgment and decision making.
- What you have previously learned will take on new meaning as you begin to apply it.

Use the checklist to assist with organizing information. When you arrive on the clinical site, use the checklist to *fill in the blanks*, so to speak. This is the first step in preparing for patient care. Along with reviewing the medical record, this step serves as

Figure 4-14 Patient problem list collection tool.

Page 1

Date:	Student Name:		
Patient Initials:	Age:	Room/Unit:	Admitting Diagnosis:
HPI:	PMH/PSH:		
IV Access Device/Size:	Large Volume Fluid/Drip:		
Allergies:	Code Status:		
Medications:	Laboratory & Diagnostic Test Results		

Figure 4-14 Patient problem list collection tool. ***(Continued)***

Page 2

	Problems	Concerns
Physical		
Mental		
Psycho-social		
Cultural/Spiritual		
Medication Related		
Laboratory Test Related		
Diagnostic Test Related		

(Continued)

Figure 4-14 **Patient problem list collection tool.** *(Continued)*

Page 3

Nursing Diagnoses:

Notes/Problem Associations/Preliminary Actions:

the preliminary phase of planning care. As you research and collect necessary information, your mind is beginning to make associations not only between your findings and potential nursing actions, but also between the facts you uncover. Once that is completed, you will be ready to receive report and begin caring for the patient. By that time most of your questions should have been answered. More questions will form throughout the day, but those initial questions stimulate problem solving thought processes.

You can also see that this form considers holistic information to be used in planning care. A complete plan of care must always include this as an integral focus of care.

Summary

Each stage and step used in concept map creation helps you to explore your knowledge base. Within that base is the foundation of nursing practice. This chapter has made you think a great deal about how knowledge impacts critical thinking and all other components of concept mapping theory. But knowledge in and of itself is not all you need to create a concept map or practice at an appropriate standard. Recognition of patient problems and how to formulate a plan of care related to them is the process that reinforces knowledge application. Application can occur only after those problems are identified and a plan of care is formulated. Using the nursing process, nursing diagnoses are created that lead to nursing actions.

In order to create those actions, this chapter has focused on methods to collect information from which patient problems can be formed. A problem or area of concern can be anything related to the patient that requires a nursing action, ranging from simple monitoring to multiple-staged interventions. One action is rarely enough to fully address any patient problem. Additionally, at any one time, multiple problems or concerns are occurring simultaneously. This, of course, requires the constant identification, evaluation, and reevaluation of problems and actions. In this way, the nursing process and plan of care are continually evolving. Problems, actions, and interventions are constantly overlapping. This entire process is multitasking at its most advanced. One problem is never fully resolved before another begins. This is one of the biggest challenges to nursing practice. Use of concept mapping theory and concept mapping will be extremely helpful to refining your critical thinking abilities and allowing you to meet this challenge. It will also assist you in developing self-confidence and better problem-solving skills. Another benefit is improved organization and prioritization. Problem recognition and nursing action formulation must employ prioritization to ultimately provide the best and safest standards of care.

Critical Thinking Questions and Activities

1. Discuss the following questions:
    a. What makes a patient problem an active one?
    b. How does it then become part of the plan of care?
    c. What defines an inactive problem?
    d. What nursing actions are taken for inactive problems?

2. Name three sources for nursing actions and formulate answers for the following questions:

   a. What part do rationales play in creating nursing actions?

   b. What are the origins for nursing rationales and how do they help to define them?

3. Create a chart showing possible origins for main patient problems and how related problem lists are derived.

4. Discuss how SBAR notes improve communication. Then, answer the following question: How are care standards affected by the use of SBAR notes?

Case Studies

Directions: Read through each case study and answer the questions using the chapter material provided.

1. D.G. is a 70-year-old female admitted with a diagnosis of pneumonia. She had complained of sneezing and cold-like symptoms for about 5 days before admission and then began with a cough and fever of 101°F. She waited 3 more days before contacting her physician. At that visit, D.G. was coughing frequently—a hoarse cough productive of thick green sputum—and her temperature was 102°F. Her physician admitted her immediately and began IV antibiotics. Her vital signs on admission are: BP: 100/50, P-95, R-30, T-102, Pulse oximetry: 88% on room air. Her current orders are:

   - Diet as tolerated
   - Bed rest with bathroom privileges
   - Oxygen as needed to maintain saturation of 90%
   - Large volume IV dextrose 5% and ½ normal saline to infuse at 100 milliliters per hour
   - Chest x-ray stat
   - Ceftriaxone (Rocephin) IV piggyback 1 gram every 12 hours
   - Basic metabolic profile, CBC, and blood cultures times two now; call physician with results

   a. Identify D.G.'s problems and concerns.

   b. Discuss additional information necessary to complete the problem list for this patient.

   c. Identify where this information would be obtained.

   d. Make a list showing subjective and objective data for this patient.

   e. Discuss interrelationships identified between all data and problems.

2. J.N. is a 50-year-old female admitted with dysfunctional uterine bleeding. She is not yet menopausal and has had heavy periods, with bleeding between periods for 1–2 years. A trial of hormone replacement therapy did not benefit J.N., and she had become anemic and experienced an altered quality of life. She is now admitted for a total abdominal hysterectomy. Her surgery is scheduled for tomorrow at

10:00 AM, so she will be NPO after midnight. She has a scheduled IV (D51/2 NS at 120 milliliters per hour) and has been complaining of intermittent burning at the site. Her main complaint otherwise is occasional moderate to severe lower abdominal cramping and pain rated 8–9 on a scale of 0–10. Her pain has been fairly well controlled with morphine 4 mg every 4 hours as needed. At this point, J.N.'s vaginal bleeding continues and she has used 6 pads during this shift. As you prepare your SBAR note, think of the best ways to effectively communicate what you want the next shift RN to be aware of and what additional information may be necessary as well as helpful.

    a. Using this scenario, create an SBAR report for your report to the next shift.

3. S.A. is a 70-year-old patient you are caring for who was admitted with dizziness causing her to fall and fracture her right wrist. Since admission she has been confused intermittently but crying in pain. She frequently touches her right upper arm while crying but cannot answer questions regarding pain with accuracy. S.A.'s responses are inconsistent but she appears to be in great pain. The physician has ordered Percocet every 4 hours as needed, but the patient will not take it.

Using this case study, create an SBAR report for a physician. When preparing your note, consider/include the following questions and concerns:

    a. What other orders might you anticipate?

    b. How does this note advocate for the patient?

    c. What other factors need to be included?

    d. What other orders might you ask for?

WWW For a full suite of assignments and additional learning activities, use the access code located in the front of your book to visit this exclusive website: **http://go.jblearning.com/schmehl**. If you do not have an access code, you can obtain one at the site.

References

Brown, R., Feller, L., & Benedict, L. (2010). Reframing nursing education: The Quality and Safety Education for Nurses Initiative. *Teaching & Learning in Nursing, 5*(3), 115–118.

Eisenhauer, L. A., Hurley, A. C., & Dolan, N. (2007). Nurses' reported thinking during medication administration *Journal of Nursing Scholarship, 39*(1), 82–87.

Institute of Medicine. (2011). The future of nursing: Leading change, advancing health. Washington, DC: National Academies Press.

Levett-Jones, T., Hoffman, K., Dempsey, J., Jeong, S. Y., Noble, D., Norton, C. A., . . . Hickey, N. (2010). The 'five rights' of clinical reasoning: An educational model to enhance nursing students' ability to identify and manage clinically 'at risk' patients. *Nurse Education Today, 30*(6), 515–520.

Thomas, C. M., Bertram, E., & Johnson, D. (2009). The SBAR communication technique: Teaching nursing students professional communication skills. *Nursing Educator, 34*(4), 176–180.

5

Constructing a Concept Map

Learning Objectives

- Identify and demonstrate the necessary steps for creating a concept map
- Discuss how concept mapping theory is evident within the problem list and complete concept map
- Explain how concept map formatting demonstrates relationship analysis
- Analyze and explain how problem identification defines nursing actions

Introduction

Information prepared for use within a concept map is important. There is no doubt about that and indeed it is part of the process. However, collection is only part of the process. It is taking that information and placing it within a concept map that gives it meaning. Placing information into a map breathes life into it. Separate and isolated facts form associations, clarify concepts, and are valuable to analyze our thought processes. So, formatting and layout are as valuable as what the concept map contains. These two components allow a story to flow demonstrating the factual information, how it relates to main and related concepts, and how it leads to actions. The bonus result is that specific thought processes are mapped out as well, providing insight into abilities reflecting judgment, decision making, and applying knowledge.

While the purpose of this text is an emphasis on nursing applications, let's first consider a nonnursing example. Concept mapping theory places a great deal of emphasis on forming links and associations between concept. Many times, this can take place more easily at first when associations are made using familiar concepts, examples, and exercises. From there, we will move on to nursing examples. These examples will reinforce the inclusion of previously learned materials into newer theory to allow us to compare what we have learned to how it can be used as part of patient care and nursing actions. This layering of information—blending past with current knowledge—is necessary in the theory application process. Formatting the concept maps will pull all of this together. It will also give you great insight into the degree to which you can critically think and make associations between concepts. At the heart of concept mapping theory is application: taking what you know and what it means in terms of defining actions, anticipating patient needs, and considering cause and effect. You will use this knowledge in exactly this way throughout your nursing career. Now is the time to establish an expansive database of knowledge and, additionally, the critical thinking thought processes that assist you in applying it. This chapter applies concept mapping theory. It also affords an opportunity to delve more deeply into knowledge application.

Key Terms and Definitions

- **Nursing-based concept maps:** concept maps containing information based on applying nursing knowledge through analysis of skills and nursing care–related actions
- **Concept map formatting:** physical layout of concept map construction to demonstrate critical thinking and relationship analysis
- **Learning continuum:** the process of learning that begins with attaining simple knowledge and continues to comprehension and ultimately application
- **Concept map uniformity:** use of one style throughout a concept map for clarity and interpretative ease
- **Open copy templates:** blank, pre-formatted concept maps adapted to a student's preferences based on learning style and mental processing
- **Symmetrical concept map formatting:** balanced symmetry within a concept map for visual appeal and interpretation

Setting Up a Concept Map

Now that you have an idea of what a basic map looks like, we need to explore how to set one up. We will use all of the information we have gathered to select the required components and starting point. Remember, each step is simple in and of itself. It is sometimes the construction part that gets confusing. We will address this and it will become clearer. I will begin with a nonnursing example that any student can relate to. This allows for an easier beginning, because we are dealing with simple and easy recall of a common situation. There are more known facts than unknown ones, which makes problem identification and relationship analysis a bit easier.

Using a familiar example makes for easier links and the ability to see where each applies and fits into our final product, which is a completed concept map clearly demonstrating concept mapping theoretical components. Proceeding in this way may make it easier to transition to a nursing example. Although the following example could be expanded, we are going to keep it simple for better demonstration. In any given situation, there is a possibility for a large number of problems or considerations. We will limit the list to about five considerations. Let's say we are having our relatives over for a holiday meal. We will create a map from that scenario.

Step 1

Ask: What is the main concept? What are other, smaller concepts that relate in some way to the main concept?

Do: Create a list with the main concept as the heading and the related concepts listed below it.

One of the most confusing elements for students is the creation of this list, especially when research related to its creation involves abstract concepts. What you have to remember is all learning involving nursing theory progresses along a continuum. That **learning continuum** involves taking knowledge and analyzing how it fits into what was previously learned and making associations. Because the process becomes easier and clearer with more exposure to knowledge and experience, creating the problem list will become easier over time. A major step in this process is to use links and associations with *all* learning and studying. Linking and associating concepts will ensure more meaningful learning and enhance critical thinking skills.

The main concept is usually very clear, depending on the map's focus. The list of related concepts requires some deeper thought processes and may stymy you at first. Review of theory or skill knowledge may be required for accuracy and completeness of the map. Instant recall of previous knowledge occurs with repeated exposure and processing of it. Although this may be viewed as time consuming, it is in reality a part of the whole concept mapping theory described earlier in the text. As any educator is aware, repeated exposure to factual knowledge aids in the comprehension process. As stated earlier, comprehension is essential if progression to application can occur. Also, because relationship analysis is a major ingredient in the process, simply thinking about what related concepts to include and how they might fit is a big step in stimulating the critical thinking spark, where one question leads to many more.

Related concepts may further be subdivided into primary and secondary related concepts. Primary concepts usually have a more direct relationship with the main concept. They are necessary to direct the actions that will be taken next. Often, secondary related concepts have an indirect connection with the main concept but are still important to the actions taken. Separating concepts into these categories assists with the analysis process and reinforces conceptual information.

So, we know that our main concept is the dinner itself. Easy, right? Now visualize the situation as if it were really happening and you were hosting this get-together in a week. Next, think of everything else you will need or need to consider that relates to having a dinner for a group of people. (Note: if you are doing this exercise with a class, you may want to limit the list to five things because of time constraints.) Your list would look something like this:

Dinner Party

- Number of guests
- Menu and courses
- Invitations
- Special dietary needs?
- Supplies

As you see, once you start thinking of things, many more possibilities pop into your head. You might choose other considerations such as time of day to host the event, the dinner theme, beverage supplies, whether to serve alcoholic beverages or not, and seating arrangements.

Once this has been completed, take a moment or two to determine what interrelationships exist on the related concept list. We can immediately take note that the supplies we need and the number of invitations necessary directly relate to the number of guests. Any special dietary needs among the group of guests directly relate to the supplies, as well as the menu and courses. Being aware of these relationships will help when we begin placing the data into the shapes. It will help to either record these extensions of the related concepts alongside each one or create small boxes near each one to establish relationships and to prevent omitting necessary information. Writing it out in this way allows you to see the interconnectedness of everything needed to plan and host a successful dinner. If not all relationships are clear, you will want to either draw lines or color code the categories. This will make you think through how each factor is linked to reinforce it. This will be especially helpful when you begin to create a **nursing-based concept map**. As you progress in this process, you will begin to look at everything you learn and encounter clinically as having an association or interrelationship with something else. *This is an important goal to set for yourself.*

The first list you see in **Figure 5-1** is a general listing of the main and related concept list. The left-hand side of the chart would be considered the main problem or consideration concepts. The remainder of the list would signify the related concepts.

Figure 5-1 **Main and related concept list for the dinner party example.**

Dinner Party	
Main List	
Number of guests	Consider: seating arrangements, relationship to host, facility size
Menu/courses	Consider: special dietary needs/restrictions, prep time, cost
Invitations	Consider: design, number of guests, postage costs, mailing date
Special dietary needs	Influences ingredients, menu, and costs
Supplies	Consider above information plus table decoration, favors, place settings

Before we proceed, let's take the list and identify related concepts according to their primary or secondary status (see **Figure 5-2**). Then we can begin to think about actions we need to take.

As you can see, each time you consider a problem area, there are many things you could think of in addition to what is listed. Let's now focus on the list we have created.

Dinner Party Guests

This is the main, determining factor from which all other considerations originate. This main concept has helped us to formulate the related categories. The guests are the focus of the party and the basis for actions taken in planning the event. Thus, an association has been made between the guests and the related concepts.

Number of Guests

Our guest list is a vital part of planning and decision making related to cost, seating, and all other organizational planning. The specific number decides overall cost and number of supplies needed. The other important association to make is that having knowledge of the guests will determine the party's success. Although this impacts many things, I

Figure 5-2 **Organizing related concepts into primary or secondary status.**

Main concept: Dinner party guests	
Primary related concepts	**Secondary related concepts**
Number	Cost, room/facility size, seating arrangements, relationship to host/hostess
Menu choices	Presentation, place settings cost, ingredients, preparation time
Invitations	Cost, mailing schedule, RSVP instructions, postage, design
Dietary considerations	Knowledge of guests' dietary needs/restrictions, cost, inclusion of nutritional information
Supplies	Groceries, beverages, place settings and silverware, cost, table decorations, favors

have isolated dietary restrictions. Not considering guest dietary restrictions could lead to allergic reactions, reluctance to attend, or even a great deal of leftover food.

Preliminary actions related to all of the information gathered could include:

- Setting up a budget
- Calling guests to ask about food preferences and any dietary restrictions
- Planning a time budget for food preparation
- Preparing table cards labeled with nutritional information of the food served

So, already in the first step, we are thinking about possible actions and making associations between them and our list of items.

Using a formal tool such as a collection tool or an informal tool such as a piece of notepaper and recording the problem or concern as you research is a good plan for a rudimentary problem list. Once that has been completed, you will then refine the list as we did here. No matter the method, be sure to begin to make associations immediately. You can include notes for each category, enclose like groupings within circles, or draw a type of chart to begin making associations. Again, I have to emphasize that because everyone assimilates and mentally processes information differently, choose a method congruent with your learning and mental processing style. Some generalized questions to ask during this process are:

1. What concepts or things relate directly to the main concept?
2. What concepts or things relate indirectly to the main concept?
3. If a link is identified, in what ways is that link evident?
4. In what ways do the items on the related problem lists associate with and differentiate from each other?
5. How do cause and effect play a role in making associations?

In order to fully tease out the specific associations, it will be necessary to ask specific questions as well. Some specific questions for this scenario might be:

1. How is cost affected by guests' food preferences?
2. How many varieties of foods are necessary based on those preferences?
3. When should the invitations be sent out so that there is enough time for guests to RSVP?

In each part of Step 1, we have used critical thinking and relationship analysis to identify concepts and anticipate actions. The same process will take place within nursing-based concept map problem lists.

Step 2

Ask: What shapes can be used and what goes in each one?

Do: Begin to play with various formats, being sure the map is legible.

In general, there is no limit to the number of shapes. It is much better to have more shapes with less content in each than too many concepts lumped together in a too large shape. Using multiple shapes allows for more effective definition of concepts through isolation, makes for a cleaner and more organized appearance, and is a format that better demonstrates the path of your concept map. It is a wonderful idea to practice as we proceed for maximum benefit. You may indeed come up with a different related concept list and use different shapes. This is where your creativity and learning style come into the picture. Having said that, if your learning style has a strong verbal focus, placing small lists or even outlines into a map may work better for you. For the more visual learner, clip art may work better. (To use a Concept Map Creator, see the Student Companion Website at http://go.jblearning.com/schmehl.)

As you begin to practice and try out various formats, pay close attention to your formatting, including all basic components and avoid clumping. It may even be helpful to simply draw shapes first to see which you like best. Then, you can adjust layout and see which ones look best. For instance, **Figure 5-3** shows some possible preliminary layouts.

The left side of the diagram in Figure 5-3 shows a clear information pathway and clear links. The right side has a chaotic and jumbled appearance that would be distracting and difficult, if not impossible, to interpret and follow. When formatting, one of the goals is to show each step in your thought process. This establishes a clear pathway demonstrating the use of critical thinking thought processes and can be used as a reflective tool as well.

Step 3

Ask: What descriptive phrases and lines work best with the relationships you want to demonstrate?

Do: Use lines to link all concepts.

Do: Choose action phrases.

Do: Experiment and find those that best fit with what you want to show.

If you draw a blank, go back and review the previous information on descriptive phrases and remember that each phrase is describing an action you have either performed

Figure 5-3 **Desired versus undesired layouts.**

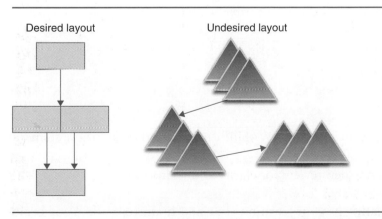

or plan to perform. The phrases assist you with demonstrating how you have linked a piece of knowledge with a necessary action. You can practice this on paper or while providing care. Let's assume you are caring for a patient with a new finding of hypotension. As you recognize that this is an abnormal finding, your mind should be linking an action. Examples of the thought patterns and possible linking phrases found below will be useful to think this through. Putting all thoughts in sentence form is another method to help reinforce information and to understand how you would "say" the same thing in a concept map.

1. *New hypotension can lead to dizziness so my action is to monitor for orthostatic vital signs and institute safety measures.*

   The phrase "can lead to" connects your recognition of hypotension to dizziness. Use of the phrases "monitor" and "institute" includes safety considerations and takes your actions a step further.

2. *My patient's blood pressure is 98/45, and this is a new finding. I will need to notify the RN and assess the patient for symptoms.*

   The first statement demonstrates recognition of an abnormal finding as well as comparative analysis of the patient's other blood pressure results with this measurement. The descriptive phrase "notify" indicates actions related to collaborative care are chosen. Additionally, it demonstrates that you recognize your own practice limitations, that the physician will be notified, and that new orders will most likely be received. Finally, choosing an action to "assess" the patient demonstrates your knowledge and critical thinking are leading you to anticipate symptoms and the possible need for further nursing actions.

3. *My patient has a hypotensive blood pressure. Before I administer these antihypertensive medications, I will need to assess for any hold parameters and then recheck the blood pressure prior to administration.*

   Several meaningful information links are evident here. Critical thinking and relationship analysis have been used to recognize the link between hypotension and administering the antihypertensive medications. In addition, past experience with these medications has created an awareness of hold parameters. The phrases "need to assess" and "recheck" reflect these thought processes.

The type of lines you use needs to connect all problems, related concepts, and actions. The lines are the roadways, so to speak, and assist with deciphering the concept map and the path your thought processes have taken. They help to show interrelationship among and between concepts.

Step 4

Ask: What layout demonstrates a clear flow of information and makes the statement I want?

Do: Fill in the layout, and then review for clarity and uniformity.

This is where you will really put your learning style and brain to work. Your brain has already absorbed, investigated, categorized, and organized the information under consideration. Now the information moves through your brain and becomes a pattern of thought processes that then move to your hands where you will express what your mind sees. While you absolutely need to have clear, in depth knowledge of your learning and brain processing methods, please know that formatting may not come easily at first. Thinking through something and then getting that information onto paper in a logical format is not always easy. Although you may think this way and carry out actions this way, there is a certain degree of difficulty at first. You need to work at it and tune in to how your brain "sees" so that the flow of information makes sense. As I stated earlier, this process is somewhat like reading symbols or thinking in a different language. It takes time and practice. Most students will choose a pattern and then continue to use it, maybe with slight variations at times. Others may experiment over several weeks until they find a format that works for them and feels comfortable. Please do not get discouraged. The work you put into this process now will most definitely reap rewards later. Give it time, be patient with yourself, seek help, and above all do not give up.

Begin with one concept at a time. Choose a shape for it, a descriptive phrase, and line style, and then link it to the main concept. Repeat this process until your map is complete. Continue to make associations as you go, just as you have done when creating the problem list.

Once you find a layout format that flows congruently with your learning style, you may choose to keep an open or blank copy of it for use in other projects. These open copy templates may need alterations when used in living maps, but can be used as is for static maps.

Open copy templates usually include shapes and formatting styles that are pleasing to the eye and flow according to how your brain sees and processes information (to use a Concept Map Creator, see the Student Companion Website at http://go.jblearning.com/schmehl). The benefit is that they lend themselves to a variety of uses because they are personalized, and all you will have to do is fill in the blanks. They can be used and stored on either paper or via electronic methods. Formatting will change little when used as a static map. At the same time, adding information when used as living maps will be very easy because you will use the same formatting. Any "add on" information will simply be an extension of the template.

Concept Map Formatting Options

In this section you will find several variations of **concept map formatting** based on the dinner party theme we explored earlier. Yours may look different, and that is fine. Remember, your personal learning style and hemispheric brain dominance in processing information is a huge part of how you see that the flow looks as it should to your mind's eye. You will know when it looks "right." Then, as long as it *demonstrates relationship analysis, contains all the components of a basic map setup, and is legible and uniform*, your concept map will have *value and meaning*. Value and meaning become evident as you follow the pathways of your map. If you take your finger and trace it along the shapes and lines of your map, critical thinking and relationship analysis should be evident. This is applied concept mapping theory.

However, this is not where everything ends. The end result of any map—what appears on the paper in front of you—is a direct result of your thought processes. It is a direct expression of how you took the information in and then processed, separated, and categorized it to create that map. It becomes a window into your mind and how it problem solves. When you are finished and are studying your map, ask yourself the following questions:

- Have I been able to see and include all necessary information?
- Did I ask enough questions and demonstrate all the necessary steps needed—whether they are skill or nursing action related?
- If I did not accomplish the above two goals, why not?

This evaluation is a form of reflection and absolutely necessary in nursing practice and nursing education.

As you move beyond creating *static maps* to creating *living maps*, you will be able to use that insight to assess your critical thinking skills as they apply to complex patient situations. Concept maps are barometers of critical thinking ability. The finished product allows you to reflect on your performance and assess your ability to apply knowledge. Faculty can assess clinical competency in addition to using each map as a teaching tool at the same time. Maps are a wonderful tool for providing feedback and guiding students toward attainment of competencies and acceptable practice standards. An extremely important component in faculty evaluation of student maps is feedback. I cannot stress that enough. Student self-assessment paired with constructive and regularly provided faculty feedback serve as reinforcement of performance and competency fulfillment.

Formatting can be carried out much more smoothly when there is an awareness and application of your specific learning style. Knowing your learning style is important because it will point you in the right direction. If you like to examine pieces of information first, your map may show a main concept in the middle of the paper, surrounded by shapes with arrows pointing back to it. If you like to consider the overall concept first, your map might show a shape at the top of the page with related concepts fanning out from it. One student might set up a map with the main concept or problem set on the left side of the page with the flow of information extending out to the right. Another may choose to place the main problem/concept in the center of the paper and then group related concepts in small clusters in each corner. *I cannot reiterate enough that there is no right or wrong way in map formatting as long as concept mapping theory is evident.* To become both proficient and comfortable with this process, you need to practice, practice, practice.

As you experiment with various formatting styles, be sure to use a pencil rather than a pen or marker. Using larger sized drawing paper or a poster board will give you more room to practice. Another helpful hint is to use small pieces of paper on which you have written your concepts/lists. You will then be able to move them around to find which layout works best. You will find that although practice is key, knowing your content is essential as well.

Figure 5-4 is set up in a sort of "T" shape where the main concept is centrally located and differentiated by color and a different shape from the others. I have altered the main concept a bit to overall planning of the party and narrowed down the related concepts because of space constraints.

The three main related concepts are outlined in gray and are the launching point for additional related concepts important to the project—signified by the cyan boxes. Interrelationships between the related concepts are demonstrated through placement of the cyan boxes against each other. This demonstrates and reinforces their links to each other

Figure 5-4 Formatting example 1.

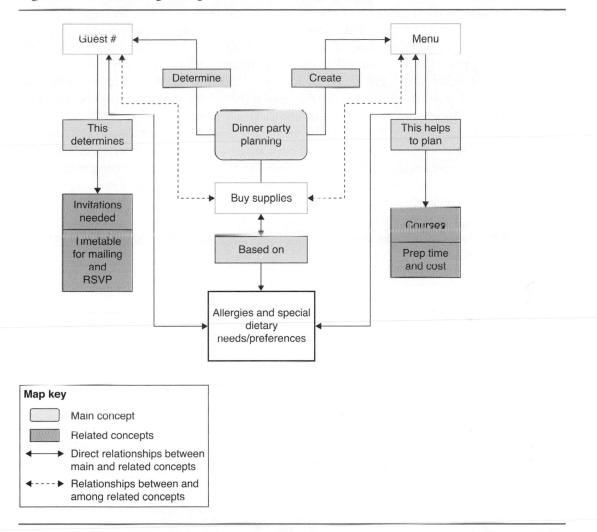

as well as the main concept. Descriptors are highlighted and connect the main focus to the related ones. Arrows show dependent relationships, and the bold black outline on the lower box stresses the importance of considering this information when planning the party. Overall, this style looks first at the main concept and then at how everything else affects it. Although it is somewhat simple, all the components of concept mapping theory are evident. This map is fairly easy to read and interpret, but the included key is helpful to reinforce the connections made.

Another thing that stands out in this map is symmetry. Though symmetry is not essential to formatting, it may make the map appear balanced and emphasize comparison and contrast within the concept map. Because one goal of map formation is creating a pathway of information that flows easily, symmetry may aid that process. Using balanced, **symmetrical concept map formatting** may also be more pleasing to look at. Just remember that the content of the map is what counts. It is not supposed to be a grand work of art. Symmetrical structure in a concept map may appear as balanced clusters of information spread out over the entire sheet of paper (often in each corner) or as divided segments of information in halves of the sheet (top and bottom or left and right). Often, this is not intentional but part of the expression of thought accompanying the learning style and brain processing method of the student. Each style has its own preference, and this will be expressed as the map takes shape. Symmetry allows for each portion of the map to be considered separately. This can assist students with analytical review and reinforce learning. It may also provide a starting point for faculty in evaluation and grading.

Figure 5-5 incorporates more visual components and a smoother format. Double-pointed arrows indicate a global interrelationship between all concepts, as do the descriptive phrases. It is also more of an action-based map. Take a moment and consider the types of descriptive phrases used in both maps. The first map has a stronger focus on planning, while this example places more emphasis on carrying out actions related to seeing the party through.

In this map, there is more of a focus on the related concepts and how they contribute to the main concept. You now begin to see how relationship analysis is accomplished in

Figure 5-5 Formatting example 2.

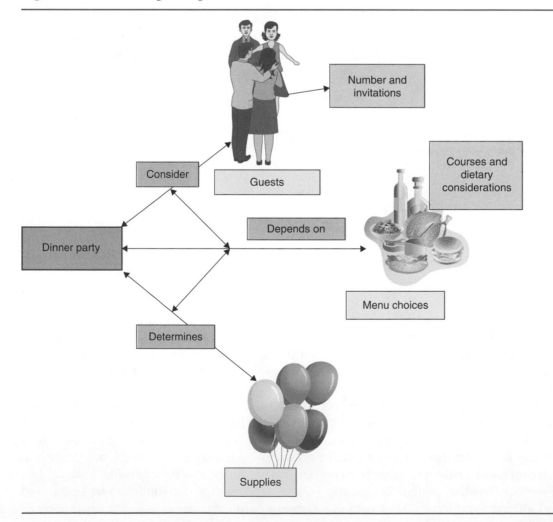

varied ways. Each of these maps is demonstrating the same thing. It is only the format that has changed. While the first map's structure appears to be very concrete and tightly structured, the second map's is looser and more open. Each map shows a starting point as well as the critical thinking and analysis allowing the endpoint to be reached. Each demonstrates the action needed to plan and host a successful dinner party. This equates to the steps of assessing, planning, implementing, and evaluating we know from the nursing process. We have assessed the needs involved in having the party. After that, we planned and implemented well-thought-out strategies. Although evaluation is not clearly demonstrated in these examples, it would occur after the host or hostess reflects on positive outcomes such as happy guests and positive comments.

There is also a much stronger visual focus with the map in Figure 5-5. Photos and clip art can have a strong impact in stimulating critical thinking for visual learners. Visualizing a situation or action can provide valuable insight into judgment and followthrough. It is important to note that if the pictures do not appear on the map a student creates, they can be mentally depicted images that aid in map creation and formatting.

For nonvisual learners, simply seeing their mental actions written on paper will accomplish the same thing. In this situation, however, that depiction may be in words, lists, or phrases. I often tell students who are having difficulty visualizing nursing actions to sit quietly and picture what they did for their patient step by step throughout the day. Then they can better create a map based on those actions. This helps all students, regardless of their learning styles. This insight then becomes integral in evaluating the knowledge application process. After you finish studying and comparing all the maps shown here, ask yourself which one looks best to you and why. Then compare that with your learning style. How does it match up?

Let's look at one more example. **Figure 5-6** is based more on a verbal learning style. It features a top-down approach, a simple format, lists, and an interconnectedness of all concepts by the *linked* boxes. The focus is the main concept and how the smaller concepts relate back to it. This is a great example of the fact that a concept map does not have to be artistically creative. This map contains all the information seen in the others

Figure 5-6 **Formatting example 3.**

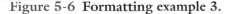

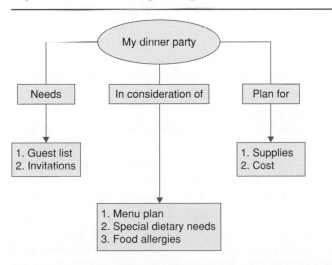

yet is short, concise, and to the point. It still demonstrates the same thing. Please do not mistake the simplicity and directness of this map as not having insight as I spoke about earlier. Simplicity and straightforwardness does not equal shortsightedness. These characteristics reflect a different learning style and mental processing and are like a snapshot of information. This map, as the others, would need to be expanded as needed to be complete and thorough.

Both simplicity and complexity in a map are determined by learning and brain processing styles, topic, subject matter, and the particular focus of the map. This is true whether the concept map is nursing based or nonnursing based.

There are other possible formatting options, personally tailored by you according to your learning style and how your brain processes information. An essential part of discovering formatting options is practice. All of the thought and reasoning processes used in creating a concept map are methods you are already using, whether in the nursing skills lab or in the clinical setting. Now you need to practice by taking your thoughts and actions and transferring them to paper. Obtaining a glimpse of your thoughts on paper is a powerful tool for self-evaluation.

All three formatting examples shown here reinforce some important points:

1. Learning styles are evidenced in completed concept maps. This is true whether a mixture is noted or one certain type dominates.
2. Creative expression is evident and reflects on critical thinking abilities. This refers to how you are able to demonstrate the connection between concepts.
3. Individual formatting styles are partially determined by mental information processing. This statement is drawn from concept mapping theory. While formatting is influenced by learning style, mental processing of learned knowledge is necessary in structuring and formatting as well.

Evaluation and Review of Your Concept Map

Once your concept map has been completed, evaluation and review are essential. The process will become faster as you go and will play an important role in the self-reflection process. A checklist is helpful in completing this process. The example in **Figure 5-7** explains how using a checklist can help ensure that you have included all necessary information within your map. It is that final step, such as you would use prior to submitting a scholarly paper or other assignment, where you check the final product for completeness. In addition to serving as a reminder of what to include, this process also reinforces learning through repetitive analysis of your map's content.

This particular checklist is not a rubric but a list of considerations for evaluation based on concept mapping theory. Please note that most students do not fully achieve all of the listed components at first. Concept mapping is a learning process and needs to be paired with theory, experience, and nurturing of critical thinking. As a student you need to know that each map should become more detailed, complex, and complete as you proceed through each week of the semester. This is not because you lack either the knowledge or the critical thinking abilities to ace this on the first try, but because you are using your thought processes in a different way. The way you think, process, and learn have not changed. What has changed may be the number of steps you use to travel

Figure 5-7 **Component checklist.**

Component	Yes	No	Notes
Is my main concept/map focus shown clearly?			
Are related concepts differentiated from the main concept?			
Do my descriptive phrases show interrelationships?			
Does my map demonstrate all connections that exist?			
Is a key necessary to interpret the map?			
Is the map legible, uniform, and easy to follow?			
Is my map comprehensive?			
Did I include all necessary components?			
Did I follow all the steps?			
Is there evidence of adequate knowledge and the ability to apply it?			

from point A to point B and how you may have to reorganize those steps and thoughts to transfer them to paper. Although you may feel you are processing information totally differently, I can assure you that this is not the case.

Now it is time to consider all we have learned so far to construct a map from a nursing example. We will use a relatively simple example. More examples will follow in subsequent chapters. Consider the following scenario: *You are getting your elderly female patient out of bed for the first time following a bowel resection the day before.* As we complete each step, please use the preceding pages to test yourself to see if you remember how to proceed. There may be a few more steps than the number listed earlier because we need to break things down a bit to thoroughly address all components.

Step 1

Our first step is to identify the main consideration or topic for our map. Although several things stand out with this patient, it is the act of getting out of bed that is our main focus. Because this patient is a postoperative patient, our *main topic*, concern, or focus can be labeled: *assisting the fresh postoperative patient out of bed.* Now we are ready to formulate the problem list.

Step 2

Our second step is to start a list and then populate it. We have an activity order to get the patient out of bed. We already have a heading. Now we need to think about all the other related considerations that have some sort of relationship to this action. Take a moment to think about this, and then look at the list I have created. If you run out of ideas, use the mini checklist in **Figure 5-8** to guide you. The mini checklist features

Figure 5-8 Mini checklist.

Component	Thought Processes/Rationales
Critical thinking	What particular factors affect this action based on: • Patient history • Safety • Communication • Related factors
Relationship analysis	How do all of these considerations affect each other and enable the action to be completed?
Application	Use all of the above thought processes and rationales to formulate a plan and complete this task. This determines specific actions listed in your map and also considers outcomes.

main components you would include, based on concept mapping theory. As stated earlier, it may help you to think about a patient you assisted out of bed in the past. What things did you think about before you completed that task? What information did you have to know? All of these things become the *related concept* listings. This step is also where *relationship analysis* should appear. Related concepts cannot be considered without a knowledge base that allows for comparison and recognition of connections that exist between actions and the factors that must enter into decision making before an action is carried out. In addition to the mini checklist, overall general categories to consider and that will assist you are:

- Safety
- Communication
- The impact of the history of present illness (HPI) and personal medical history (PMH)
- Any diagnosis or information related to patient ambulation

This checklist may be used with either static or living maps. It may need to be revised somewhat depending upon the focus of the map, particular patient considerations, the care setting, and the action to be performed. What may change is the section on thought processes and rationales. The components will always remain the same, because they embody concept mapping theory. Using this mini checklist, which can be tailored to a specific patient or situation, with the component checklist will assist you in formulating a complete and thorough problem list and concept map. In a moment we will use the mini checklist to evaluate our problem list. At this point, you should be able to determine that constructing a concept map requires use of concept mapping theory, use of all necessary components, and a knowledge base from which to draw information for analysis. Applying concept mapping theory also allows comparison and contrast between old and new knowledge in a way that reinforces the application of it.

Problem List

Main Concept: Assist the fresh postoperative patient out of bed.
Related Concepts: Considerations relative to completing this task include:

- Patient history related to any mobility/ambulatory concerns
  - Diseases/conditions causing mobility/ambulatory dysfunction
  - Sensory deficits
  - Past history of falls/PMH
  - History of syncope
  - Mental status and ability to understand teaching
- Current considerations
  - Abnormal lab tests contributing to syncope
  - Medication effects leading to dizziness/syncope
  - Pain control
  - Need for any assistive devices/personnel
  - Incisional support

Let's take a moment to analyze the list. In consideration of critical thinking, we know safety is of primary concern. We need to have knowledge of all factors that might contribute to any adverse safety outcomes. Our actions within the map will demonstrate this. If we take a closer look at our list to determine interrelationships, we see that patient history and all of its components directly relate back to our task at hand. Failure to consider any one of those items may result in undesired outcomes. Perhaps our patient has a history of ambulatory dysfunction, a fact that greatly impacts the action of assisting her out of bed.

Communication is an essential part of this task because we need the patient's cooperation. Mental status and any sensory deficits relate to our main task and goal of getting this patient safely out of bed. The presence of any deficits may mean the task will take longer and require more education as well as more reinforcement of it to ensure understanding. Splinting the incision will aid in controlling some of her pain and prevent wound dehiscence. The patient's ability to comprehend and follow directions is integral to outcomes.

The related factors under the current considerations have a relationship with critical thinking and relationship analysis, as well as application. If we are not able to recognize, consider, and research these, there is a critical thinking deficit. Pain control is essential before we begin, but we must also recognize side effects such as dizziness. Major surgery usually means blood loss equivalent to at least a half unit of blood (approximately 200 mL) or possibly more. Knowledge of hemoglobin and hematocrit levels would indicate whether the patient may experience orthostatic hypotension, which increases her fall risk. Finally, all of this translates into application, because that is the culmination of all of the considerations, relationships, and actions we have recognized. Does this all make sense? Can you recognize the nursing process within this scenario?

Our thought processes here have demonstrated both concept mapping theory knowledge and the steps of the nursing process. We have identified where each component of concept mapping theory enters into our decision making. We have also assessed our patient's needs, diagnosed patient deficits, and planned actions to complete our task.

Implementation will be the act of transferring the patient from bed to chair, and evaluation can be added to our maps as a section on how this patient tolerated the procedure. Although I have emphasized how the concept map itself will highlight your critical thinking skills, you can and should easily see that the process starts with the related concept list. If you are unable to recognize every essential concept that affects or has a relationship with the main concept, you may need to take another look at how you critically think. The same is true if you lack insight into interrelationships between items on the related concepts list as well as those that occur between that list and the main concept. Making associative learning an active process—a learning and comprehension focus based on interrelationships—will assist you in achieving goals of enhanced critical thinking.

Step 3

In this step, we are ready to choose shapes and begin formatting our map. But before we do this, we have to determine how we want to identify and label the related concepts. For this example, the related concepts' shapes will contain the necessary nursing actions relative to getting the patient out of bed. Looking at the list we have created, it is evident that there are *primary* or main concerns and *secondary* concerns. A very important consideration in this step is deciding what a prime area of focus is and what then extends off of or stems from that primary consideration, which then becomes the secondary consideration. This is what we mean by taking actions out far enough on a concept map. That process takes into consideration all steps needed to meet all requirements of mapping theory, allowing for outcomes. This is one of the steps in relationship analysis—being able to compare and contrast through isolating and examining individual and grouped concepts. Take a few minutes to think about this and give it a try. Then look at the following example.

Once you have done that, it is time to choose shapes for the main and related concepts. Choose any shapes you would like. Enter the main concept. Then, before adding the connecting lines, decide on the formatting you will use. Use large paper and a pencil with an eraser. Take your time and experiment with formats you like. Remember that those you like, that appear very pleasing to your eye, will be aligned with your learning style and mental processing methods. Draw, erase, and reformat as needed until it looks the way you want it. Once you have completed that task, add lines and linking phrases for this first section. (You can also use a Concept Map Creator from the Student Companion Website at http://go.jblearning.com/schmehl.)

Figure 5-9 is an example of the first steps utilized in creating a concept map for our patient. Color differentiates the main concept from our primary related concepts inside the heavily lined boxes. These have been identified as having a primary focus because they will guide our actions. Think back to the dinner party example. Although we had an entire list of considerations, we separated out those things that were necessary to focus on that would then include all of the others. The first sets are areas and actions that have to be satisfied before we can move forward. And so it is in this example. Everything we begin with considers factors related to safety, communication, patient history, and other related factors, as we identified earlier. Each primary related concept extends from the main concept as identified by the arrows, and the cyan linking phrase boxes explain their relationship back to the main concept. You can easily see that each linking phrase speaks to an action. Each action can be equated to a step in the nursing process. The blocks containing information on PMH and current considerations would be part of assessment,

Figure 5-9 Example of the first steps utilized in creating a concept map.

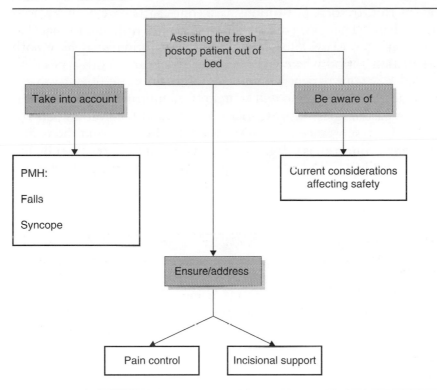

diagnosis, and planning. The boxes containing information on pain and incisional support are the implementation.

Step 4

Our next step is to complete the map by adding the secondary related concepts, along with their specific linking phrases. Use color differentiation if necessary and be sure to include a key if needed. This will include any remaining items from our list not previously addressed. Again, they are our nursing actions—things we will specifically need to perform to ensure positive outcomes related to our goal of getting the patient out of bed. Sources for obtaining some of this information may be:

- The patient's verbal statements or health history
- The nursing database
- The chart itself
- The patient Kardex
- Family members
- Vital sign graphs
- The medication administration record (MAR)

If you are not familiar with where to find valuable patient information on the chart, please take time to review this. In some institutions hard copy charts have been replaced completely by electronic charts. These may display information in a different format that makes it difficult to find and/or access information. Other institutions may have both types. Request an orientation period where you have time to research both types. You cannot have full knowledge of your patient without this information.

The history and physical (H&P) section will contain the admitting diagnosis, HPI, and PMH, as well as any past surgical history, social history, and medication listings. Psychosocial, cultural, and any substance abuse history would also be found there, and including this information in your plan is integral to providing holistic care. The nursing database will have a health history, the admission physical assessment, and religious preferences.

Step 5

Now that our map is complete, we have to review it for clarity, symmetry, all components of concept mapping theory, and information flow (see **Figure 5-10**). You may recall that your map may have a different formatting. As long as it meets all the criteria we have been discussing, that is fine. No two maps are or have to be exactly alike. The example map clearly differentiates between the main concept and the related ones. If we had more room, we could be even more specific. Let's examine each of the numbered boxes in Figure 5-10 and think about what else we could add:

1. This box addresses deficits. Things to include here would be deficits present post-cerebrovascular accident (CVA) such as a flaccid extremity, a limb with a fracture, an amputated limb, blindness, a neuromuscular disease, or generalized weakness. Any of these are important to outcomes when it comes to tolerance of the activity and its duration. Include any assistance and the number needed, as well as any assistive devices used. An inclusion and awareness of these indicate strong critical thinking skills. Getting a patient out of bed seems simple, but many individual factors must be considered.

2. In this section, other actions to be included would be the need for dangling the patient to assess for tolerance when the blood pressure is orthostatic. Identify specific lab results such as hemoglobin and hematocrit that contribute to the preceding facts. Because this affects oxygenation, including measurements such as oxygen saturation and any respiratory symptoms that occur would be an excellent idea. Any medication effects resulting in dizziness would be noted. Perhaps the medication would need to be held until the patient is returned to bed.

3. Pain must be assessed before trying to move the patient. Things will proceed much more smoothly when the patient can tolerate it. Adding a box for the medication name, dose, and effectiveness would address this. In addition, a pain score before, during, and after would indicate pain medication effectiveness.

4. I would include teaching in this section, as well as return demonstration. Also valuable would be a wound assessment, both before and after the activity.

The last element you could add would be additional lines showing the interrelationships between data groupings. For example, adding dashed lines connecting syncope with

Figure 5-10 Completed concept map.

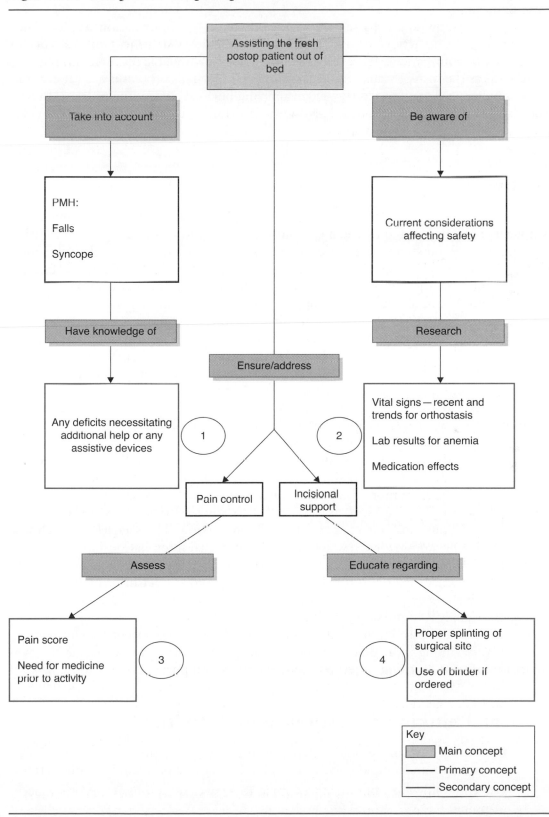

medications and abnormal labs would show that syncope has occurred secondary to those findings.

You should now begin to see the type and volume of information needed when determining nursing actions as well as their sources. Always strive to know as much as possible about your patient. Have adequate knowledge of available resources and how to quickly access them. As I stated earlier, nothing is static. This process is a great example of that statement. As you proceed, you are applying but also continuing to learn. In fact, everything you just did is application. Now, the last thing is to use the checklist provided in Figure 5-7 to review your map.

Summary

In summary, a concept map can be as simple or complex as you need it to be. Simplicity or complexity is often affected by the map's purpose but is also an indicator of your critical thinking skills. For instance, in the creation of a skill-related static map, a relatively simple style can be utilized because the relationships are simpler and the list of related concepts may be smaller. A larger, more complex living map related to nursing care, however, or a more involved skill, will be more complex because there are more concepts to consider and a greater degree of in-depth critical thinking skills is required. *A concept map is a direct expression of your critical thinking, problem solving, and clinical judgment skills.*

Following specific steps for problem list and concept map formatting, as well as applying concept mapping theory and use of basic or advanced components, allows you to blend past and present theory for the most effective and meaningful learning. This entire process also impacts and is impacted by the nursing process, standards of care, and evidence-based practice. Concept mapping is a powerful tool for blending and demonstrating all of these practice-defining nursing standards.

We have used nonnursing examples within this chapter, as well as nursing based ones. It is a wonderful way to compare and contrast knowledge. You can continue to use this idea as you gain more understanding about concept maps and their use within nursing education. Examples such as these will allow you to envision how concepts affect each other and how those effects relate to decision making. The scenarios you choose can be very simple and involve few actions and conceptual interrelationships or be a bit more expansive. The important thing is that you are thinking in terms of associations. This type of practice also reinforces how you research and extract information sources. Implementing these concepts with a nonnursing example makes it much easier to then subsequently apply it in nursing practice.

We have also discussed terms such as *symmetry* and *clarity* in concept map formatting. Style may vary among individuals, but being able to demonstrate key concepts clearly is a must for effective learning, interpretation, and reflection purposes.

Critical Thinking Questions and Activities

1. Discuss the similarities and differences in using nonnursing- and nursing-based examples to understand concept mapping theory and problem list formulation.
2. Use the following nonnursing example to answer questions related to concept mapping:

You are planning to clean out your car and wash it.

   a. Create a problem list identifying the main focus.

   b. Identify the primary and secondary components.

   c. Create a concept map demonstrating your thinking related to the supplies needed and the rationale for choosing them.

3. Create a problem list and concept map detailing nursing actions for a patient with a large volume IV infusion. In addition:

   a. Discuss your rationales for the primary and secondary concepts you identified.

   b. Compare your concept map and problem list with your classmates' maps and lists.

4. Discuss both the differences and similarities between nonnursing- and nursing-based concept maps in relation to the problem list and construction.

5. Discuss your thought process when completing the following.

   a. Identifying problems for the problem list

   b. Thinking about concept map construction

   c. How you make associations, connections, and links

6. Discuss and share ideas for other ways to think about the term *problem list*. What additional terms might be applicable dependent upon the specific patient care situation?

Case Studies

Directions: Read through each case study and answer the questions using the chapter material provided.

1. Katie has been asked to create a concept map focused on a simple nonnursing example to help her and her classmates to understand concept map construction. She decides on steps to consider when buying a new car.

   a. How should Katie begin to create this concept map?

   b. What types of things will make up the problem list?

   c. What criteria are used to differentiate between main and related problems/ concerns?

2. Katie has constructed her concept map like a wheel with spokes. She has placed the phrase, "buying a new car," in the center and all related concepts spreading out from that. How does this correlate with Katie's learning and mental processing style?

3. Todd is creating a concept map for one of his patient's main problems: surgical wound care. He is having difficulty demonstrating information flow and reasoning related to the actions he has carried out. His goal is to show his nursing actions in response to wound assessment, redressing, and care management.

   a. How does concept map construction relate to this?

   b. How do design and the use of descriptive phrases help with the flow of information and decision making?

    c. How can both design and construction reflect critical thinking?

    d. What are some other tools and techniques Todd could use to help explain his concept map and make it easier to follow and interpret?

4. Lucy has asked how the use of color can best be used to emphasize or highlight a feature of her concept map.

    a. What is the best answer to this question?

    b. Help Lucy to understand this through providing her with some basic rules for using color within a concept map.

    c. How can color and symmetry be used to make a concept map's purpose clear?

    d. How does the use of line types affect interpretation?

WWW For a full suite of assignments and additional learning activities, use the access code located in the front of your book to visit this exclusive website: **http://go.jblearning.com/schmehl**. If you do not have an access code, you can obtain one at the site.

References

Altmiller, G. (2010). Quality and safety education for nurses: An introduction to the competencies and the knowledge, skills and attitudes. Retrieved from http://www.qsen.org/teachingstrategy.php?id=148.

Conceição, I. C. O., & Taylor, L. D. (2007). Using a constructivist approach with online concept maps: Relationship between theory and nursing education. *The National League for Nurses Journal, 28*(5), 268–275.

Hsu, L., Hsieh, S.-I. (2005). Concept maps as an assessment tool in a nursing course. *Journal of Professional Nursing, 21*(3), 141–149.

Struth, D. (2009). The 60 second situational assessment. Retrieved from http://www.qsen.org/teaching strategy.php?id=89

6

Methods of Map Composition

Learning Objectives

- Discuss the various methods available for concept map composition
- Identify the advantages and disadvantages among composition methods available
- Explain how creativity plays an important role in concept map composition

Introduction

Thus far, a great deal of information has been presented on concept mapping. We have discussed the theory behind map construction, types of components, and content, and we have explored formatting. Next, we will take a look at concept map composition methods. Creativity is an important part of concept map composition and is as much determined by artistic ability as it is by learning style and brain processing. It is also a large part of formatting as well. Although formatting and composition are very similar terms, you can learn to differentiate between the two. Formatting, also known as layout, is the use of concept map components you choose to display, add content to, and link within the concept map. Composition is the method used to create the map formatting—either hand drawing it or computer generating it. The end result, your completed concept map, is a blending of these two methods.

Although not meant to be an exquisite work of art, neatness and design do count. As discussed earlier, the ultimate goal is to demonstrate concept mapping theory and an easily interpreted map of your thought processes within the concept map. So concepts such as clarity, symmetry, and arrangement each have a role to play in composition.

This chapter explores methods of composition as well as the advantages and disadvantages of each. The purpose is for you to be introduced to various methods and to then find the one most comfortable to use and that is most compatible with your style of learning and mental processing. As you learn more about concept mapping and utilize maps for various assignments and learning situations, you may have an opportunity to use a variety of methods. Initially, you may need to use a particular method as dictated by either the assignment or faculty preference. Later, you can experiment until you find your own preferred method.

Key Terms and Definitions

- **Hand-drawn concept map:** concept maps composed via use of pencil and paper
- **Computer-generated concept map composition:** concept maps composed via use of a computer
- **Software-based concept map generator:** software designed specifically for concept map composition
- **Free-form method:** creative concept map composition via sketching or drawing and the use of nonconfigured concept map components
- **Structured method of concept map composition:** creative concept map composition via computer generation and the use of preconfigured concept map components
- **White space:** unfilled spaces within pages, lines of text, and words or drawings that aid in separating words, drawing, and ideas
- **Realism:** utilization of life-like situations and content in learning

Hand-Drawn Concept Maps

Concept map composition can be achieved through two methods, hand drawing and computer generation. Each method has advantages or benefits that will be discussed in this chapter. No matter which method you use, the following standards apply and must be part of your checklist with each and every concept map you create:

- *Legibility.* An illegible map has no meaning and makes no statement. It will not lend itself to interpretation, and all of the work put into it will be for naught. Problems or difficulties with legibility not only stem from unreadable writing, but also from use of tiny lettering and cramped space.
- *Use of white space.* Reminding yourself that some space on the paper used for your concept map needs to remain unfilled will aid in legibility of it. This also allows room for adding notes, editing sections of the concept map, and adding lines or arrows for the purpose of linking concepts.

- *Uniformity*. Uniformity refers to use of similar colors, shapes, lines, and content themes throughout the concept map. Using like colors, for example, and indicating their meaning with a coded key not only adds to interpretability, but also reinforces conceptual links within your own mind. In this case, creativity used in this way reinforces theory. Uniformity of content refers back to the focus of the map. If the focus is based on nursing actions, for example, then design, descriptive phrasing, and linking need to be focused in that particular direction. This would be an appropriate method within a static concept map, where the entire concept map has the same focus. Content uniformity can relate to sections of a map as well. This would be particularly important when composing a concept map based on nursing actions for a patient's problems. In another way, this term refers to formatting concepts the same way within a map. If you are using squares with lists of actions, for instance, then you would use that format for all action groupings.

- *Clarity*. Using all of the above standards consistently will ensure clarity. See **Figure 6-1**. Each standard affects the others and overall clarity as well.

The first method under consideration is the hand-drawn method. As the preferred method for use when learning about concept mapping theory and for use with your first attempts at concept mapping, it is also the easiest and cheapest. **Hand-drawn concept map** generation is a **free-form method** where the basic concept map components are sketched and can have any dimensions you choose for them. All you really need to get started are a pencil, an eraser, and a piece of paper. If your artistic skills are less than precise, you may want to add a ruler to ensure straight lines for your shapes and connecting

Figure 6-1 Composition standards.

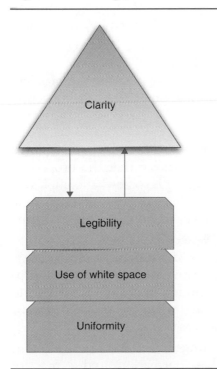

lines. When you are first practicing, it is best to do everything in pencil. If you experiment with a coded key, it too can be completed with pencil. Simply use shading and different line weights to show differentiation. The point is that you can erase and reconstruct very easily and that process is what contributes to the most effective learning.

As far as paper is concerned, you need paper that is large enough to allow you to include necessary information while allowing white space to remain at the same time. Regular sized 8.5″ × 11″ paper will not be sufficient. Extra space allows you the freedom to create while allowing you to follow the thought patterns of your content at the same time. Appropriate sizes are 16″ × 20″ or larger. Some examples of larger sized paper are:

- Large drawing paper
- Poster board
- Blank newsprint
- Larger-sized construction paper
- Larger-sized art paper tablets

Most of these can be found at craft, office supply, dollar, or department stores. If your budget does not allow for specialty paper (although most of these are inexpensive), take four sheets of printer paper or construction paper and tape them together. The main thing is that you do not want to run out of room to express yourself. Some students prefer graph paper. Draw lightly with pencil so that you are able to erase and reuse, thus conserving paper. Practicing repeatedly will help you to become more comfortable with the process and give you more confidence. Once you are comfortable, you may want to add color using erasable colored pencils. Permanent colors should be used and added only once you are comfortable and sure of your content. If you do use permanent colors, complete your line or shape edges in light pencil first, and then trace them with a marker or pencil. Markers are not always the best choice because they may bleed on the paper and distort the map's appearance. Additionally, if you made a mistake, you would have to begin the concept map all over again. Plain pencil and paper offer the best advantages for experimenting with formatting and composition. They are also appropriate for the problem list because you will want to include notes and other information to associate concepts.

Other free-form practice ideas include the following:

1. Practice by focusing on parts of a concept map prior to attempting a completed map. From all that was previously discussed, you can see that the process of beginning to practice and understand concept mapping is somewhat complex. It involves understanding and applying multiple, complex concepts and takes time to master. Separating the map into segments and working on each one at a time can make it easier to learn, analyze interrelationships, and apply theory.

2. Practice by using a dry erase board. A dry erase board can be used in two ways. You can use it to practice formatting before transferring ideas to paper. This provides a preliminary view without wasting paper and is very easy to use over and over again. A classroom dry erase board can be used when you desire to review with friends and experiment with formatting ideas as a small group.

3. Practice with movable shapes. Cut basic formatting shapes and lines from felt or construction paper. Then use a poster board as your background to practice various layouts. Because not everyone may desire to erase and re-erase, this serves

as an alternative, especially if your learning style is not strongly visual and you are having difficulty with formatting.

4. Take advantage of verbal practice. Remember that aural learning styles benefit from listening and auditory learning methods. Sounding out your ideas in content and formatting assists in audio recognition of concepts and associations. Whether you do this individually or as a group, you will benefit. Please be sure to complete the drawing along with the auditory practice for reinforcement. In a way, verbally reviewing is a bit like talking to yourself or thinking through nursing actions you take in the course of bedside care.

5. Practice while visualizing real patient situations. Aligning your thoughts and thought processes with the care of real patients and actual patient situations when composing concept maps injects **realism** into learning and makes it more meaningful. This signifies direct application of theory. Any time you personally perform a procedure, assessment, or other nursing action, you are applying what you have learned, and it is making an impact on critical thinking, clinical judgment, and decision-making skills.

Free-form, hand-generated concept maps have many advantages. Supplies are very easy to obtain and are not costly. Each method discussed lends itself to uncomplicated editing as well as multiple learning styles and mental processing types. This allows for expression and creativity that is not restricted in any way. This does not mean there is no structure—that is supplied through the inclusion of the various concept map components and formatting that demonstrate concept mapping theory. It simply means that open creativity goes into each and every shape, line, and layout used within the concept map.

One disadvantage noted is that the entire process can be quite time consuming. To clarify, there are many types of concept map foci that are not time consuming. Simple, static maps and segments of concept maps may not take longer than an hour or so to complete. It is the more complex living maps that can take as much as several hours to complete. Practice, along with knowledge and critical thinking development, can diminish time requirements. One thing to keep in mind is if you are completing a patient-related complex concept map, you may encounter problems and potential actions of which you have limited knowledge. This adds to the research time necessary to complete the assignment.

When formatting and composing, be sure to include all concept map components. Every concept map needs to have descriptive phrases. There is no exception to this rule. These can be written along lines that connect concepts. You can also draw small boxes for descriptive phrases that run parallel to the page edge if you wish.

Computer-Generated Concept Maps

The second method for composing concept maps uses computers. **Computer-generated concept map composition** can be considered more structured in that preconfigured shapes and lines are already supplied. All you need to do is choose the ones you want. Creativity is influenced by program type. The several types available include:

- *Microsoft Office software based*. Many computers these days come out of the box with preloaded software allowing for a degree of free-form creation of concept maps. Though not designed solely for this purpose, they lend themselves to use for this purpose quite well. One example is Microsoft Word, which is typically preloaded on personal computers (PCs) (though it is usually for a limited time before a license will need to be purchased; Apple users can purchase Office for Mac). The library of shapes and lines offers a variety of types and colors to format as you wish. The advantage of this is that you have more creativity than with some programs, but it may take longer to format a concept map this way until you become more comfortable and familiar with the process.

- *Textbook based.* Some textbook companies now include concept mapping software on companion websites (a Concept Map Creator accompanies this text as well: See the Student Companion Website at http://go.jblearning.com/schmehl). This allows you to practice not only concept mapping but also computer-based concept map applications. You may find that many of these are tightly structured, with not only a preconfigured format, but also preset content. In other words, you may have a list of problems and from which actions to choose.

- *Commercial concept mapping software.* **Software-based concept map generators** will have a cost associated with them that may or may not begin with a free trial. Some are available only as a download and others are downloads with back-up discs available for a fee. Many of these are great programs and allow varying degrees of free-form creativity; many are also moderately structured and perform other business-based tasks. This may mean you are paying for more than you will ever use.

- *Free concept mapping software.* Very few programs are actually free. Many may have limited version access until the full version is purchased. Others offer limited function overall.

To summarize, there are advantages and disadvantages to all of these as well. Using software for a more **structured method of concept map composition** is not all negative. If it is not highly structured, you will be able to supply your own content for maximum opportunities with relationship analysis. In comparison, highly structured software programs do not allow a student to recall, review, and reinforce theory enough to be truly beneficial. With the free options available, you have no need to purchase an expensive program. When evaluating software, consider the following: computer system compatibility, download size, ease of use, program features, and whether or not there are any fees involved.

Another thing you need to consider when composing a computer-based map is paper size. Using regular sized 8.5″ × 11″ paper translates into very tiny print for your map and very limited legibility and clarity. If you are going to use the computer for your concept maps, then you will need to invest in rolled paper, larger sheets, or complete your map in segments so that you meet the standards mentioned earlier.

Another advantage is that you will be able to store, print, and resize your maps on the computer. If electronic submission is allowable, this avoids extra travel time to deliver them. You will always need to be aware of compatibility between your file types and those of the school or faculty.

As mentioned earlier, one option is to create a computer-generated map using Microsoft Word. The program is user friendly although somewhat time consuming depending on map complexity. The disadvantages are time and expense regarding the specially sized paper and purchasing the software. You also need to be aware of compatibilities between software versions. Newer versions of Word use a .docx file format, while older versions use .doc. The newer file types cannot be opened in the older software versions unless the user of the older version installs a macro to convert .docx files to .doc. This becomes important if you are submitting assignments electronically.

Here are a few simple steps to get you started. Refer back to this section as needed. (Please note: These instructions pertain to Microsoft Office 2010, PC version.)

Step 1: Create a new blank document by clicking on *file* and choosing *new*.

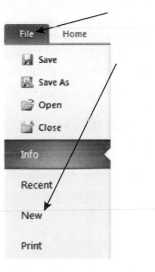

Then choose *blank document* from the list of templates.

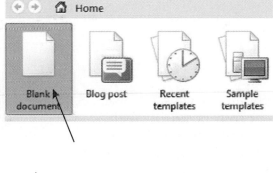

Step 2: Under the *page layout* tab, click on *orientation*, and choose *landscape*.

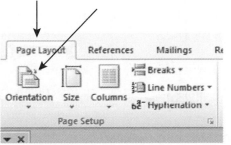

Now you will be able to begin your concept map by choosing shapes. Although there is a preconfigured shape library, there are many to choose from. They are also easy to edit for sizing and color.

Step 3: Click on the *insert* tab and choose *shapes.*

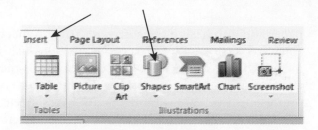

You will see a wide array of shapes and lines available for your use. Click on the shape of your choice, and then move the mouse back over your document. A + sign appears on your blank document. Click the mouse and pull the shape to the desired size. The shape appears as a color-filled one. To change this, right click the shape and select *format shape* from the bottom of the pull-down menu. Select the color fill you want or choose *no fill* if you want a clear shape. Options also exist to change line color and line width. Right click within the shape to choose the *add text* option. Clicking within the shape brings up a series of border dots along the shape. Use the dots to move or resize the shape.

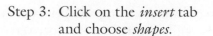

Step 4: Repeatedly use the *insert shape* option to add both shapes and lines as needed.

To insert text, simply right click on a shape and choose the *add text* option. To move shapes around, hover over the edges of a shape, click, and drag. To repeatedly use a desired shape, just use the cut and paste options. Then you can reposition it wherever you want. If you are unfamiliar with this program, you may need to take some time to practice until you feel comfortable. Keeping shapes simple, cutting and pasting, and using the preset colors will save time. As a nursing student, you cannot afford to waste time. Time is like gold and every moment of it is precious.

With this method you will find that your paper fills quite quickly. Please be sure to make the shapes and text large enough to be legible and clear. If necessary, divide your map into sections, and complete each on separate pages.

Do not forget to use all concept map components in this method. Adding descriptive phrases is slightly more difficult than with pencil and paper. In order to maintain text alignment, it is best to use a text box. Follow these steps:

Step 1: Under the *insert* tab, choose the *text box* option.

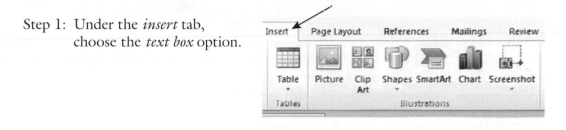

When that option opens, you will see a list of templates. Below them there is an option for *draw a text box* that you need to choose. Just as with the shapes, a plus sign appears when you move your mouse back over the document.

Step 2: Drag the text box to the size you want and right click it to add text. Formatting for color is completed the same way as with a shape. Remember the standard of uniformity and choose the same color for all text boxes. This will make them stand out as signifying descriptive phrases. Editing options do exist for changing text direction. As you become more familiar with this process, you can experiment with them. Text color sometimes changes automatically, depending on the shape color. If you want to change it to a different color, right click within the text box and look for a color bar under the letter A. You can click either on the bar itself, which will change text to the color shown, or click the down arrow next to the letter A to choose a different color. An example of this process is shown in **Figure 6-2**.

And that is all there is to it! To add a coded key using this method, simply add a shape and choose the *no fill* option. Then add mini boxes filled with the colors matching those in the concept map, along with the matching lines.

Figure 6-2 **Example of formatting color.**

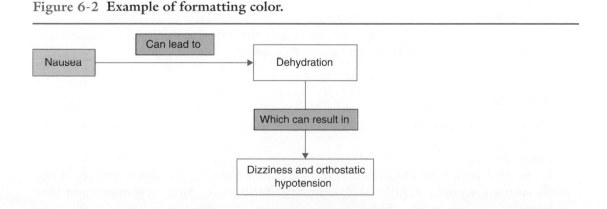

Summary

No matter the method chosen to compose a concept map, in addition to practice and knowledge as well as all of the other important factors we have discussed, patience is a must. Each method has its advantages, but it takes a while to become familiar with the process. It will be beneficial if you set small goals for yourself. Remember that many types of learning are occurring simultaneously. Recall of past theory is continuously compared to new theory. Relationships are being established, and in addition to all of that, you are considering how concept mapping theory fits into the picture while being mindful of critical thinking and perhaps realizing what your learning style is and how to use it. Setting both long- and short-term goals will give you time to process all of this information in sections. Make reflection a daily and active part of this process as well. Reflection and review should occur individually and with a group of your classmates to allow for an exchange of ideas.

Every concept map you create, even if it is only a portion of a map, will enable learning for comprehension, reinforcement of theory, and thought processes related to application. This is such a valuable tool and you should be excited that you can participate in this type of learning. Celebrate your growth along the way and share it with other students too.

Critical Thinking Questions and Activities

1. Create a static concept map on the evaluation of patient laboratory results using pencil and paper. After that is completed, repeat the process via computer and answer the following questions:
   a. Which method seemed easier to complete and why?
   b. How does your learning style relate to the method you preferred?
   c. What advantages and disadvantages have you identified with each method?
   d. What has this taught you about the following:
      1. Concept mapping theory
      2. Making connections
      3. Use and application of nursing knowledge
2. Research various concept mapping software sources, including those any of your textbooks contain. Examine the features and structure. How do more structured programs affect learning?
3. Compare and contrast the methods you have practiced with. Which method is easier in terms of mentally processing and thinking through how to construct the concept map? Why do you think that is?

Case Studies

Directions: Read through each case study and answer the questions using the chapter material provided.

1. Sarah is reviewing the concepts related to constructing concept maps. She is not sure exactly what white space, legibility, clarity, and uniformity mean and how

Figure 6-3 **Sarah's concept map.**

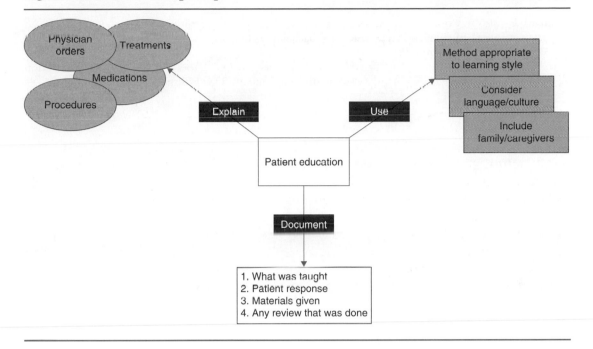

they relate to constructing a concept map. She has constructed a concept map focused on patient education and would like some feedback (see **Figure 6-3**).

a. Critique Sarah's concept map for clarity. Is the purpose of this concept map clear?

1. Does it really tell how this skill might be completed adequately and thoroughly?

2. Is there a clear starting and ending point?

3. Does the map flow smoothly and is it organized?

b. Do you think this concept map is legible and uniform? Why or why not?

1. If not, what would help make it so?

c. Help explain white space to Sarah and how it could best be used in this map.

2. If Sarah continues to have difficulty, what are some methods of practice she can use to help understand these concepts and improve?

3. Does this concept map make a statement about Sarah's critical thinking and if so, what?

a. How does this compare to your critical thinking?

References

Bruillard, E. (2000). Computer-based concept mapping: A review of a cognitive tool for students. Retrieved from http://129.194.9.47/tecfa/teaching/bachelor_74111/Cours_2010_2011/semestre1/cartes_conceptuelles/Bruillard.pdf.

Novak, J. D., & Cañas, A. J. (2006). The origins of the concept mapping tool and the continuing evolution of the tool. Retrieved from http://ivi.sagepub.com/content/5/3/175.short.

7

Use of Concept Maps in Nursing

Learning Objectives

- Demonstrate understanding of how concept mapping theory is used in nursing-care applications.
- Verbalize how the use of concept mapping contributes to critical thinking skill development.
- Discuss how concept mapping theory and the nursing process are demonstrated within nursing-based concept maps.
- Identify the ways a nursing-based concept map demonstrates thought processes related to nursing actions and outcomes.

Introduction

Concept maps in nursing lend themselves to use in a wide variety of ways. The focus of this chapter is to explore those uses and further explain what each use can accomplish. Although the goals of concept mapping theory continue to be inclusion and demonstration of critical thinking, relationship analysis, and application, each focus area allows achievement of each of those concepts in a different way. As mentioned earlier, student learning always proceeds on a continuum. Each component mentioned within concept mapping theory is achieved along different timelines and depends upon a variety of factors. How concept mapping theory and utilization of it occur also depends on many factors.

This chapter focuses on nursing-based application of concept maps, how concept mapping can be used as a plan of care, and how concepts such as the scope of practice, the nursing process, nursing actions, and outcomes are reflected within concept maps. Your critical thinking abilities will be put to the test, allowing many opportunities for reflection. With every concept map you complete, you will be able to trace the pathway of your thought processes and evaluate them in terms of competency, in knowledge level and knowledge application. While this is something you need to perform on an ongoing basis along the continuum of your nursing education, the process of composing a concept map emphasizes self-evaluation because you can actually see your thought processes on paper. In order to make this a positive experience, set goals along the way and do not think in terms such as weakness or inadequacy. Learn to think in terms that inspire action and change. Instead of saying, "one of my weaknesses is . . . " say, "to make that action more effective I will need to . . . " This statement and others like it will help you to maintain a positive focus and raise your performance bar. Through positivity you can set meaningful goals that will better guide your learning as you progress as a novice in nursing education.

This chapter contains a great deal of material. In order to ease navigation, it is separated into several sections. Each section is full of several concept map examples and rationales that can be directly applied to practice. As stated earlier, practice as we proceed and your critical thinking can only benefit. Question yourself regarding association between concepts and actions. Test yourself regarding past knowledge and how it fits into how you are now using it. Practice also allows an opportunity for reviewing basic terminology and concepts threaded through all nursing care. Associate, link, and connect for the most meaningful learning.

Key Terms and Definitions

- **Purpose-based nursing concept map:** concept map composition emphasizing components of concept mapping theory as they relate to nursing actions, reasoning, and judgment
- **Process-based nursing concept map:** concept map composition concentrated on core processes affecting nursing standards, planning of care, and patient care outcomes
- **Focus-based nursing concept map:** concept map composition concentrated on a specific patient care concept

Another Look at Concept Mapping Theory

Critical thinking has been integrated into all levels of nursing education. Although it may not always be presented as a formal lecture, it is certainly mentioned by faculty during orientation, within nursing textbooks, and as an important component in performing nursing skills. It is also one of the elemental goals in performance objective achievement. For students, familiarity and employment of critical thinking occurs on a continuum along with other nursing knowledge and concept mapping theory components. In recognition of this, you will need to make critical thinking a major part of all areas of nursing education so that is becomes second nature and ensures transition to the analytical processes paving the way to eventual application. You will be introduced to the concept early on in your education. Recognition is the first step in the process. From that point, you need to research it within all resources available to you. Nursing articles written from a critical thinking focal point are wonderful resources, as are the Internet and your textbooks. Another important piece of information is that relationship analysis is itself a component of critical thinking. One of your short-term goals should be to reassess your critical thinking ability each week.

Recall that critical thought processes are composed of multiple questions. So, another goal would be to create a list of questions that could then be used to evaluate your critical thinking skills. Use these either along with lecture review, lesson readings, or both. Some examples of general questions are:

1. How does the concept, disease, or skill I am studying relate to nursing actions?
2. In what way do the symptoms I am learning about reflect this particular disease process?
3. What is the link between this lab result and what is happening in the body?
4. If I carry out this action, what will need to happen next?

There are many more questions you might ask, and you can choose your own to fit specific situations. Any questions you create must consider cause and effect as well as links and associations.

Along with lecturing and other learning and studying strategies, concept mapping can and should be utilized to demonstrate and reinforce critical thinking. This process associates and layers critical thinking skills with theory and nursing actions. This will stimulate the growth and continual enhancement of critical thinking skills. As time passes, you will begin to recognize and demonstrate critical thinking in all aspects of nursing care. As an educator I have learned that consistently reinforcing this information yields the best results for students both in terms of understanding and developing the skill as well as enabling demonstration of it.

As critical thinking skills become established and consistently practiced, relationship analysis follows naturally. Refinement of both skills makes it almost impossible to consider one fact or bit of information without thinking about how the two are related. The degree of growth and depth evidenced by these two abilities increases along with an expanding base of nursing knowledge. Awareness leads to inquisitiveness, which leads to comparisons, which leads to an elevated level of learning that is meaningful and far surpasses basic learning. Cultivating this knowledge is essential for long-term use and retention, especially within a profession where ongoing analysis and application of knowledge are critical to maintaining standards of care.

As stated earlier in this text, application is the goal of nursing knowledge. While each component of concept mapping theory overlaps with the others, critical thinking and relationship analysis are mental activities; application is the "physical" outcome of those thought processes. Information obtained or recalled through critical thinking allows reasoning through analysis of relationships and both of those processes equal application (see **Figure 7-1**).

In nursing this thorough process translates into our actions related to providing bedside care, whether it is giving a bed bath, performing patient teaching, or completing a skill such as bladder scanning. This aspect of application is fairly easy for you to

Figure 7-1 Concept mapping theory and clinical reasoning.

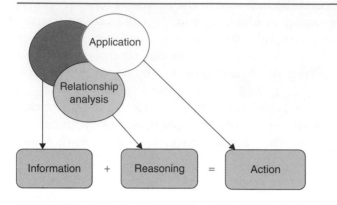

understand. What sometimes poses more difficulty is recognizing that this process also comprises decision making as a nursing action. For instance, if you note that a patient's morning hemoglobin is 8.0, then obviously an action is required. It is not enough to recognize the laboratory value as abnormal. You must also recognize how that value influences care decisions and other nursing actions.

Students often think in terms of tangibility. However, application of nursing knowledge includes the ability to consider the intangible things that affect nursing care. All pieces of data must be considered for the best outcomes. Application reinforces the need for more information before acting, forcing you to draw on past knowledge, ask more questions, and compare facts to draw conclusions. It also reinforces the need for research of new knowledge. Not every action is based on previous knowledge. Many actions, especially in the clinical areas, are based on either new knowledge or prior knowledge that students have not yet had an opportunity to apply fully. While this can be somewhat stressful for you, it does ensure comprehensive learning. Research introduces and reinforces knowledge, allowing for application.

Application also mandates collaboration in achieving the desired outcomes. This is another intangible concept you might have difficulty comprehending even if you do understand the need for it. However, you might not fully understand your specific role and responsibility in the process. Through student feedback I have found that this stems from several things: 1) a student's lack of self-confidence, 2) a student's knowledge deficit regarding his or her role as part of the care team, and 3) a student's perception of feeling dismissed by co-assigned registered nurses. Nursing care does not occur in isolation. Collaborating with and updating the co-assigned registered nurse, as well as the rest of the care team, is an action itself and promotes awareness of the scope of practice. One of the solutions to this would be to reinforce the need for collaboration through each level of nursing education. Making collaboration a part of the clinical competencies and reinforcing the concept in teaching sessions can assist students with developing these skills.

The following concept maps demonstrate and validate all that has been addressed. Both clinical and nonclinical examples are provided. Each example demonstrates how critical thinking is expressed as well as the evolution of thought process involving relationship analysis and application.

The next section describes how concepts maps are used within nursing education and provides examples. Use of concept maps in nursing education is valuable whether the educational focus is an emphasis on theory or related to clinical skills. In general, I would say that most education and concept mapping utilization has an emphasis on actions. The main categories of emphasis used to address both areas are *purpose*, *process*, and *focus*.

Purpose-Based Concept Maps

We have spent a great deal of time discussing the purpose of using concept mapping in nursing education. I would like to spend a bit more time on this, because the purpose leads to the processes and focus areas chosen to achieve that purpose. The sections that follow describe the main areas or purposes for which concept mapping is used.

Enhanced Critical Thinking

Critical thinking abilities are usually present in some degree in each nursing student. The degree of development may be different for each student and depends upon many factors. Those factors are as varied as the students themselves and may be difficult to assess. Nursing programs and faculty normally base this ability, at least partly, on grade point average (GPA) and current academic standing. Other factors that may impact this but which are difficult to assess are previous exposure to critical thinking application in prior educational settings, age, and life experience. Once the student enters the nursing program, the degree and depth of critical thinking are measured via competencies related to skills testing, verbal exchanges, clinical performance, and theory grades. Concept mapping will allow you, as well as nursing faculty, to combine all of these factors in one tool for complete critical thinking assessment. We will discuss this further within each map example. Competency in critical thinking skills leads to effective practice and eventually to independent practice in the graduate nurse role.

Remember that critical thinking occurs when questions are asked and associations are made. You could create a concept map solely concentrated on critical thinking itself, focusing on one or two concepts that would demonstrate it (such as a disease and its symptoms) or highlight the sections within a large concept map that demonstrate it. It is also important to realize that you can "think out" or "talk out" steps in the critical thinking process as well. This is part of the reasoning and mental processing that occurs as part of critical thinking. You will see this appear in your maps as associations, concepts connected with descriptive phrases, and actions. In this way, the express purpose for using the maps is also demonstrated within them.

Suppose your instructor has asked you to create a concept map on assessing a peripheral intravenous (IV) site. One of the objectives is to demonstrate your critical thinking abilities related to this nursing action. You proceed to formulate a problem list and then compose a concept map (**Figure 7-2**). Now, take a moment to study this concept map, keeping in mind the mini checklist created earlier (with thought processes relating to critical thinking, relationship analysis, and application). Formatting of the map is adequate and the reader can clearly interpret what you are assessing and how you will carry it out. The content is lacking, however. The main reason we assess an IV site is to assess for infiltration or infection. Those two objectives or assessments are not listed and there is very little subjective and objective data. Another way to assess the site, as well as to ensure patency, is to flush it with sterile saline.

Figure 7-2 Use of critical thinking during IV site assessment.

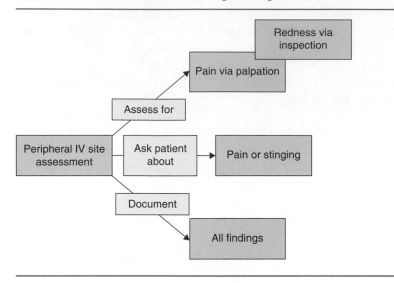

So, the proper steps for IV assessment include:

- Checking the order for whether the site should be capped or an IV infusion should be in place
- Palpating and inspecting during the assessment for signs and symptoms of infection or infiltration
- Combining thorough subjective and objective data to complete a thorough assessment
- Noting the insertion date and assessing for an intact dressing
- Documenting the site assessment on the appropriate form or page of the medical record
- Performing follow-up assessments of the site

Therefore, there is not adequate demonstration of critical thinking or its components in this concept map. There is incomplete relationship analysis as well as inadequate application.

This is how you evaluate your abilities and thought processes reflectively. Thus, a growth in critical thinking skills when you realize that, as you follow the pathway of the concept map, steps and pieces of information that are integral to the assessment's completeness are missing. You now need to reevaluate your knowledge regarding IV site assessment and be sure that you are providing complete and safe care.

Improved Organization and Prioritization

Although actions are important at all levels of nursing education, organization and prioritization are important as well. As you progress through the nursing program, more emphasis is placed on independent function and the ability to manage more complex patients and multiple responsibilities. So, along with growth in critical thinking, there must also be an improvement in organizational skills and the ability to discern which actions take priority and why. If you think about this, nursing actions are carried out through a series of steps. If you need to carry out step A first, before proceeding to steps B and C, you must have organization and prioritization in order to do that. While many nurses may feel that organization and prioritization have much to do with managing multiple patients and multitasking, it also has to do with prioritizing and organizing specific actions.

The purpose of using concept maps to obtain this goal is that students have direct visualization of their actions, which helps show how organizing and prioritizing those actions allow for appropriate outcomes. Analyzing this process also establishes a knowledge base of action rationales. Clinical judgments and decision making are clearly demonstrated through this process as well because they stem from all of the above.

Linking Theory With Practice

This is also known as application. Although we have emphasized nursing actions as the ultimate evidence of this, a huge part of accomplishing the theory-to-practice link is student recognition of its definition. In the early weeks and months of nursing education, students may tend to see actions and theory as isolated from practice. Or, they may see a simple link but not realize this means application. The critical thinking and relationship analysis abilities necessary for application take time to develop and fully integrate into practice. Concept maps can be useful early on to focus in on and accentuate the importance of this process and its development. Although critical thinking will be demonstrated in all map examples, it can also be isolated as a map focus, as discussed earlier.

Consider the following scenario. Suppose you are a freshman student and have been instructed to create a concept map on proper medication administration of an oral medication (see **Figure 7-3**). You would most likely include the necessary information presented in one of a variety of formats, dependent on your learning style and mental processing abilities. This formatting and assignment may be simple, but it indicates whether or not you are able to comprehend information recalled from theory. The map demonstrates all the proper steps, and the linking phrase in the cyan box states the number of checks needed to safely administer an oral medication. A deficit in critical thinking would

Figure 7-3 Theory application and nursing actions.

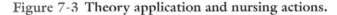

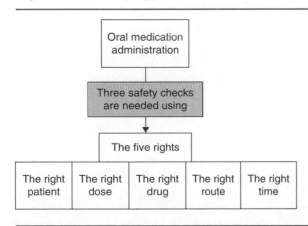

be noted if you were unable to recall an important step, were unaware of the number of checks needed, or omitted one of the five rights. Remember that recall of past theory combined with new theory and then using all of it to determine nursing actions is application. The concept map in Figure 7-3 is simple and yet accurate. It demonstrates recall of important facts related to oral medication administration as well as safety checks related to this skill/action.

Now, let's suppose that you have progressed to the middle of freshman year and are asked to create a concept map demonstrating one or two nursing actions used in implementing the five rights of medication administration for any medication other than IV push or piggyback. This is somewhat more involved because in addition to theory recall, you need to consider information sources as well. This adds to time management and organization. Your concept map will exhibit some variation of the first map and look something like the one in **Figure 7-4**. The recall you complete will reinforce previously learned information and link theory with actions as well as one action with another one. No action a nurse takes is really simple when thought of in this way. Thinking through

Figure 7-4 In depth relationship analysis and knowledge application.

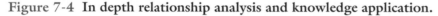

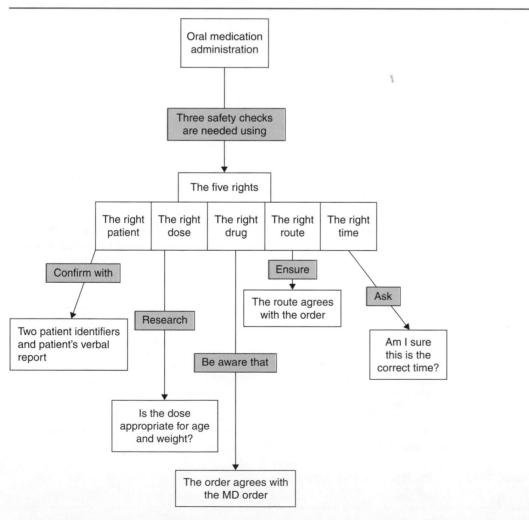

actions by using concept mapping helps you to constantly reflect on and evaluate your ability to satisfy course competencies and provide safe, effective nursing care.

This sample shows progression and advancement in critical thinking ability. These nursing actions indicate thinking through extra steps concerning safe medication administration. Relationship analysis is evident in the comparison of various information sources to find important information. Application is apparent because all decisions are based on previous knowledge. Now, if this map were to be evaluated in terms of the nursing process, then some actions would need to be added. **Figure 7-5** describes where the nursing process was included and where information could be added to include all steps.

Simple, static, skill-related maps that ask only for the steps to follow may not appear to strongly evidence the nursing process; however, appearances can be deceiving. Each step of a skill is based on an assessment of a body system process, a symptom, or evaluation of a medical treatment. Every procedure is focused toward a patient problem. Therefore, the nursing process steps are threaded throughout. Whenever nursing actions are the focus, the nursing process should be strongly demonstrated. This includes each and every

Figure 7-5 **Additional information about the nursing process.**

Nursing Process Step	Evidence	Additional Information Needed
Assessment	Refers to safety in medication administration. This is included in both the primary and secondary related concepts.	None at this time
Diagnosis	None are included here, but may not always be needed in a simple, skill-oriented map.	Information could be added on medication education or evaluations needed prior to administering it, such as pulse or BP.
Planning	This is addressed somewhat with timing of the medication.	An altered administration time because the patient is NPO could affect time management and could be added. If the patient has difficulty swallowing, planning could include crushing the medication or putting it in applesauce. Basically, anything affecting completion of the administration could be included here.
Implementation	In this case, this step is inferred because we know once all checks are satisfied the medication will be given.	Some of the information listed above within the planning section overlaps into this area. If that does not apply, then nothing needs to be added.
Evaluation	Skill evaluation regarding following the correct steps has been accomplished. If outcomes are asked for, then follow-up information would have to be added.	Additional information related to outcomes would include medication tolerance, side effects present, etc.

BP = blood pressure; NPO = not by mouth

step, and especially outcomes and any required follow up as they lead to nursing actions as well. All components of concept mapping theory are also evident in this map. Refer back to the previously supplied checklist to review.

Our map thus far has demonstrated critical thinking of various depths, as well as application, which is our link between theory, or previously learned knowledge, and practice. Now let's look at prioritization and organization. Suppose we use the same situation, but now state that the focus is on the order of the steps, including the nursing actions listed in the previous map example. The map in **Figure 7-6** now shows all components of concept mapping theory, plus the nursing process. It also speaks to anticipation. As you grow in your critical thinking skills, you will also see progressive growth in clinical judgment and reasoning abilities. This includes the ability to anticipate not only patient problems and needs, but also the ability to detect signs of patient compromise or deterioration.

More space would be needed to add information on outcomes and follow up as mentioned above. As far as the correct steps, we have included each step from point A to

Figure 7-6 Blending the nursing process with concept mapping theory.

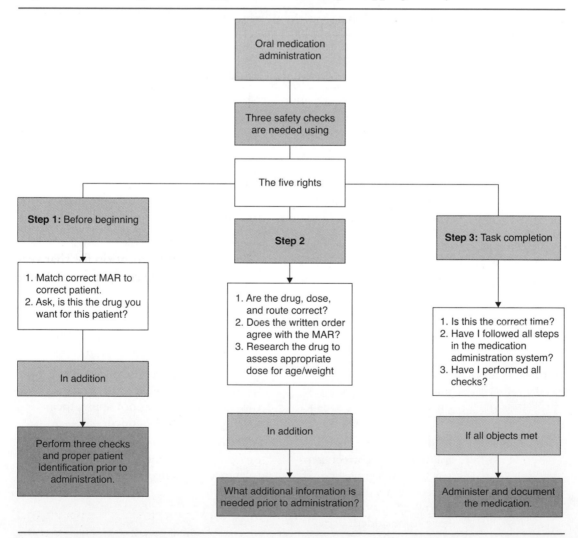

MAR = Medication Administration Record

point B—safety checks, through administration to documentation. Within all content included in the map, we can clearly see reinforcement of previously learned information; how information was recognized, clustered, and prioritized; and some evidence of independent thinking.

Being able to look at one main concept and then figure out how to identify all the related data applying to it is a major accomplishment for freshman nursing students. While most students can select at least a few things, many are not able to select each and every piece of information that applies. While a strong base of foundation knowledge enables this, I cannot mention enough times that repetition cements knowledge. This repetitive reinforcement is not only the student's responsibility. Faculty assist with this process through verbal examples, case studies, questions and answers, and many other methods. All of these methods embody concept mapping theory with accompanying reinforcement of critical thinking and relationship analysis. Application then follows and is as much a mental process as it is a physical one.

Walking through the steps of concept map construction—from identifying the main concept, creating the related problem list, clustering, and so on—fosters critical thinking as well as all components of concept mapping theory. This is true whether the student can immediately recall previously learned information or must research it to complete a map. Repetition equals reinforcement, which equals meaningful knowledge, which can then be applied. Knowledge building also leads to confidence building and fostering independent thought and preparedness for the graduate nurse role.

Process-Based Concept Maps

Processes are another pathway to link critical thinking with application. Processes specific to nursing must be integrated into practice to ensure adequate care standards. A process can be chosen as the focus of a map in isolation or included as a related area. These identified processes provide structure and outlines for care, regardless of care setting. They are universal and describe what nursing care is and what it means. They are woven through the fabric of nursing and introduced early on in nursing education for that very reason. These valuable processes also appear in program and course competencies. Some of these are:

- The nursing process
- Nursing diagnosis
- Safety standards
- The medication-administration process
- Functional health patterns/holistic care practice processes
- Communication and documentation
- Cultural competence processes
- The process of interventions, nursing actions, and outcomes

While each of these processes is important in its own right, it is also apparent that overlapping and blending of the processes occur. This is because, as I like to say, "nothing is static"—not pathophysiology, decision making, or nursing actions. All of these processes has important places in nursing care, and, in fact, are requirements to maintain a high-quality standard of care. Let's discuss each one of these.

The Nursing Process

The nursing process has already been discussed and used as an example to demonstrate how to include this information within the concept map. Because of the varied methods available to produce concept maps, we are able to create an assignment that focuses on the entire nursing process or just one portion of it. While inclusion of the entire process would be most valuable, especially for more advanced students, taking the time to examine each portion of it may be valuable for first-year students who are just learning about the nursing process. You might also create an assignment where each student creates individual maps of each step and then analyzes how they meld together. Another alternative would be to have individual groups of students work on separate portions of the nursing process and then present each section to the class so that everyone participates in how it all blends together. Endless possibilities exist!

Let's use the following case study to show examples of each nursing process step:

> You are caring for a 70-year-old patient admitted with moderate to severe abdominal pain. It began 1 week ago and is centered in the midabdominal region, sharp and stabbing and occurring intermittently. It is also associated with nausea. The patient has been unable to tolerate any food or drink except toast, milk, and water for the past 4 days because the pain becomes worse when eating. She continues to have nausea but has not vomited. She states she has lost 8 pounds over the week, and now the pain is continuous and radiates to her mid-back area. She states she has had a BM daily since the pain began. Over the last 3 days, the stool character has changed to black and tarry instead of her normal brown. She complains of feeling weak, thirsty, and in pain—rated 9 on a scale of 0–10.

For educational purposes as well as because of page size, we will limit this example map a bit. We will limit the related concept list and include a debriefing session at the end. For this example we will not focus on specific abnormal data such as findings from the examinations. We will create a general map for a patient with this problem.

Before we begin map construction fully, we need to create a related problem list. My list is provided below. Remember, if you are completing this with me, yours may look different.

MAIN PROBLEM: ACUTE PAIN

Primary related problems	Secondary related problems
• Nutritional deficit	• Weight loss
• Dehydration	• Weakness
• Nausea	• Volume deficit
• Probable GI bleeding	

Now that we have a problem list, we can begin map construction. We'll begin with a small map focusing on the part of the nursing process dealing with assessment (see **Figure** 7-7).

The next step in the nursing process is diagnosis. Let's use pain, nutritional deficit, dehydration, nausea, and probable GI bleed in our map for this step (see **Figure** 7-8).

So, our assessments and patient information have provided us with the means to formulate priority nursing diagnoses. This will enable us to plan care. Planning nursing care is not focused solely on nursing actions. The planning of care considers all care the patient will receive, all of which is overseen by nursing, including:

1. Nursing care and actions related to short-term problems and concerns
2. Nursing care and actions related to long-term problems and concerns
3. Actions and interventions related to collaborative problems and concerns
4. Actions and interventions related to anticipated problems and concerns

Figure 7-7 **Including assessment findings within the concept map.**

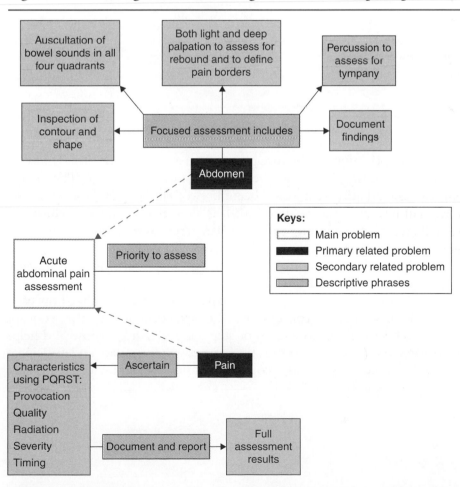

Figure 7-8 **Connecting nursing diagnosis with nursing actions.**

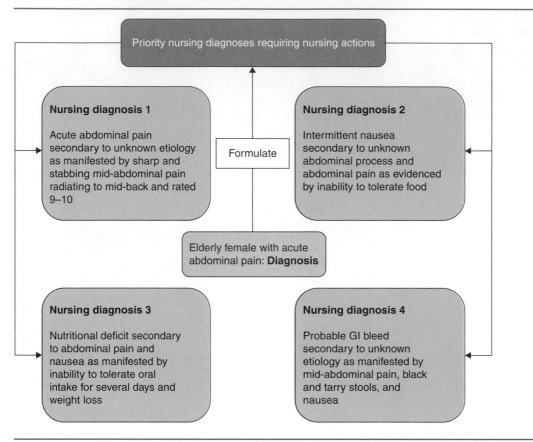

The emphasis here is that planning by the discipline of nursing does not occur in isolation but rather by necessity must be collaborative to be holistic and complete. The map in **Figure 7-9** considers collaboration that would occur between nursing and the attending physician, consulting physicians, and the dietician. It is also refers to and is inclusive of all of the necessary pieces of information needed to plan care and nursing actions.

So far we have addressed our patient's problems, created a problem list, formulated nursing diagnoses, and considered planning care. Our next map must focus on nursing actions related to all we have addressed thus far.

Building a concept map in steps and stages may help you to better visualize how each phase adds to the whole or sum of the concept map. Construction of the entire concept map is influenced by each section. Each section or step has a specific purpose and helps to build on and reinforce the other. As a result, the actions you formulate and anticipate are derived from past knowledge as well as recognition of how to employ or utilize that knowledge in patient care (see **Figure 7-10**).

Figure 7-9 Formulating a collaborative plan of care.

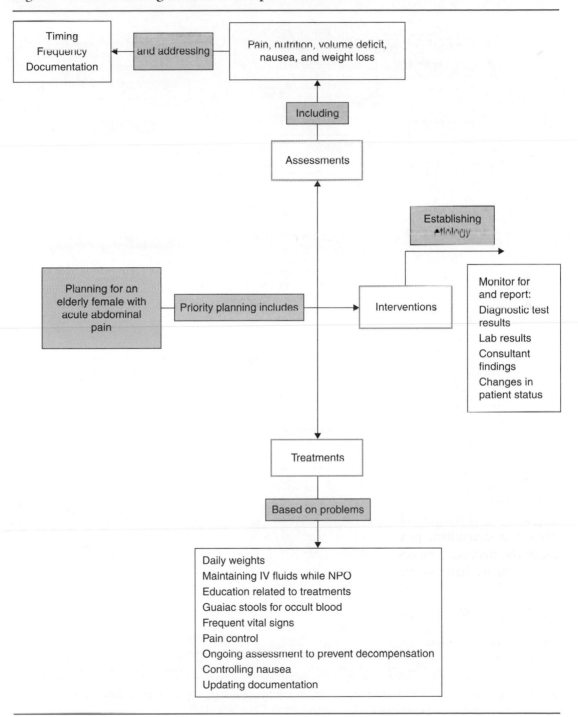

Figure 7-10 Implementing a concept map driven plan of care.

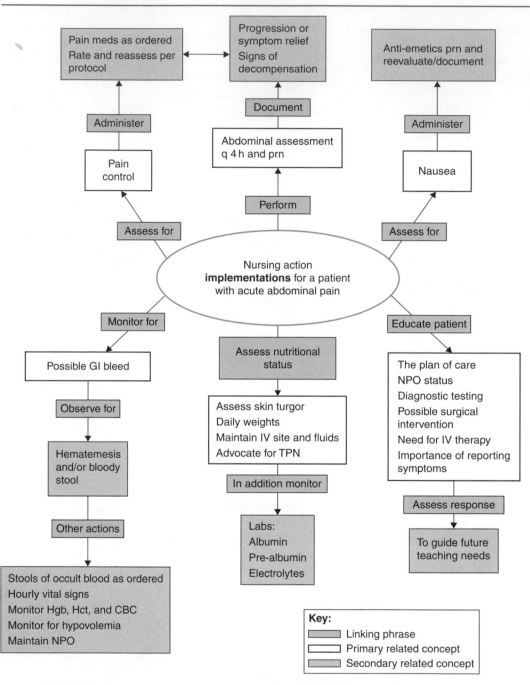

prn = as needed; q = every; h = hour; NPO = not by mouth; CBC = complete blood count; TPN = total parenteral nutrition; Hct = hematocrit; Hgb = hemoglobin; IV = intravenous; GI = gastrointestinal

Hopefully, you can now recognize that a strong foundation of knowledge along with strong critical thinking and relationship analysis abilities are necessary for application. This is not just true of concept maps. It is true for any patient contact and in all bedside care. If you sit and think about it, you are already performing with all of this in mind. As you progress in your nursing education, you just have to hone these abilities. Now is the time to set goals that will enable you to build and perfect these essential skills.

Before we can debrief, we need to address the last step in the nursing process: evaluation. Because I have not provided any facts within the scenario, I have invented a few for our use here (see **Figure 7-11**).

Debriefing of the Nursing Process

We have completed maps for each step of the nursing process. Separating the steps and presenting them from the perspective of an actual patient scenario demonstrates how all aspects and components of concept mapping theory appear, have a place in, and are utilized to complete that process. For students along any point of the education continuum,

Figure 7-11 **Evaluating outcomes using concept maps.**

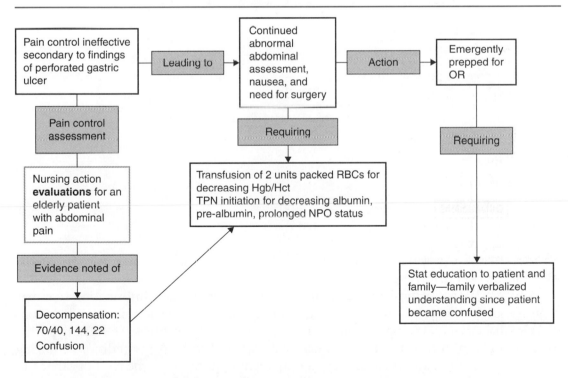

NPO = not by mouth; RBCs = red blood cells; Hct = hematocrit; Hgb – hemoglobin

this would be a very valuable exercise. Being able to separate the various pieces and portions used in map construction allows for control in altering the simplicity or complexity of your practice. For many learners, breaking it all down has some advantages in considering the entire process. An important point to note here is that there is no wrong way to practice or complete maps, as long as you are utilizing concept mapping theory and all of its components.

Did you notice how easy the steps make it for you to create a problem list and then transition to formatting? At the same time, it may seem difficult and even overwhelming to then have to bring in all other necessary information such as nursing actions, safety, the nursing process, and so on. Trust me when I say this entire process as a whole becomes easier the longer you work at it. The difficulty eases with an increased knowledge base and clinical exposure, allowing application of your knowledge. This is why I recommend an early introduction to basic concepts within concept mapping theory and reinforcing them by using them at every opportunity in nursing education. It then becomes second nature much more easily. Also, using an actual patient or scenario enables mental "picturing" of the patient, which often makes recall of patient facts and nursing actions much clearer. Many companies offer video-based scenarios where students can actually see the patient as they continue through the case study.

A thorough map would include much more information if we were going to deal with all nursing actions. Important information to add would include:

1. Past medical history (PMH)
2. Past surgical history
3. History of present illness (HPI)
4. Current medications
5. Specific abnormal laboratory tests and diagnostic testing data
6. Collaboration in care
7. Advocacy
8. Psychosocial factors
9. New events in hospital
10. Patient decompensation

Although we have previously addressed data collection, let's take an opportunity to review that information before we continue.

A patient's past medical and surgical histories contain valuable information that may apply to our problem list. Medically, long-standing diseases necessitating nursing actions include: diabetes (DM), hypertension (HTN), coronary artery disease (CAD), hypothyroidism, and chronic obstructive pulmonary disease (COPD). Any condition requiring ongoing monitoring and treatment as an outpatient requires the same level of care as an inpatient. Some examples of actions are listed in **Figure 7-12**.

In short, many nursing actions are all about anticipation. Past surgical history may or may not be pertinent depending on the nature of the procedure and the length of time since it was performed. For instance, a history of appendectomy 10 years ago will most likely not be pertinent to any nursing actions. However, if a patient who had surgery 2 weeks ago now presents to the emergency department (ED) with lower abdominal pain, this history of recent surgery has important implications.

Figure 7-12 Examples of nursing actions related to the past medical history.

Condition	Action
DM	BG monitoring
	Monitoring for hypoglycemia/hyperglycemia
	Oral medication and insulin administration
	Monitoring renal function
HTN	Assessing maintenance of normal BP
	Education regarding holding meds or instituting new meds
	Initiating hold parameters
CAD	Assessing for chest pain recurrence
	Need for telemetry monitoring
	Recognition of disease states potentiating chest pain
Hypothyroidism	TSH level monitoring
	Ensuring med doses are maintained as condition changes
	Being alert for myxedema or thyroid storm
COPD	Monitoring ABG levels
	Assessing oxygenation
	Weaning/titration of oxygen therapy

DM = diabetes mellitus; HTN = hypertension; CAD = coronary artery disease; COPD = chronic obstructive pulmonary disease; BG = blood glucose; BP = blood pressure; TSH = thyroid-stimulation hormone; ABG = arterial blood gas

The HPI always has implications necessitating nursing actions because it tells us about all the surrounding events that lead a patient to seek health care. It is through those events that we can determine how ill a patient really is or what potential problems we can anticipate. One example is a patient who has been admitted post-fall and who is currently taking warfarin (Coumadin). The admitting diagnosis may be a fractured wrist, but much more might be happening. The patient could be experiencing a subdural hematoma or extensive bruising. This is a situation that may lead to new, untoward events or patient decompensation.

Medications also require their own nursing actions. Often this is based on treatment effects, such as in the patient using insulin, but may also include side effects or effects related to nontherapeutic drug levels.

Each lab finding in the abnormal range should be investigated for the need for nursing actions. If a student notes abnormally low hemoglobin levels, this indicates some degree of hypovolemia in many cases. This affects safety when getting the patient out of bed or ambulating him or her. It often requires that orthostatic vital signs be performed as well.

Advocacy usually accompanies cultural and psychosocial factors concerning the patient. Some examples include language barriers, economic status affecting the ability to pay for and comply with treatment, homelessness, psychiatric history, and substance abuse. This further necessitates collaborative care with social services and case managers.

To learn the most and get the most out of creating concept maps, it is essential that students isolate all problems and refrain from lumping and consolidating information without linking it appropriately. Lumping all abnormal laboratory results together, for instance, does not allow adequate relationship analysis to occur. Students need to be able to identify and reason through why the laboratory result is abnormal, what body system and disorder it reflects, and what that in turn means in terms of their nursing actions.

Nursing Diagnoses

Now let's move on and consider a map based on *nursing diagnoses* (see **Figure 7-13**). Although we have addressed this to some degree in the previous section, we need to take a closer look. Diagnoses lead to nursing actions. The following map uses nursing actions that stem from a patient's nursing diagnosis related to COPD. An advantage of setting up a map from this perspective is that a student has another view of how to get from point A to point B in regard to nursing actions. This is true whether the problems are actual, potential, or anticipated. In this example, we can see that safety can be a focus for one of our nursing actions. It is something that should be addressed in each and every patient, no matter the care setting. The skill and action related to nursing diagnosis formulation

Figure 7-13 Nursing actions resulting from nursing diagnoses.

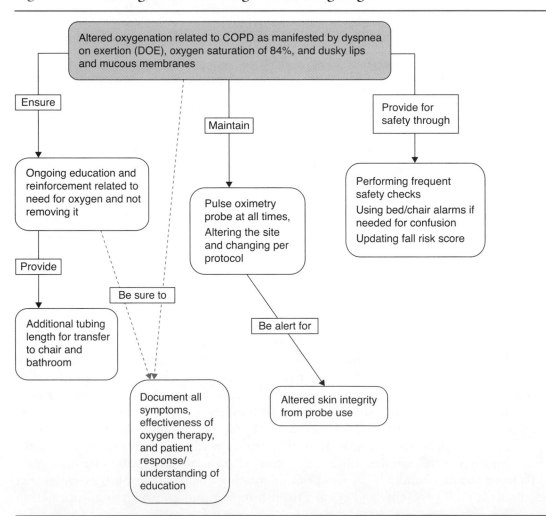

are a process within a process. Although part of the nursing process, it is also its own process in planning care and nursing actions.

Because of limited space, I have grouped nursing actions. If one action leads to other related ones, I would suggest placing them into different shapes. This will make the map appearance neater and enable the reader to follow it more easily. If your comprehension and ability to apply knowledge will be enhanced by taking a nursing diagnosis and using it to identify problems and actions, by all means do that. Many students identify strongly with nursing diagnoses in this way and derive more meaningful learning from this method.

Safety Standards

Safety and safety standards are additional processes important to nursing actions that can and should be incorporated into concept mapping. Although we have touched on safety, let's look at a map example where safety is our main concern (see **Figure 7-14**). This is a general example. A more general example such as this one helps to show where safety standards originated, how they are utilized, and how they are incorporated into nursing actions. More intricate examples can also be used. Safety considerations should be part of every nursing-based concept map. You will see it is a main focus throughout the examples in this text.

Figure 7-14 Emphasizing nursing actions related to safety within a concept map.

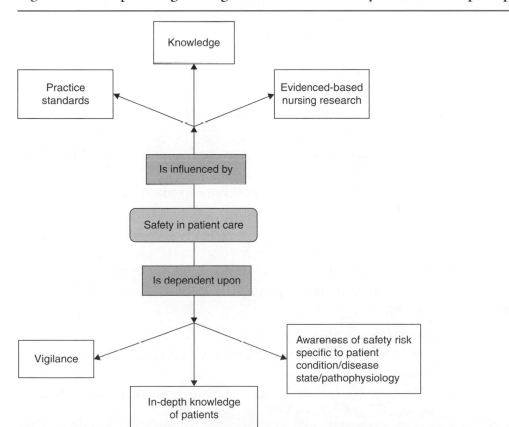

Medication-Administration Process

Medication Administration is another area where concept maps are extremely valuable for use within nursing education. Whether the process is broad or narrow, detailed or generalized, each and every aspect of medication administration can be addressed. Common uses are highlighted as follows:

1. Static maps
   - Medication administration by route (e.g., procedure for intramuscular [IM] medication administration)
   - "The five rights"
   - Safety check steps for medication administration
   - A particular medication, along with actions, usual dose, etc.
2. Living maps
   - Medication purpose specific to the assigned patient
   - Nursing actions specific to the medication side effects this patient is experiencing
   - Patient education related to a particular medication
   - Monitoring drug levels

Administering medications is never just about being able to identify the five rights and then administering the medications. Examples of other things we need to think about before handing medication over to patients include:

1. The patient's ability to swallow
   - Has anything changed since admission?
   - Has a swallowing study been completed to address preexisting swallowing difficulties?
   - Does either a current or past diagnosis play a role in swallowing difficulty—whether current or potential?
   - Must oral medications be split or crushed prior to administration?
2. The number of pills to be administered at one time
   - Are there similar types of medications ordered at this time that should be separately administered to avoid adverse effects? (For example, three of the five medications ordered are for HTN. Is it appropriate to give all at once?)
   - How should the ordered medications be prioritized?
3. Dietary considerations
   - Has the patient been ordered to remain NPO?
   - Are there fluid restrictions in place that limit the intake allowance when giving the medications?
   - Should the medications be held because of patient complaints of nausea?

These considerations play an integral role in medication-administration safety. They also represent only a few of the considerations related to our nursing actions, because only oral medications were considered. This should prompt you to think of many more considerations.

Versatility, simplicity, and complexity need to be kept in mind when using concept maps because the myriad ways maps can be used make them a very valuable educational tool. Consider a living map for the following patient scenario:

> Your patient is a 60-year-old male who has been prescribed atenolol for HTN. He was admitted 24 hours ago with possible transient ischemic attack (TIA) and accelerated HTN. He was not previously aware of having HTN and has never taken any medications for it before. His blood pressure was consistently around 180/100 prior to the start of the medication, has been steadily decreasing, and has now dropped to 110/50 after only 2 doses of 100 mg daily. There are no other contributing factors precipitating the hypotension. The patient does complain of dizziness even when lying in bed.

This example serves as realism within nursing education (see **Figure 7-15**). Situations such as this one, as well as the others used throughout the text, are very likely to occur

Figure 7-15 A living concept map based on an acute patient problem.

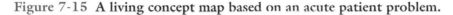

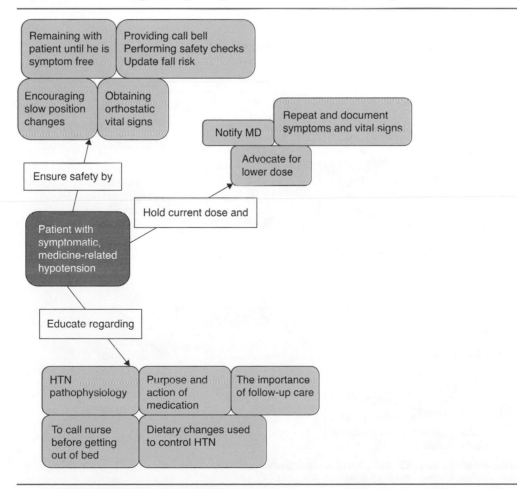

in practice. Considering either a case study or actual patient example provides preparatory and reinforcement opportunities that are valuable to meaningful practice and study.

This map includes all components of concept mapping theory as well as the nursing process. As stated earlier, to add in information regarding evaluation, we would have to expand the map and address outcomes from our nursing actions. It is a great demonstration of another perspective that can be utilized to address critical thinking in nursing care and reinforce information.

A recurrent theme in the most recent map examples is documentation. Documentation is necessary and is the endpoint of all skills. Many times, however, I find that students have difficulty formulating even simple notes. I cannot emphasize and reinforce the importance of this skill enough. It is an art form and so very important in many aspects of our profession. I will continue to use it within the examples and give it a special mention under the focus section later in this chapter.

Now that we have seen a living concept map highlighting medication administration, consider an example of a static map dealing with administration of a single medication (see **Figure 7-16**). Let's say that your students have just learned about phenytoin (Dilantin) and you ask that a map be created about the medication's use.

Static maps of a medication are wonderful to study from. Early on I mentioned **open** or **blank copy** maps. Once a student is comfortable with a static type of formatting, that same copy can be used over and over again. This is just one example of a situation for

Figure 7-16 **A static concept map based on medication administration knowledge and actions.**

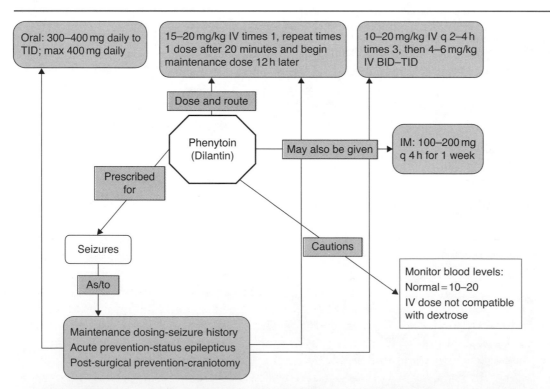

BID = two times per day; TID = three times per day; q = every; IM = intramuscular;
IV = intravenous; h = hour; mg = milligram; kg = kilogram

this type of concept map. Most maps such as Figure 7-16 would also include pharmaco-kinetic and pharmacodynamic information as well. A variation on the entire assignment would be to begin the static map as freshmen and then build on the maps progressively throughout the program.

Holism

Holism is an important aspect of care that is integrated into all nursing education programs. Whether a program utilizes Gordon's Functional Health Patterns to address this or some other method or theory does not really matter. As long as it is addressed throughout the program, the goal has been achieved. Providing holistic care means we are concerned about the entire person's health status—both the mental and physical. While we may want to focus on the physical aspect of the body's response to illness and disease, we always need to consider mental and emotional responses to illness as well. In addition, we need to consider factors influencing the patient's ability to cope and properly heal. From a holistic standpoint these factors can include concerns such as:

1. *Health maintenance and compliance* with prescribed treatment regimens. This category includes disease-prevention efforts, follow up with a primary care provider for management of ongoing healthcare needs, keeping current with flu and pneumonia vaccines, taking medications as prescribed, and so on.

2. *Support systems.* While this usually means the patient's family, it may be any individual or group of individuals who care about and support the patient.

3. *Employment and place of residence/living conditions.* Individuals who are homeless and/or out of work may be unable to cope with illness. They may also tend not to seek medical care because of cost.

4. *Personal value systems and religious beliefs* may strongly influence a patient's health-care maintenance practices, as well as adherence to and acceptance of medical/nursing treatments.

5. *Altered psychosocial factors* such as a mental health illness, mental retardation, substance abuse history, and patient abuse in the home are also major factors to be considered when planning care.

6. *Acute and chronic illnesses* affect the body and the mind.

7. *Perception of illness and wellness* affects and is affected by all of the above.

In essence, within this category we are focusing on somewhat intangible factors at times. We are also focused on a patient's advocacy needs, ensuring collaborative care as part of providing holism, and other patient support systems. As a student, these areas may not seem to be concrete. You may be uncomfortable and unsure of how to both recognize and address these types of needs. Many occur on a lifelong continuum and have no specific endpoint. Most actions you have knowledge of are related to concrete things: assessment findings, abnormal vital signs, post-procedure care, and other things with such straightforward and established actions that they can be complete fairly independently. For instance, if a patient's mental status has changed, the student follows the nursing process to determine the nursing actions and a plan for following up that includes evaluating outcomes. This example and many others similar to it are how student nurses see their scope of practice. They see a problem or concern and they act on it. There is a starting point, an action, and a conclusion. In contrast, concepts such as advocacy, collaboration, and a patient's psychosocial needs are multifaceted and very complex. While you may partially recognize and agree that these matters are important in nursing care, there may be times when you have difficulty recognizing that addressing these needs is part of your scope of practice. In addition, it is sometimes difficult to ascertain how advocacy and alterations within the categories mentioned earlier become part of the plan of care necessitating nursing actions. It is not that faculty are not teaching this; it just takes a certain amount of time for you, as a student, to fully recognize and integrate this theory into your care. As with other more advanced concepts that we spoke about, this knowledge must be layered in along with all other theory so that it becomes ingrained and automatic. It becomes an additional component in application. Concept maps will assist with reinforcing nursing actions related to holism.

In addition, this area of nursing care has a strong focus on developing rapport with others and improving human interaction skills. Communication skills are important in every patient interaction, but especially so when psychosocial problems are being addressed. Various factors play a role in these situations that may impede nurse–patient communication. Some examples are severe anxiety and depression, altered patient perceptions, and ability to respond—as in mental retardation or post-stroke aphasic patients. Another factor to consider is that as a student's role expands, important communication interactions take place between various collaborators as well as the bedside nurse. Therefore, in addition to learning about therapeutic and professional communication techniques, students also need to be educated about collaborator roles. We have emphasized communication in many ways within this text, and it is certainly integral to providing complete care. I am re-emphasizing it here because of the degree of multidisciplinary communication that must take place to provide complete care in this area of practice. **Figure 7-17** illustrates these concepts and ties them all together.

This may be an area where a strong focus needs to be placed on the problem list, because students have difficulty recognizing problems in this area. More opportunities to peruse and apply these concepts will allow in-depth consideration and application. It would not be inappropriate to focus on this portion of map construction alone because it enables thought associations and comparative analysis to occur. Let's look at a problem list related to holism.

The following case study illustrates these concepts:

You are caring for a 35-year-old male admitted after being found lying on the sidewalk by police. There was a strong odor of alcohol on the patient and he was barely responsive. On his arrival to the ED, no significant injuries were found. His blood alcohol level was above normal, and he was admitted to the critical care unit.

The facts in **Figure 7-18** were discovered after his transfer to the medical-surgical unit.

One thing that stands out from this list is that many of the patient's problems not only originated outside of the acute care setting but may also need to be addressed in that setting as well. It is fairly clear that nursing as a discipline will be unable to meet every one of these needs during his hospital stay. For one thing, many of the behaviors, such as lack of a belief system and substance abuse, do not occur quickly. Many are developed and continue over a long span of time. Deep-seated, ingrained characteristics and beliefs

Figure 7-17 Holistic care focus.

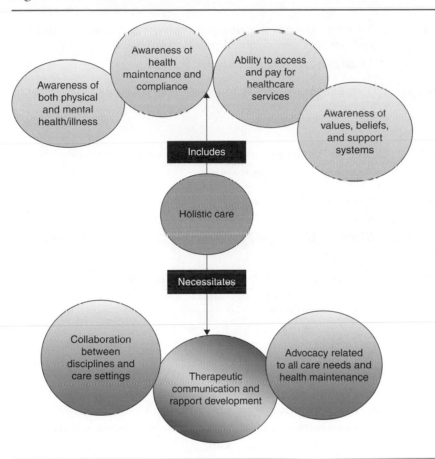

Figure 7-18 Psychosocial factors impacting patient care.

Primary Related Concepts	Secondary Related Concepts
Patient is frequently ill and has no insurance.	Patient refuses flu vaccine.
Patient has stated that he is homeless and "no one cares about me."	No next of kin has been listed—lack of advocacy.
	Patient denies having a support system.
Patient is unable to pay for healthcare services.	Patient has potential for health complications.
Patient has a knowledge deficit regarding healthcare maintenance.	Patient is unable to fully comprehend education because of mental status.
Patient states he feels hopeless: "I don't believe in God anymore."	Lack of a belief system contributes to hopelessness.
Patient has a history of cocaine and alcohol abuse.	There is concern for safety.
Patient's medical history includes hepatitis C.	Knowledge deficit is related to current illness.

Figure 7-19 **Categories of problems.**

Actual Problem (A)	An active and possibly ongoing problem occurring currently and needing nursing interventions *Example: severe abdominal pain*
Potential (P) Problem	A problem that is likely to occur based on patient condition and abnormal assessment/diagnostic findings *Example: The patient may need surgery.*
Primary Problem (PP)	An acute problem that requires priority actions at this time *Example: Need for pain control*
Secondary Problem (S)	A problem that impacts the patient's condition but is not acute and does not need to be addressed immediately *Example: The patient has a history of HTN and the BP is stable currently.*
Tertiary Problem (T)	An identified problem that does not directly impact current care and can be addressed later (either during hospitalization or as an outpatient) *Example: The patient has a history of insomnia.*

embody and strongly influence a person's perceptions and interactions. What this means for nursing students is that these are considerations that lead to nursing actions as they greatly impact the plan of care. Also, nursing diagnoses can still be formulated based on these problems, and although some of the patient's care related to these problems will take place outside the acute care setting, both short- and long-term goals can be created specific to the acute care setting.

When considering nursing actions for the problems listed earlier, we need to assess our thinking ability concerning some basic concepts. We need to cluster the list as we have done previously, separating and isolating acute problems needing immediate attention from those that are chronic and necessitating attention over a longer span of time in other healthcare settings. This is what we have been doing all along, although our focus was on a more acute setting. If you review previous education you have had on patient problems, you may remember that problems affecting patients and their care can fall into several categories: actual or potential problems and primary, secondary, or tertiary problems. This may help you to determine how to more completely identify and cluster problems for nursing diagnosis formulation and care planning. **Figure 7-19** defines/reviews these terms.

Now take a few minutes to study the case study patient's problem list before proceeding. Next, let's divide the patient's problems into type based on Figure 7-19 (see **Figure 7-20**). It may also help to take the problems and convert them into nursing diagnoses. The goal is for you to find some method that enables you to associate these types of problems with nursing actions.

It may take some time to digest all of this information. If you are still having difficulty, think about questions you can ask yourself that may help to direct problem

Figure 7-20 Identifying which categories the patient's problems belong in.

Problem	Type	Rationale
Frequent illness with no insurance	A/PP	The patient's state of health is impacting his current problems and may determine whether or not he completes this admission or leaves against medical advice.
Refusal of flu vaccine	A/PP	The patient is in an overall poor state of health and homeless, placing him at high risk for influenza.
Homelessness and lack of a support system	A/PP	The patient needs his basic needs to be met and a place to live when discharged. Collaborative care is needed to address these issues.
Inability to pay for medical services	A/PP	Affects patient compliance, access, and willingness to seek care. Case management may be able to arrange for funding and care programs.
Health complications	P/S	At this point in time there is no stated evidence of a complication. We have identified that he is at high risk for this. At this time we need to focus on other problems.
Knowledge deficit/inability to comprehend	A/S	While this may be of concern, the patient's mental state and feelings of hopelessness indicate that education would be ineffective. This would not prevent goal setting for the immediate future.
Hopelessness	A/PP	This is no doubt a manifestation of depression and despair. A psychiatric care collaborator would provide valuable insight into treatments and outpatient treatment programs, as well as detoxification.
Lack of a belief system	A/T	From the information we have, this is something that has been in place for some time. Although pastoral care and emotional support could be offered, the patient would have the right to refuse those offerings. Once an advocacy system is developed (if that is possible), his current views may change.
History of drug/ alcohol abuse	A/PP	Although no toxicology screen results have been reported, the patient does admit to use of illicit substances so withdrawal is an area of high concern. The patient should be monitored for delirium tremens, and physician collaboration is essential to prevent this. Long-term care goals for drug and alcohol rehabilitation should be set.
Safety concerns	A/PP	The patient is at high risk for elopement, acting out, possibly exhibiting suicidal behavior, falls, and other medical safety risks related to his hepatitis C.

(Continues)

Figure 7-20 (*Continued*)

Problem	Type	Rationale
Hepatitis C	A/PP	Obviously this patient has had no ongoing treatment for the hepatitis and may have comorbidities associated with this disease. This must be investigated, along with a complete workup of his liver function.
Knowledge deficit related to his current illness	A/PP	Although we stated the patient may have difficulty processing education now, we do need to explain what is being done for him so that he is somewhat involved in his care.

A = actual problem; P = potential problem; PP = primary problem; S = secondary problem; T = tertiary problem

identification and decision making related to these types of problems. Follow this template:

1. *Is the particular concern affecting physiological functioning?* If the answer to this is yes, nursing actions are needed to ensure maintenance of homeostasis.

2. *Is the particular concern affecting psychological functioning?* An answer of yes to this question indicates deficits related to safety, communication, agreement to care, and compliance, all of which necessitate nursing actions.

3. *What is it about this concern that makes it an alteration in physiological or psychological functioning?* For instance, how does not having a belief system affect psychological function? How does that affect nursing care and lead to a nursing action? Belief systems strongly affect a person's perception of health and illness and can also affect mental health. If a person has nothing to believe in, this often results in feelings of depression and hopelessness. This affects response to healthcare related treatments, education, and compliance. As I said before, "nothing is static."

4. *Who is responsible for an action related to this problem?* If you are confused by this, remember that the discipline of nursing has many collaborators. Each discipline's scope of practice is specific to their actions and all disciplines blend that scope to attain the goal of complete, collaborative care. This team effort is advocacy in action. Although nursing oversees all care and consults collaborators, not every action is actually carried out and followed through on strictly by nurses. Other collaborators include:
   - Social services
   - Case management
   - Pastoral/spiritual care providers
   - Mental healthcare teams
   - Physician consultants
   - Respiratory care
   - Wound care teams
   - Patient educational teams

- IV therapy teams
- Pharmacists
- Physical therapy teams
- Hospice care
- Ethics teams and committees

5. *Where else will patient care take place?* Because patients many times have shorter lengths of stays than ever, more care within the healthcare continuum takes place beyond the acute care setting. In order to effectively collaborate as well as educate our patients, we need to have an adequate understanding of each facility, each care provider, and their roles in care provision. Knowledge regarding this is an essential part of addressing evaluation and outcomes within the nursing process.

Advocacy is a common thread woven through all nursing actions and processes. It is the act of supporting and defending patients and their rights. It assists in raising the bar to set the highest quality standards of care and ensure holism in care. Advocacy itself is an action and may be carried out in a wide variety of ways. Nursing actions—resulting from critical thinking, relationship analysis, and application—that result in advocacy in patient care include:

- As you read through your patient's morning labs, you notice his potassium level is 3.0 mEq/L. No potassium has been ordered on the medication administration record (MAR). You assess the patient for symptoms and then place a call to the physician for a potassium order.

- As you complete your patient's assessment, you notice a small, reddened area over his right scapula and are worried about the potential for skin breakdown. You complete wound documentation and add your finding to the plan of care. In addition, you recalculate the patient's skin integrity score.

- Your asthmatic patient has increased wheezing along with increased respiratory effort. You collaborate with the respiratory therapists to ask for an as-needed aerosol treatment.

- Your patient is getting out of bed for the first time after surgery. Because of the current circumstances as well as a history of rheumatoid arthritis, you recognize the patient is at increased risk for falls. You inform the physician on rounds and request a physical therapy consult for strengthening and ambulatory assistance.

- Your patient with end-stage liver disease has decided he no longer wants treatment and requests that nothing more be done for him. You notify the physician, ensure that he completes the do not resuscitate (DNR) form, request a pastoral care visit for patient and family support, and arrange for a consult to hospice care.

Advocacy can be addressed through direct and indirect nursing actions related to any aspect of holistic nursing care.

All nursing care is about prioritizing and organizing. Identification of problems in terms of acuteness or chronicity allows us to better plan when there are multiple complex problems. Planning by this method also forces us to think about the total continuum of care a patient may have to experience and our role in that care. This process guides our collaborative efforts as well. Let's identify our case study patient's nursing actions with the actions of the collaborative team and advocacy in mind. Placing them into concept map form allows you to visualize them in a different light, helping you make connections and associations (see **Figure 7-21**). It has been proven that learning anything by making associations makes learning more meaningful.

To sum up all of this, holism as it is applied to nursing care practice does not focus solely on the physical, mental, and psychosocial needs of a particular patient. Its other main focus is how that care is accomplished using communication, advocacy, and collaboration. All of these areas are essential to ensure holistic care.

Advocacy

Figure 7-22 is an example of a static map about advocacy. When we look at advocacy in this way, it is transformed from a few words on paper or what may seem to be a rather simple concept into a complex concept that touches on and affects every area of our practice. It also emphasizes to students that nursing care cannot be isolated from collaboration—that all members of the healthcare team have valuable input into the care

Figure 7-21 Demonstrating advocacy within the concept map.

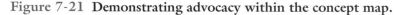

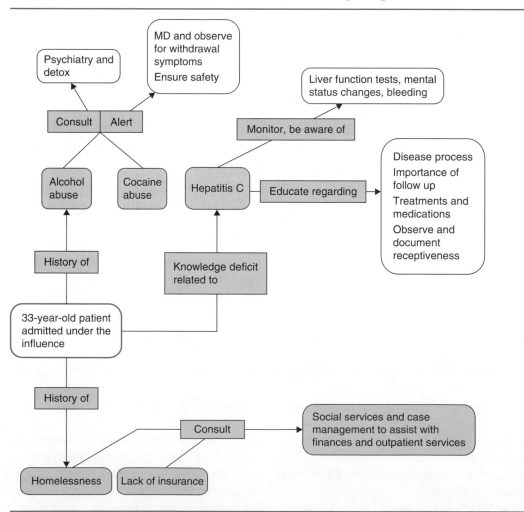

Figure 7-22 A static concept map related to advocacy and nursing actions.

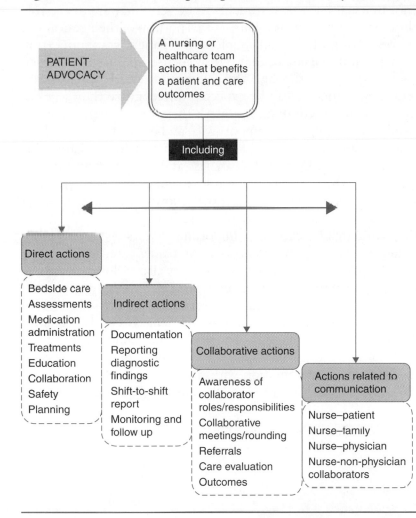

and patient outcomes achieved. What a wonderful lesson this is. Whether an instructor is presenting this in a class or a student is creating it, the same lesson is learned. One small concept map can say so much! This map defines nursing practice, promotes awareness of collaborative roles, and incorporates the nursing process. I know of no other tool that is able to accomplish so much.

Communication and Documentation

Another area that both holism and advocacy in care touch on and are greatly affected by is *communication*, which we examine more closely here. Communication skills are as essential in professional, collaborative relationships as they are in bedside care. Often, when a nursing student learns about therapeutic communication, a link is automatically made between the nurse–patient relationship and this concept. While that is extremely important, communication among and between healthcare team members is just as important, because care would be incomplete without it. Students just beginning their nursing education may have difficulty recognizing this because they are focused on the patient and may have little opportunity to communicate with anyone besides the faculty and bedside nurses. It is not unusual for novice students to be very unaware of the role other disciplines have within the healthcare team. During this portion of their education, these students are focused on learning tasks and simple nurse–patient communication skills. It is difficult for them to think outside of that tightly focused framework to even consider collaborators. As they progress through their education and role expansion occurs, this changes. At this point students can be expected to recognize the scopes of practice of various collaborators and to communicate with them on an ongoing basis. From these interactions, students develop both a rapport with and understanding of how each discipline interacts with nursing to provide the most thorough and safe care. This process can also assist students with an increased awareness and clarity of the student nurse role and how it compares to the graduate nurse role. More experienced students attain a comfort level with their overall roles and skills that allows them to develop an awareness of the entire healthcare team and each member's responsibilities.

Written communication skills are also extremely important in nursing care. Written communication, which includes the documentation that accompanies care, accomplishes several important things (see **Figure 7-23**). Today, this category also includes electronic documentation. Many healthcare facilities now use some type of electronic system for all documentation, including that of collaborators and for order entry by physicians. This necessitates additional preparatory time for student clinical experiences as well as collaborating with staff educators within clinical facilities. Nursing faculty and students must be prepared to understand and navigate the computer charting programs of all chosen clinical sites to be able to complete documentation within the set guidelines. Because nursing is the discipline overseeing all care, we need to be aware of what is being charted

Figure 7-23 **The role of documentation in communication.**

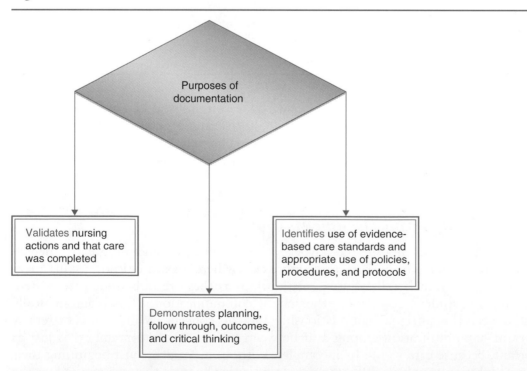

by other disciplines and how that affects our care. Concept maps, both static and living, can be developed for explaining any portion of the documentation process.

Validation of nursing care means that if something is not charted it was never done. Suppose a patient tells the student that he has pain around his IV site. If the site is checked and determined to be problem free, but this is never documented, imagine what could happen should the patient develop phlebitis requiring a prolonged hospital stay and other complications. This has implications from a legal perspective. Legal consequences could result if the patient stated the nurse never inspected the site.

Demonstrating planning, outcomes, and critical thinking shows application of the nursing process in care. Both types of communication skills are reflective of the other categories as well. The nursing process is an essential part of practice, identifies role responsibility, and is normally included in nursing position performance objectives. Thus, it implicates the nursing scope of practice.

Identifying the use of standards, policies, and protocols not only reinforces the nursing role in ensuring quality care, but implications also exist from an accreditation perspective. Accrediting agencies take this very seriously. This also addresses that nursing competencies such as cultural care and holism are satisfied. Documentation of these standards ensures that accreditation mandates are achieved and that care standards are adequate. Documentation is not only the nurse's responsibility but also the nursing student's.

Documentation examples related to nursing and healthcare team collaborators may include but are not limited to:

- Nursing
  - Patient education
  - Medication administration
  - Wound care
  - Admission and discharge
  - Post-procedure care
  - Addressing language barriers
  - Pain
  - Psychosocial concerns
- Respiratory therapy
  - Aerosol treatments
  - Chest physiotherapy
  - Patient tolerance of therapies
  - Supportive device settings and management such as BiPAP and patient-owned CPAP machines and ventilators
- Physical therapy/occupational therapy
  - Fulfillment of prescribed therapies as ordered by the physician
  - Patient tolerance and ability to complete ordered therapies
  - Patient readiness for discharge
  - Adaptations or alterations necessary to the current plan of care based on the above
  - Input into patient placement post-discharge

- Social services/case management
  - Patient readiness for discharge
  - Decision making related to power of attorney status
  - Assessing patient financial needs
  - Liaison notes to family and support systems

As you can see, not all collaborators chart on the medical record, but we need to be aware of those who do and what it is they are documenting. The entire process of multidisciplinary documentation becomes a communication pathway—explaining, justifying, and validating multidisciplinary care provided to a patient throughout the hospital stay.

The narrative note is an important component of complete documentation that complements assessment documentation. Most charting referred to up to this point takes place on specific forms, whether computer-based electronic forms or handwritten. Form charting may be appropriate for assessments but does not always address or allow for an expanded recording of events and follow up. Narrative notes, also known as progress notes, do allow for inclusion of "the rest of the story" that begins within other charting formats. Before we examine this type of charting more closely, let's look at some examples. **Figure 7-24** will assist you to understand the meaning and usefulness of narrative notes and to encourage you to think of more examples. These

Figure 7-24 **Narrative notes.**

Event/Originating Form	Required Narrative	Rationale
IV infiltration/IV flow sheet	As a follow up to care needed after an extensive infiltration	Proves ongoing monitoring of the situation, effectiveness of treatment, and outcomes
Patient received post-conscious sedation/flow sheet	Receiving note and care protocols	Shows adequate recovery, response, oxygenation, and safety measures instituted with the use of conscious sedation
Physician visit	Communication	Indicates data reported to the physician as well as patient concerns
Wound care/wound care flow sheet	Descriptive elaboration	Wound characteristics are varied and need in-depth description or there are significant changes requiring physician notification and new orders
Change in vital signs	Patient status	Requires a call to the physician regarding status and any decompensation
Need for stat aerosol treatment/nursing and respiratory flow sheets	Explanation of need and effectiveness	Demonstrates nursing process, collaboration, and outcomes

are only a few examples of when a narrative note is required. Each example reinforces that safety, the nursing process, collaboration, and advocacy have been addressed in some fashion.

Narrative notes are free-form notes for the most part, but electronic medical record (EMR) documentation programs usually include preformatted notes, too. These normally include documentation events such as admissions, discharges, patient transfer and receiving notes, and several types of treatment-related notes. Often they are brief and uniform, somewhat like a form letter. Free-form notes provide the best opportunity for in-depth explanations and rationales as referred to earlier. Several formats can be used. Some facilities require the use of a certain format that must be demonstrated in the note while others allow a nurse to decide which format to use. In any case, several important components are necessary to include in any narrative note: the *information or event*, the *action taken* and the *response to that action, follow up* of that action, and *patient progress/ response*. The general rule of thumb is to use these important elements to elaborate on some event or unit of data that requires more information. We can also look at this process as a set of questions:

1. What happened? What is it that needs to be communicated?
2. What action(s) resulted?
3. Was the action effective?
4. Have I completely addressed this event/information?
5. What was the end result?

Let's examine each of these in more detail. Then we can consider static map examples.

Information/Event

This category can include:

- An abnormal laboratory test
- A change in patient status
- A medication reaction
- Refusal of a medication
- Report of a diagnostic test
- Transfer, admission, or discharge
- A patient treatment initiated via protocol (e.g., bladder scanning)
- A physician visit
- A behavior or symptom

Each of the items listed here requires a narrative note because each has the potential to change the current plan of care. In addition, a nursing action is needed to address them as part of the nursing process. They refer to both assessment and diagnosis, reflecting the nurse's critical thinking and clinical judgment abilities. Narrative note examples will be included at the end of this section.

Actions

Actions taken might include:

- Calling the physician
- Reassessing or performing a more focused assessment of the problem
- Initial nursing actions taken for an event
- A statement of patient comments/concerns
- A statement of orders received
- A direct action resulting from a nurse-initiated protocol (e.g., straight catheterization)
- A statement that the physician was aware of an event/information
- A note outlining actions regarding a patient or symptom

This part of the note demonstrates progression of the event—what the nurse did to address it.

Action Response

This portion addresses the immediate responses to the actions taken. It may include statements such as:

- "New orders received"
- "Vital signs reassessed"
- "Patient assisted back to bed"
- "Medication held"
- "Respiratory therapist paged to administer stat aerosol treatment"

Thus far we have seen that an event or information was the catalyst for requiring a note. An action was taken based on the event/information, which then required an action response to describe what was done about it.

Follow Up

Follow up is necessary to demonstrate that we follow the nursing process as well as to address other factors such as advocacy, communication, and safety. Many events are patient problems or condition changes so that one action by itself is not enough to adequately address or correct the problem. Including follow up addresses legal concerns and shows that the nurse did everything possible to achieve resolution. Some examples are:

- Continued assessment
- Repeating physician calls
- Administering repeat medication doses
- Pain reassessment

Follow up can be short term or long term depending upon the event or problem. In some instances, follow up occurs over several shifts and involves collaborators.

Patient Response and Progress

Patient response and progress can also be short or long term. Some events resolve quickly while others reoccur. At times, this portion accompanies the previous portion.

Let's look at some examples. In each one, the following key will identify the format portion in parentheses: **I/E** = Information or event; **A** = action; **AR** = action response; **F** = follow up; and **PR** – patient response/progress.

1. 11/2/11, 0800: Patient's morning potassium level is 2.8. (**I**) Call placed to physician. Patient assessed for signs and symptoms of hypokalemia—none noted. Patient states he "feels fine." (**A**) 0815: Physician returned call and new orders received—see MAR. (**AR**) Potassium level to be repeated at 1300. 0830: Patient tolerated oral potassium without nausea. Remains stable. (**F, PR**)

   This example has a long-term component in that the patient may develop signs and symptoms of hypokalemia if the replacement potassium dose is ineffective and also because of the future order of a potassium level.

2. 11/2/11, 1000: Dr. Jones visited and examined. Aware of patient complaints of dyspnea on exertion and normal assessment findings. (**I/E**) New orders received for V/Q [ventilation/perfusion] scan to rule out pulmonary emboli. (**A**) 1100: Patient transported to nuclear medicine via litter accompanied by transport. (**AR**) 1150: Patient returned in stable condition and without new complaints. 1215: Call received from nuclear medicine regarding V/Q result of high probability for pulmonary emboli. Dr. Jones made aware and new orders received for heparin therapy. Patient aware. (**F, PR**)

   As this note continues and patient teaching is added, the format would repeat itself. Follow up would consist of patient tolerance of the therapy as well as how teaching was carried out and the patient's receptiveness to it.

3. 11/2/11, 1200: Patient admitted from the emergency care unit via litter with a diagnosis of right lower extremity ulcer. (**A**) See nursing database. Patient states that currently she only feels mild discomfort rated 4 out of 10 on a scale of 1–10 in the right lower extremity, along with occasional burning and stinging. Area undressed and ulcer over right ankle measures 2 cm × 2 cm × 0.5 cm. Ulcerated area erythematous with darkened edges and serosanguinous exudate. Cleansed with saline and redressed with a sterile non-stick dressing, followed by a dry sterile dressing and gauze wrap secured with paper tape. Patient oriented to room, staff, and unit routine. Bed in lowest position with bedrails up times 3 and call bell in place. (**AR**) 1300: Patient condition unchanged. Continues to state pain rating is unchanged and acceptable to her. Database completed. (**F, PR**)

   Although many admission notes are pre-formatted and seem somewhat routine, this is a good example where emotional needs and physical symptoms need to be expanded upon. Patient education and any communication between the nurse and the patient's family could be added here.

Now let's take what we have learned and take a glance at a few static concept maps regarding documentation (see **Figures 7-25, 7-26, 7-27,** and **7-28.** With any narrative note documentation, you will see communication layered in. Most notes also have collaboration incorporated. Advocacy is, of course, included in the entire process as well.

Figure 7-25 Static map #1 on documentation.

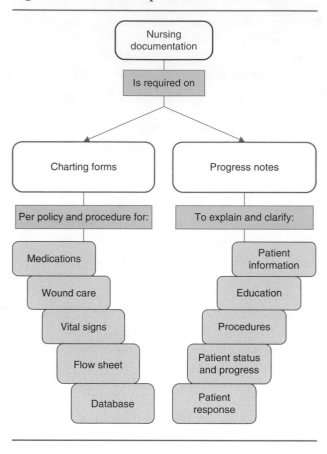

Figure 7-26 Static map #2 on documentation.

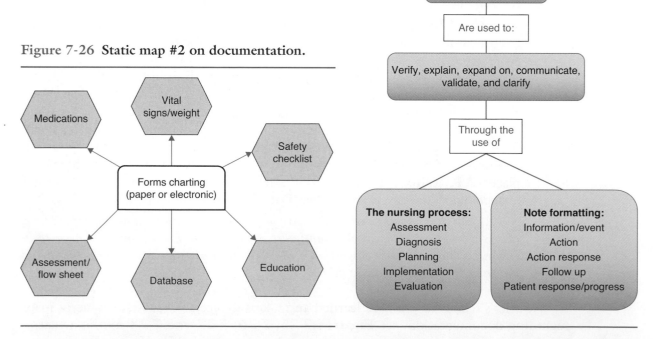

Figure 7-27 Static map #3 on documentation.

Figure 7-28 Static map #4 on documentation.

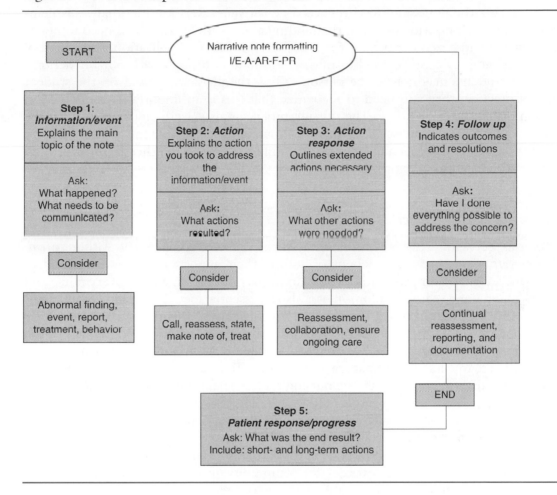

Remember that advocacy is not usually stated specifically in a treatment plan or note, but rather inferred directly and indirectly through actions. Each member of the healthcare team plays a role in patient advocacy.

Now we can refer back to an earlier scenario (case 1) to consider what a living concept map regarding documentation might look like (see **Figure 7-29**). An assignment such as this reinforces critical thinking through application. It is especially valuable when completed after care of a patient on the clinical site. The information and actions are fresh in the student's mind and can also be used for reflection purposes. While the focus here is on the documentation, please remember the same situation could be used to focus solely on nursing actions.

11/2/11 0800 Patient's morning potassium level is 2.8. (1) Call placed to physician. Patient assessed for signs and symptoms of hypokalemia—none noted. Patient states he "feels fine." (A). 0815 Physician returned call and new orders received—see MAR (AR). Potassium level to be repeated at 1300. 0830 Patient tolerated oral potassium without nausea. Remains stable. (F, PR) This example has a long-term component in that the patient may develop signs and symptoms of hypokalemia if the replacement potassium dose is ineffective and also because of the future order of a potassium level.

This example reinforces concept map theory. Critical thinking allows the student to recognize that the potassium level reflects a deficit state. Relationship analysis is demonstrated by an association between that finding along with an identified need to notify the physician and assess the patient for untoward symptoms. Application is using all of the knowledge previously learned to initiate and follow through with nursing actions. Although students may not be the person calling the physician, based on the student scope of practice, they still need to recognize that this is an important component in problem resolution in this case. The nursing process is also clearly implicated here. The student identifies and assesses a problem, formulates a mental diagnosis that includes awareness of symptoms that may stem from it, initiates actions, and then follows through on the problem to completion.

Cultural Competence Processes

Another aspect within the process category is cultural care competency. Although *cultural aspects of care* are a component of holism, their importance deserves individual treatment. Cultural competency is a Joint Commission requirement for every nurse and must be maintained yearly. In addition, it is also an essential focus point for meeting standards required for Magnet status. In addition, we must be able to understand and provide care for the various cultural populations in our communities. The demographics of the United States have changed a great deal over the years. Most U.S. communities today contain large segments of multicultural populations. To be able to address the healthcare needs of such diverse populations, the nursing profession must have an awareness of each culture's perception regarding health and illness. The ability to cross language barriers is also necessary for establishing rapport and an environment of trust where members of each population feel comfortable seeking care. So, cultural competency begins with awareness of other cultures and extends beyond hospital walls to the community. Competence also includes nursing advocacy for community agency establishment as part of the entire continuum of care and enabling access to care.

Concept maps can be used to introduce students to cultural care through the use of static maps on various cultural groups or living maps involving nursing actions according to an individual patient's culture. Cultural care is an area where we need collaboration and advocacy to be built into the plan of care. Integrating cultural concerns into nursing care may include concepts such as:

- Culturally therapeutic communication techniques
- Inclusion of the patient's family members in education
- Ensuring accuracy in translation
- Awareness of attitudes and perceptions related to health care and health maintenance
- Legal concerns related to informed consent
- Respecting cultural boundaries within the realm of care provision
- Understanding hierarchy in family roles

As far as bedside care is concerned, concepts such as eye contact, personal space, caregiver gender, and communication are some examples of these concepts stated. It

Figure 7-29 Living map on documentation.

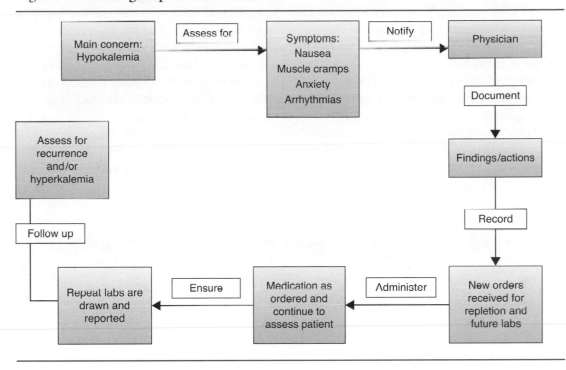

may seem impossible to know everything about every culture, but activities focusing on common cultures within one's community are a good place to start. This will lead to the creation of a resource database that can assist all nurses to achieve and maintain competency. This is a great area for use of both static and living maps. Blank copies of static maps can be created for simple maps on basic introductory information pertaining to various cultures. They will lend themselves to reuse for study. Personalized according to learning style, this makes them absolutely wonderful resources.

Living concept maps defining nursing actions in regard to cultural care demonstrate the competencies developed from the static maps. This allows a student to see the depth of cultural knowledge attained and whether or not it is effective when applied to nursing care. In some ways, concept maps serve as checklists for critical thinking and application abilities.

A toolkit for ensuring nursing-related competencies in cultural nursing care should contain:

1. Curriculum objectives relative to attaining cultural competency
2. A text for each educational level on culture
3. Integration of assigned readings on culture
4. Inclusion of cultural care aspects within classroom, nursing lab, and clinical settings
5. Presentation and use of concept maps in that education

Using culturally therapeutic communication techniques is important in any nurse–patient interaction. Applied to cultural care, however, we also have to consider tone of voice, eye contact, and personal space in our approach. Addressing these concepts will assist the development of trust and rapport. Often, the extended family plays a strong and important role in the patient's care, so they must be included as well. Sometimes one family member will dominate as a leader and other times this responsibility may be shared, depending on the culture. Perceptions of the patient related to health care, wellness, and illness greatly impact acceptance of treatments and future compliance.

Translation should always take place through a professional interpreter or the use of an interpreting phone. This ensures that accurate information is being relayed in words the patient can understand. Family members may help at times but should not be the main source because they usually have no medical background. All of this takes on special meaning legally and ethically when informed consent is obtained. We must be sure that the patient fully understands and accepts what he or she is signing and is not coerced in any way. All of these concepts comprise the knowledge base needed to understand, achieve, and apply cultural competence.

Let's examine some examples of concept maps related to culture. The first is very basic and will help to guide students in understanding the basic information required when caring for various cultural populations (see **Figure 7-30**). The second example stems somewhat from the first and assists with guidance related to research of the required information (see **Figure 7-31**). This is the beginning of establishing an educational base eventually used in application.

Figure 7-30 **Cultural care map #1.**

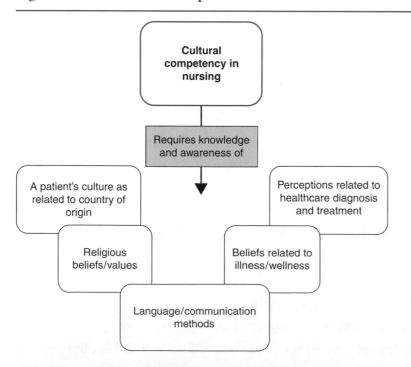

Figure 7-31 Cultural care map #2.

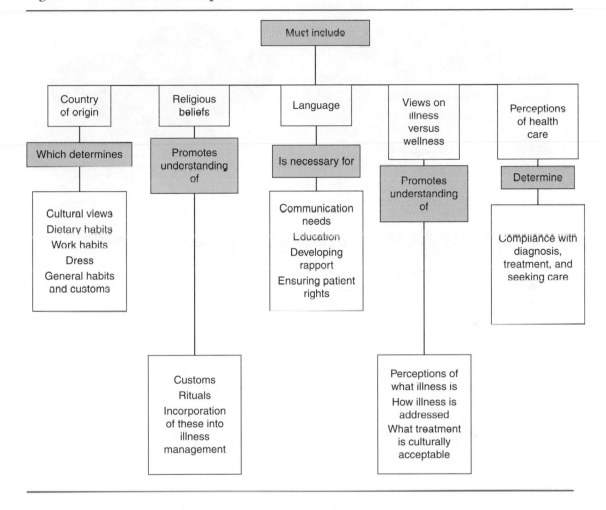

The third map is an example of a complex static map (see **Figure 7-32**). Each main component is related to the other, reflecting critical thinking and relationship analysis. The nursing process is included in the nursing actions.

Effective uses for this type of concept map include:

- This type of map would lend itself to generate discussions related to cultural nursing care and competency, as well as to addressing the need for collaboration in providing culturally competent care.

- A map such as this would also be a great study tool.

- It could also be incorporated into a post-conference setting after students have cared for a patient of another culture because it would reinforce the care standards. An exercise involving comparison and contrast between current standards and the actual care provided would be extremely valuable.

- An exercise could be used where each student would have to add examples of the secondary related concepts.

Figure 7-32 **Cultural care map #3.**

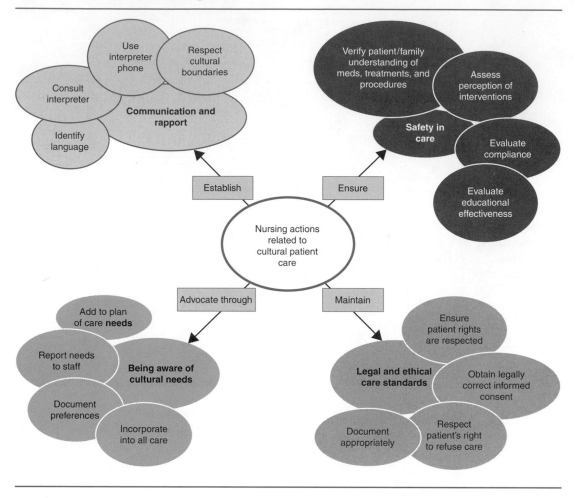

The list of uses is truly endless and limited only to our creative imaginations.

Interventions, Nursing Actions, and Outcomes

We will complete the process section by discussing *interventions*, *actions*, and *outcomes*. Although each of these is used and addressed as part of concept mapping theory and the nursing process, as previous examples have shown, further explanation will assist students in better understanding these concepts and their origins. Interventions and actions originate from all members of the healthcare team, and all affect patient outcomes (see **Figure 7-33**).

Nursing actions comprise anything and everything done for patients by nurses. From giving a bed bath to administering a medication and providing education, to collaborating with the care team or documenting—all of these things comprise our nursing actions. Some actions are directly related to physician orders. Others are enacted as preventive measures or secondary to nursing orders. Each action has a meaning within the nursing process, concept mapping theory, and standards of care within the nursing care

Figure 7-33 **Origin and application of interventions, actions, and outcomes.**

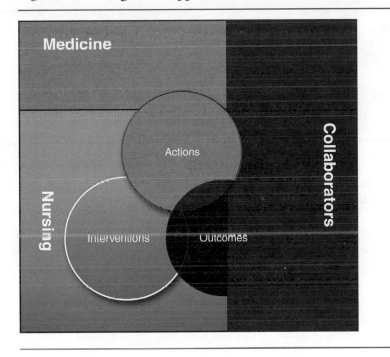

continuum. Some actions can be carried out independently using nursing judgment, while others require physician collaboration. Still others necessitate interdisciplinary collaboration. Complete care addressing all patient needs necessitates a team approach. Examining all of these concepts gives meaning to our actions. Origins often determine rationale and assist us with understanding what actions are necessary for problem resolution.

Nursing *interventions* are actions. In most cases, using this terminology signifies that the origin for such interventions is nursing based. In other words, the entire decision-making process used to carry out the order is nursing based. Established nursing practice–based policies, procedures, and protocols are examples of this. Some types of nursing interventions are completely independent and part of nursing judgment. As we have learned, adequate critical thinking is necessary to build effective nursing judgment and clinical decision-making skills. It is extremely important to mention here that independent actions originate from nursing standards based on nursing research. Every action taken has meaning and follows these set standards. Students must learn to recognize this. Evidenced-based nursing practice defines and guides all nursing actions in patient care. It is also integral to setting standards in care regardless of location or practice area.

Other independent nursing interventions must interface with those actions originating from physician collaboration. While this means the nurse may initiate an action, the physician needs to be involved as well. In this case, the action initiated may affect a physician order and thus must be reported. In addition, the event precipitating the action may require multiple actions necessitating physician orders. Some of these actions are independent but actually stem from an order. You may be asking, "How can this be? Isn't an order either independent or interdependent? Can it fit into both categories?" Yes, it can. The reason for this is that sometimes actions are an extension of a physician order and not directly related to it. Part of the action is nursing judgment based and part is enacted as a direct result of the physician order. One simple example would be: The physician orders sequential compression devices (SCDs). Nursing policy states that these devices must be removed once per shift to assess the patient's skin or when the patient is out of bed. The nurse makes the independent decision to remove the devices as needed during these times and then reapplying them.

Scope of practice as defined by state boards of nursing regulates these actions as well. Both nursing students and licensed nurses must always be aware of the scope of nursing practice guidelines. More detailed examples of independent nursing interventions are provided in **Figure 7-34**.

Interdependent nursing *actions* originate from direct physician orders. These orders may be in electronic format, handwritten, or given directly in verbal or telephone exchange. Institutional policy will dictate whether verbal or telephone orders can be accepted. To avoid errors with this process, specific instructions must usually be followed. These may include repeating the order back to the physician for confirmation, having another registered nurse listen and verify the order, or a requirement that the order must be signed by the physician within a certain timeframe. Again, it is extremely important to be aware of scope of practice and policy related to this. Most states prohibit students from taking either verbal or telephone orders. Nursing actions stemming from physician orders are any actions other than the independent interventions stated earlier. What this means is that these particular types of orders cannot be carried out in the absence of a

Figure 7-34 **Independent nursing interventions.**

Intervention	Rationale
The nurse provides information on diabetic education classes.	This is an independent intervention based on nursing judgment concerning health promotion, complication prevention, and advocacy for compliance.
The patient complains of an inability to void and is assessed for a distended bladder. The nurse initiates a bladder scan.	This is an independent intervention based on safety. Findings from this will now interface with physician orders if either a Foley or straight catheterization is needed.
A patient's beta-blocker is held even though no parameters are in place when the blood pressure reads 88/46.	This was a nursing judgment decision. It is somewhat interdependent in that the physician must be notified and the nurse should advocate for parameters.
A patient complains of diaphoresis, dizziness, and "not feeling well." The nurse obtains vital signs, initiates a rapid response team call, and has the nurse aide obtain a fingerstick glucose reading.	This is an independent nursing judgment based on patient decompensation. Further actions will be interdependent and in collaboration with the physician and care team.
The nurse completes preoperative education teaching.	Independent actions to provide education advocate for patient understanding and a choice in care decisions.

physician order, although there is a component of independence that will be addressed later. Orders generating these actions include, but are not limited to:

- IV fluid therapy
- Diet and nutritional supplements
- Initiating consultations
- Vital sign frequency
- Medications
- Activity
- Diagnostic and laboratory testing
- Wound and dressing care
- Notification parameters relative to vital signs
- Invasive procedures and line placement

Hopefully, this explanation allows adequate comparison and contrast regarding nursing actions. While students are able to carry out both types of actions, practice scope limits and prohibits certain actions. It stands to reason then that new graduates experience stress not only with their new roles, but in having to complete nursing actions (and nursing judgments related to those actions) that they were not allowed to carry out as students. Promoting awareness of this fact during nursing education will allow students to set goals related to it and hopefully decrease anxiety over it. Static concept maps outlining these types of actions can be created for use upon graduation.

To summarize, nursing actions may be independent, interdependent, or contain components of both types. Static concept maps can also enhance learning related to determining and thinking through whether an action is independent or interdependent. As stated earlier, this goes along with critical thinking and clinical decision-making abilities. Honing both and blending them with concept mapping theory allows for more complete learning outcomes in this area.

Before we examine concept map examples related to nursing actions, let's look at a scenario to further clarify all the facts. Patient-related case studies or scenarios are another valuable way to put everything into perspective. If students are able to mentally walk through an action or patient care scenario, they can derive much deeper meaning from it because they can relate it to their own actions and thoughts related to those actions.

Suppose your patient's chart contains the following orders:

- Admitting diagnosis: acute abdominal pain
- NPO [no oral intake/not by mouth]
- IV 1000 mL [milliliters] NSS [normal saline solution] at 125 mL per hour
- Bed rest
- Stat obstructive series—call me with results
- Vital signs every 4 hours—call for temp greater than 101°F
- Telemetry
- Obtain CBC [complete blood count], basic metabolic profile
- Anti-embolism stockings with SCDs

- Tylenol [acetaminophen] 650 mg every 4 hours PRN [as needed] pain/fever
- Dilaudid [hydromorphone hydrochloride] 2 mg IV every 2 hours PRN pain

Now, let's look at each order and try to determine whether it is an independent nursing intervention or an interdependent nursing action.

NPO Status

This is an *interdependent* order but does have some independent actions. The order is placed in the computer to alert dietary and on the plan of care to alert nursing staff. The nurse then makes the patient aware. The independent part relating to nursing judgment is to remove all food and beverages from the room and to place a sign above the patient's bed.

Intravenous Fluids

The action relating to hanging the fluid as ordered is *interdependent*. A nurse would never hang an IV fluid without a physician order. The independent portion here involves an IV site assessment and completing the order in a timely manner.

Bed Rest

This order would have strictly interdependent actions. Enforcing bed rest is a direct follow through of a physician order, and even if a protocol is in place to get the patient out of bed on the second postoperative day (or some similar order), it is still interdependent because it can only be done with that order in place. I think it is important to mention here that nursing judgment always plays an important part—no matter the order origin. For instance, if there would be an order to get the patient out of bed at a later time, judgment must be exercised by taking into account the patient's diagnosis, vital signs, and ability to tolerate that action.

Stat Obstructive Series (With Results To Be Called to the Physician)

Again, this is fairly straightforward and is an interdependent order. Any independent action would originate from calling the physician if the patient was not able to complete the testing or refused it, or other need for independent nursing action.

Vital Signs With Notification Parameters

In large part this is interdependent. Independent actions could result if the vital signs happened to be abnormal and needed to be repeated. Nursing judgment would determine whether or not orthostatic vital signs should be obtained and when to call the physician.

Telemetry

Telemetry would be an interdependent order. Some examples of independent actions related to this order would be changing the patches as needed to maintain tracings, mounting and interpreting strips, and changing the battery as needed.

Laboratory Testing

This particular order is interdependent. Independent actions would be ensuring the blood draw is completed by the phlebotomist as ordered and that the results are available as needed.

Anti-Embolism Stockings and Sequential Compression Devices

Application and maintenance of the stockings and devices are interdependent, but as discussed earlier, nursing protocols allow for some independent actions related to their use and removal at certain times.

Medications

Medications must be administered as ordered. However, nursing judgment dictates that independent actions are utilized when it is prudent to hold the medication. If the patient is nauseated, acetaminophen (Tylenol) would *not* be the best choice here. If you are going to administer it because of fever, another order for an alternate route of administration would be needed. Dilaudid dosing may be affected by the patient's blood pressure. If the patient would not tolerate the ordered dose, further orders are needed.

Let's examine a few concept maps focused on nursing actions. Static maps can be created for specific order sets and used to demonstrate order/treatment patterns. Living concept maps may be used based on a case study or actual patient assignment from the clinical setting where the student must create a map based on the nursing actions provided

Figure 7-35 Nursing action map #1.

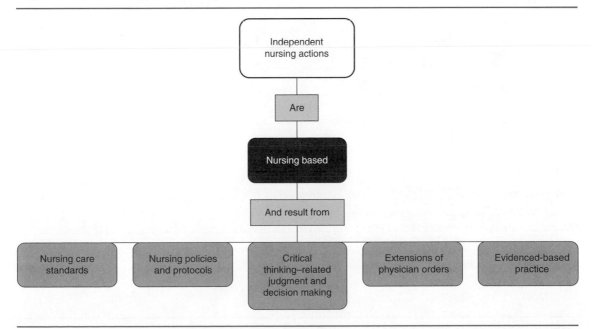

in response to patient problems or concerns. (To use a Concept Map Creator, see the Student Companion Website at http://go.jblearning.com/schmehl.)

The first nursing action map promotes reflection on where nursing actions have their origins (see **Figure 7-35**). Because nothing is static or occurs in isolation, it provides rationales for not only the actions but also for how protocols and policies come into being. This example could even be used to introduce evidence-based practice (EBP).

The second map is somewhat more detailed and includes some examples of independent actions. It can be used as a more in-depth example of action initiation (see **Figure 7-36**).

Before we take a look at a living map example, we need to discuss *outcomes*. Each action we take leads to an eventual outcome. Outcomes are the result of our actions; they are nursing care outcomes. Although, as discussed earlier, outcomes are part of the nursing process—a component featured in nursing diagnosis formulation and also addressed within concept mapping theory. Students are not always fully aware of the

Figure 7-36 Nursing action map #2.

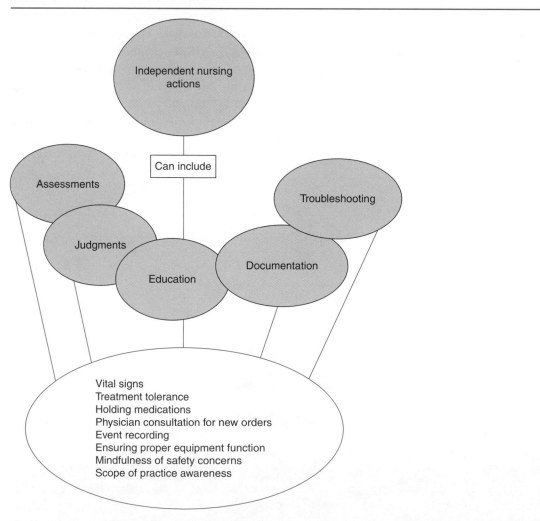

depth and breadth of all outcomes. The term *outcomes* relates to total care outcomes resulting from team collaborative care as well as smaller outcomes assessed as part of daily care in response to the patient problem list.

Nursing actions are paired with outcomes, and one nursing action may address more than one outcome. Actions and outcomes necessitate goal setting in patient care, along with the multidisciplinary team. As far as the nursing process and nursing standards are concerned, the goal of nursing care–related outcomes is a positive result. This is true whether the action is nursing based or has its origin within the physician orders. A positive result means that EBP decisions, actions, and standards have been followed and utilized for the best results. Realize that within this process that not all problems are resolved in the acute care setting. In addition, some problems have no resolution, depending on the disease, complications, health status of the patient, and many other factors. This topic is a very broad one that could certainly fill an entire book. For the purposes of this text, we are talking about events that students will deal with in the patient care setting for which goals can be set and resolutions attained. Actions plus goals equal outcomes.

To address outcomes from our actions, we will have to narrow our focus a bit. To simplify this information and demonstrate a more focused link between actions and outcomes, let's classify actions and outcomes using the following scale: *simple, complex, short term*, and *long term*. Narrowing the focus will enable the process of not only identifying the action but also recognizing multiple steps that are needed to reach an outcome. These concepts also overlap with those of nursing actions as discussed earlier. Action type also stems from the type of problem or concern needing to be addressed.

> Students need to know that each problem or concern a patient has requires a nursing action. An awareness of outcomes means that each problem must be followed through on with as many actions as are needed until resolution can be achieved. Every action has an outcome and becomes part of the overall outcome of successful patient care.
>
> Concept maps focus on actions and the follow through necessary to realize outcomes.

Simple Action

A simple action has several key features or components:

- It occurs in response to a simple problem or concern.
- It requires only one or two actions and simple goal setting to be attained.
- It is able to be achieved quickly.

If an IV site becomes infiltrated, the nursing action is to remove the site. The desired outcome of the IV therapy would be to have zero complications. However, if a complication does occur, the goal becomes addressing the problem and achieving resolution without further complications. Removing the site, performing a focused assessment for any complications such as infection or tissue extravasation, and then dressing the site and documenting appropriately achieves this goal for a positive outcome. An additional action may include the need for a compress. Ideally the site would begin to improve rapidly. Worsening of the site appearance or suspicion of infection would necessitate notifying the physician.

Complex Actions

In contrast to simple actions, complex actions result from more complex problems/concerns. In this case, multiple actions are needed to reach a resolution. Assessing outcomes in this case could occur over a longer period of time or even be delayed.

Suppose your patient has developed new-onset atrial fibrillation. The ventricular response is a tachycardia at a rate of 140–160 and the patient becomes hypotensive but asymptomatic. The desired outcome in this case is for the heart rate to be controlled and the patient to then be asymptomatic. From a student's perspective, some nursing actions to achieve our goal of patient stability would be:

- Have the patient remain in bed and obtain vital signs every 15 minutes.
- Notify the co-assigned registered nurse who will notify the physician.
- Assist with obtaining an electrocardiogram.
- Assess the patient for any other untoward effects.
- Administer medications as ordered for heart rate control (if within the student's scope of practice).
- Document and monitor frequently.

Stable vital signs would signify one of our goals but may not be able to be achieved until the heart rate is controlled. If IV push doses of medication are ineffective, a medication drip may be necessary. Often, several doses of an IV push medication may need to be given before results are seen, and they will need to be spaced several hours apart. This prolongs current actions and outcomes assessments and may lead to many more nursing actions. If the patient develops additional complications such as chest pain, the whole picture of care may change. Outcomes in this case may take many hours over several shifts.

A common theme evidenced throughout this discussion is following up and following through on a nursing action, which includes outcomes. I can tell you from personal experience that concept maps are excellent for explaining and demonstrating this. When a student addresses a problem or concern on a concept map, the thought processes involved are clearly visible. Each step in an action shows the pathway from the first action chosen to the last. If the student stops short of considering all actions or the outcome, faculty need to determine why.

Short-Term Actions

Short-term actions will usually accompany simple actions and are utilized with less complex problems where outcomes are easily achieved. For example, your patient complains of a headache, acetaminophen is already ordered, and so you administer it. When you reassess the pain, it has improved. Thus, your goal or outcome has been achieved.

Long-Term Action

In contrast, long-term actions are usually linked with more complex problems or concerns that need multiple actions and possibly multiple collaborators as well to achieve resolution. A great example of this is the patient who has had a hip replacement. One of the outcomes desired is to have patients return home to their previous level of functioning, able to complete all activities of daily living (ADLs) and quality of life. Because many of these patients move on to a physical rehabilitation facility to complete all of the steps toward this goal, multidisciplinary actions must take place. Many of the actions also take place at the rehabilitation facility and thus are long term.

Long-term actions also refer to repeated actions that occur in the ongoing monitoring and follow through of a patient problem. Nursing actions that require ongoing application may be necessary over several shifts or days, as well as during the entire hospital stay. Some examples of this include:

- Recurrent hypotension with repeated orthostatic vital signs
- Ongoing assessments for dehydration in the patient receiving fluid replacement or fluid challenges
- A patient with a complex wound requiring complex wound care daily
- A post-surgical patient experiencing complications
- A diabetic patient whose blood glucose levels are difficult to control

If we look at outcomes separate from actions, they could be identified as either general or specific. For each patient in the acute care setting, the general goal or outcome is to maintain the current level of function and plan for discharge to the appropriate setting without complications. While under normal circumstances this is to the patient's home, there are many times when that is not possible. In that case an alternative care setting must be chosen. Specific outcomes are then set according to diagnosis and active patient problems. Origins for active problems can be found in the admission diagnosis, complications and new problems occurring during admission, and finally from the PMH. We will briefly examine each of these areas in regard to outcomes.

The main diagnosis usually takes center stage. Specific outcomes related to this may be goals such as stabilization of the disease process, maintaining the patient's baseline function, and preventing complications. Outcomes are then reached and achieved through physician orders, treatments, and nursing actions.

Any complications or new problems are undesired outcomes related to treatments and actions. Outcomes desired in this case are that the patient does not deteriorate or pass away. Ongoing assessments and actions are employed to address each problem and area of concern, no matter how minor.

Each patient's PMH must be carefully examined because it is often as important as the main diagnosis, and sometimes more so. If care is focused solely on the main admitting diagnosis, important findings relative to the history will be omitted from the plan of care. That would be similar to saying that patients leave all past diagnoses at the door when they enter the hospital, which is of course not true. Many chronic illnesses are affected and exacerbated by the physical stress of disease and may even be the reason for the hospitalization. Two examples of this are: 1) the patient with COPD who develops community-acquired pneumonia with resultant exacerbation of the COPD; and 2) any patient with DM and acute illness will have elevated blood sugar, which is frequently difficult to control. So, just as with concept mapping theory, we need to consider and see the bigger picture so that we are providing complete care at a high standard.

To summarize, every patient situation is different and each type of action described in this section may be utilized and employed in various ways, sometimes for the same patient. The important thing is that each problem or concern is addressed with actions and that actions follow through to desired outcomes. **Figure 7-37** also summarizes this discussion.

Another word about actions: In most cases we have been speaking about nonurgent actions based upon the assertion that the patient is stable. For any patient who is developing active problems and acute decompensation, emergent, urgent actions would be required. This would include initiating a code blue or rapid-response team notification.

Figure 7-37 **Problems and outcomes.**

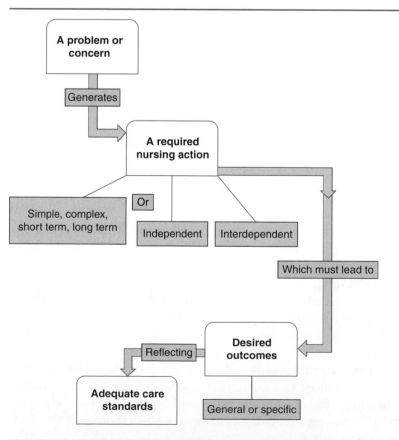

Living Concept Maps

Living concept maps focused on nursing actions can become rather large and involved. While an expansive map of this type may not be suitable for beginning students, it could be used to emphasize application for students in the latter part of the first year and definitely in the second year. Guidelines would have to be set and limitations agreed to before instituting this process so as not to overwhelm students.

To better illustrate what we have been discussing, let's pull everything together and construct a concept map based on nursing actions by using the following scenario:

You are caring for a 65-year-old male admitted with pneumonia. He lives at home with his wife and has been under the care of a physician for COPD, HTN, and DM type 1 for the past 4 years. His medications include regular onsulin according to a sliding scale, lisinopril 10 mg daily, Advair (fluticasone and salmeterol) 250/50 2 puffs daily. He was feeling well and in his usual state of health until 5 days prior to admission when he developed a frequent cough productive for thick white sputum, a slight fever, and slight burning in his chest. As the next few days passed, he began to feel worse, coughed more frequently, and expectorated thick green sputum. His fever rose and he was unable to eat adequately because of frequent coughing. He called his primary care physician who admitted him. The patient is complaining of chest wall pain secondary to coughing. Other pertinent data include:

- Oxygen is in place at 2 L via nasal cannula and an oxygen saturation of 92%
- Blood pressure 156/90
- Heart rate 98
- Respirations 24
- Noted dyspnea with mild exertion
- Chest x-ray (CXR) indicates bilateral lower lobe pneumonia
- Abnormal laboratory levels: potassium 3.3 mEq, fasting glucose 240 mg/dL

Additional orders include:

- Oxygen titration to maintain saturation greater than or equal to 90%
- Sliding scale insulin orders
- Lisinopril
- Advair
- Kdur 20 mEq orally single dose now
- Repeat potassium level in 4 hours
- Prednisone 20 mg orally daily
- Ceftriaxone (Rocephin) 1 g IV daily
- Acetaminophen 650 mg orally every 4 hours PRN pain/fever
- Daily CXR every morning for 3 days
- Bed rest
- 50-g carbohydrate diet
- Out of bed with assistance

- Large volume IV NSS 100 mL/hour, begun after peripherally inserted central catheter (PICC) line placed
- Teds and SCDs when in bed
- Telemetry

All of this patient-related information provides us with a problem list that would look like the following table.

Primary Problems (Main Concepts)	Secondary Problems (Related Concepts)
COPD exacerbation Pneumonia	Dyspnea Need for oxygen Tachypnea Cough productive for sputum Activity intolerance Need for steroids Poor appetite Need for frequent CXR
Hypertension	BP not controlled
Pain	Tachycardia Inadequate chest expansion
Diabetes Steroids	Uncontrolled blood sugars
Fever	Need for IV fluids Possible mild dehydration
Hypokalemia	Need for potassium repletion
Potential for bed rest complications	Need for Teds and SCDs
Potential for further infection secondary (2nd) to . . .	Infectious process and invasive line

Let's Debrief

Wow! We really need to debrief after that one. Using a case study or scenario is so valuable in this type of learning. Many times the diagnoses and actions are common, and students can relate to and recognize them. Within the learning continuum, this also provides additional exposure and opportunities to link ideas for progressive learning. As we have already learned, that process signifies meaningful learning, including comprehension and application.

First, let's start by thinking back to the steps used in formulating a concept map. In the previous example (see **Figure 7-38**), we have taken the facts about our patient and

Figure 7-38 A complex, living concept map.

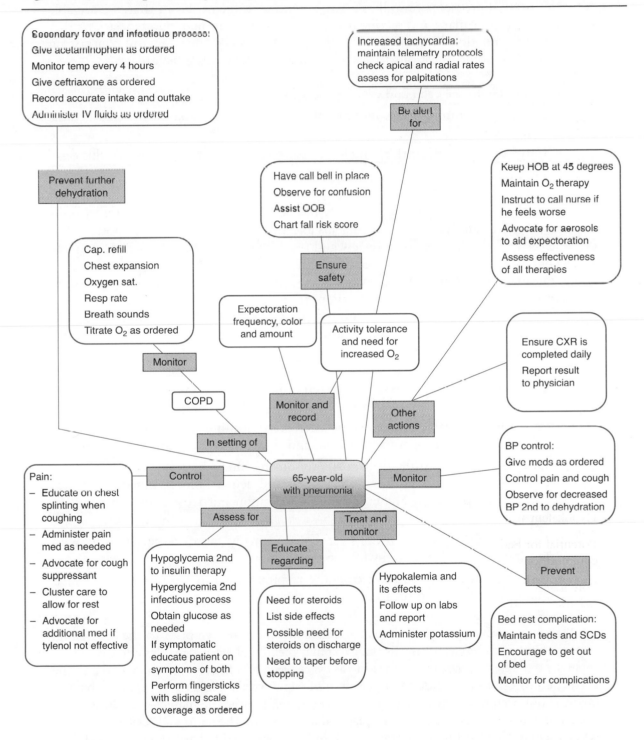

created a problem list. Reviewing the admitting diagnosis and PMH allows us to see the active and actual problems as well as a few potential problems. From that, we are able to create a list of primary and secondary problems and begin making associations that lead us to true relationship analysis. Within this process is comparing and contrasting of information. Some questions to ask yourself as you review the list are:

- Am I able to see each and every association?
- If I had a scrambled list, would I be able to successfully make all the connections that exist?
- Can I see how critical thinking is necessary to arrive at the correct conclusions?
- Do I need further review of concept mapping theory?

This is the start of everything, and it should be clear that a sound knowledge base is necessary to successfully recognize problems and their connections to one another. It is often necessary to complete some review and research with your textbooks. As you can see, a concept map of this type goes way beyond simple knowledge. Application is where you are headed, and your thought processes must be utilized effectively to achieve that. As mentioned earlier, connections are so important because focusing in on and studying them allows common patterns concerning actions to emerge. This is another valuable part of active, comprehensive learning leading to application. Let's look a little deeper at the connections. Test yourself as we go.

- COPD is a chronic illness characterized by ineffective air exchange and shortness of breath (SOB).
- Any other respiratory illness can exacerbate it, leading to increased symptoms, altered quality of life, hospitalization, and the need for antibiotics and steroids.
- Diabetic control is difficult to maintain during illness because cortisol and catecholamine release increases system stress and demands more glucose. Steroids add to this problem. Hyperglycemia is common but treatment can result in hypoglycemia.
- Dehydration can result from fever. This normally causes hypernatremia with resultant hypokalemia. Rehydration usually normalizes electrolyte levels.
- Pain is contributing to the worsening respiratory status because the patient is unable to take a deep breath.

Please remember if you have been creating a map of your own prior to the debriefing, it may look very different from this one. You may recall that learning styles and brain processing vary. The format can vary as long as every piece of information is included and the correct connections are made. A larger piece of paper would allow us to expand a bit and separate out each problem and some of the actions. Examine the map closely. Each component of a map is present and has its place. Shapes contain the main and related concepts, text boxes contain the linking phrases, and slight color variation has been used for definition. Expanding the map would most likely necessitate using a key to explain the map, especially if separate shapes were used to define the problem separate from the actions.

The descriptive phrases chosen indicate that a nursing action is needed. Some of the phrases speak to the type of action needed. Here is a summary of the phrases:

- "Prevent" refers to ongoing nursing actions employed with an active problem that does not have immediate resolution
- "Control," "assess," and "be alert for" are phrases that refer to ongoing problems classified as actual and potential
- "Education" and "safety" are common themes throughout the map
- "Treat" and "monitor" also indicate ongoing, collaborative nursing actions

The nursing process is clearly evidenced, as it must be, because it is a necessary process guiding all care. Let's examine each part of this valuable process.

Assessment

For each problem or area of concern, there is a statement of assessments necessary. Some are general and others are focused. Assessment skills must improve along with critical thinking for effective and adequate care provision.

Diagnosis

Nursing diagnoses formulated from patient problems are a necessary part of care as they help us to recognize actions leading to outcomes. Examples of nursing diagnoses in this case would be:

- Ineffective air exchange secondary to COPD exacerbation as evidenced by the presence of pneumonia on CXR, dyspnea, activity intolerance, and the need for oxygen therapy
- Risk for significant dehydration and hypovolemia secondary to fever and infectious process as manifested by hyperthermia and need for acetaminophen, antibiotics, and rehydration
- Hyperglycemia secondary to DM and acute illness requiring steroids as evidenced by a blood glucose of 240 and the need for sliding scale coverage
- Risk for potential hypoglycemia related to insulin coverage
- Uncontrolled blood pressure as manifested by HTN and the need for medication therapy
- Activity intolerance secondary to acute illness and pain as manifested by dyspnea, fever, and chest wall discomfort

Planning

Indications of ongoing nursing actions related to patient problems demonstrate the planning phase.

Implementation

Space limitations may make it seem as if this phase has not been properly addressed. There actually is evidence that implementation will be carried out in the mention of fingersticks and ongoing monitoring. In an actual patient case, you would list actual actions and their outcomes.

Evaluation

Evaluation is addressed when it is stated that an assessment will occur to ensure that treatments are effective.

There is strong integration with laboratory and diagnostic testing within the problem list and as part of the nursing actions. This is another necessary step to include in care and which becomes easier as critical thinking develops and expands in depth. Abnormal laboratory tests lead to symptomatology, which necessitates actions, monitoring, and reporting. The nursing knowledge base must include that of normal laboratory values and coexisting symptoms necessitating assessments. Diagnostic testing results may lead to further procedures or additional testing and so are part of collaborative care and interdependent nursing actions.

Holism could easily be included as we recognize the patient's mental status, religious needs, family involvement in education, or cultural needs.

Nursing actions reflect the various types discussed earlier. Let's review each for reflection and analysis.

> • Capillary refill • Chest expansion • Oxygen saturation
> • Respiratory rate • Breath sounds • Titrate O_2 as ordered

These are independent, long-term, complex actions. Although each one in and of itself seems fairly simple, this patient is at risk for deterioration because pneumonia will complicate his COPD. All of these actions are ongoing and will occur throughout the patient's hospital stay. As each assessment is performed, comparison and contrast occur between the patient-based findings and normal findings. Choosing these actions indicates that critical thinking is occurring. A change detected in these assessments for the worse shows progression of the infectious process and the patient's deterioration.

> Expectoration frequency, color, and amount

Choosing these actions indicates critical thinking and consideration of outcomes. If the ceftriaxone is effective and the correct medicine for the organism involved, then the patient's cough should diminish fairly quickly in frequency and severity, expectoration should cease, and fever should subside. Any remaining cough or expectoration would indicate the patient has returned to his baseline state of health. Nonresolution signifies that another medication may be more effective. Alerting the physician to this finding would be an interdependent action. Otherwise, these actions mirror those above because they require multiple, ongoing assessments.

> Activity tolerance and need for increased O_2

We often take the need for oxygen therapy for granted, but not everyone walks around with oxygen on. So, the need for it is a problem or concern and requires nursing actions. Oxygen therapy may be short or long term. Many patients use it in the home. In addition, in many cases oxygen is ordered as needed for a certain oxygen saturation maintenance level. Thus, this is an interdependent action because it requires physician collaboration. Please recognize that any type of respiratory therapy–related order also alerts the respiratory therapist who then becomes our collaborator as well.

> • Keep head of bed at 45 degrees • Maintain O_2 therapy • Instruct to call nurse if patient feels worse • Advocate for aerosols to aid expectoration • Assess effectiveness of all therapies

This action grouping is both independent and interdependent. The first three are independent and help to ensure effective oxygenation and air exchange. The last two are interdependent in that collaboration with both the physician and respiratory therapy personnel may be necessary. If the patient is weakened to the point that airway clearance becomes difficult, aerosol therapy with a bronchodilator and expectorant would be in order.

> • Ensure CXR is completed daily • Report result to physician

Following up on order completion is an interdependent action and part of our standard of care. Other than sending the patient off the unit for the test and seeing that he returns, most facilities require the radiology technologist to sign a form or initial that the test has been completed. If there is some reason that prohibited this from happening, the physician must be made aware. This is a relatively simple, short-term nursing action.

> • Have call bell in place • Observe for confusion
> • Assist out of bed • Chart fall risk score

Safety surfaces in almost every nursing action in some way. A patient with COPD complicated by pneumonia usually has some degree of altered perfusion and may easily become confused. With any active confusion noted, a bed alarm would be added, along with frequent observation and even restraints or a sitter. Although this may be more of a potential problem at this point, it is highly likely to occur. So, at this point we could say that this problem is simple and short term but could easily transition to a complex, long-term one as additional actions are required.

> Increased tachycardia:
> • Maintain telemetry protocols • Check apical and radial rates
> • Assess for palpitations

Telemetry and the protocols accompanying it make this a complex, long-term, interdependent action. Monitoring is initiated and maintained with a physician order, and part of nursing's responsibility is to run and interpret rhythm strips and be alert for arrhythmias.

The tachycardia here may have causes rooted in dehydration and hypovolemia, as well as anxiety and mild respiratory distress.

> **2nd fever and infectious process:**
> • Give acetaminophen as ordered • Monitor temperature every 4 hours • Give ceftriaxone as ordered • Record accurate intake and outtake • Administer IV fluids as ordered

These actions have relationships with the symptoms of fever and dehydration. They are all interdependent, as well as complex and long term. All of them will need to be followed through on until the patient improves and symptoms are resolving.

> **Blood pressure control:**
> • Give meds as ordered • Control pain and cough • Observe for decreased blood pressure secondary to dehydration

Any time the patient has a PMH (which is almost every single patient), the nurse must be aware of it. That is the simplest action there is related to the PMH. The other component to look at is how that particular PMH either affects or is affected by the current disease process. This is critical thinking and relationship analysis. Always, always address these on the concept map. If the blood pressure were stable, you would state actions such as: "Administer the antihypertensive and assess medication effectiveness." Because the blood pressure is elevated in this case, we need to include more frequent monitoring and physician notification if the BP control is lost with current therapy. As far as comparison and contrast are concerned, we are always looking at balance. If we have elevated blood pressure, it stands to reason that treatment in the setting of dehydration may lead to hypotension. This would be an undesired outcome because it threatens safety and must be addressed. This is the yin and yang of our profession.

> **Pain:**
> • Educate on chest splinting when coughing • Administer pain med as needed • Advocate for cough suppressant • Cluster care to allow for rest • Advocate for additional med if acetaminophen not effective

Pain is always a symptom necessitating ongoing monitoring. Rarely do we achieve pain control with only one dose of a medication or via one alternative method. Nursing actions related to pain assessment, monitoring, and control lead to long-term, complex actions. Another important action is to determine whether or not the medication and dose ordered are adequate to address the pain. Advocacy plays a major role in this situation. If physician collaboration is required, please have all the facts. These would include the pain rating both before and after medication administration, the patient allergy history, any medication intolerances, and objective data.

> • Hypoglycemia secondary to insulin therapy • Hyperglycemia secondary infectious process • Obtain glucose as needed if symptomatic • Educate patient on symptoms of both • Perform glucose fingersticks with sliding scale coverage as ordered

Despite what is commonly stated regarding assumptions, a nurse can always assume that any diabetic who is ill will experience hyperglycemia. In contrast, and looking at that balance idea again, hypoglycemia frequently results with treatments and as the disease process and symptoms evolve. Education is an action integral to the entire treatment process. Not all diabetics need insulin as outpatients, yet within the acute care setting it is utilized more often than not with acute illness of the diabetic patient. So, education addresses the patient's fears about remaining on insulin indefinitely as well as providing us with educational opportunities regarding DM management. It also serves to remind us that the PMH always plays a role in nursing actions.

> • Need for steroids • Side effects • Possible need for steroids on discharge • Need to taper before stopping

The need for steroids is clear, given the patient's condition and degree of exacerbation. You now need to recognize the impact of steroid administration on the patient's blood glucose. In addition, there is a great impact on educational needs related to both acute and chronic steroid use. While the patient is under your care, you will be assessing for elevated glucose levels and the symptoms of hyperglycemia. When the patient is discharged, however, he and his family members will need in-depth education regarding this, plus information regarding the side effects of steroids. The other important consideration is education regarding the dangers of stopping the medication without physician collaboration and tapering.

The method used for breaking down and interpreting specific areas of a concept map is what you should use as well. Completing that process allows you to meaningfully reflect on your critical thinking skills. It enables the question-and-answer process so important in assessing critical thinking abilities. Examples of reflective questions are:

- How does this fact affect or help me decide my nursing actions?
- What are all the connections this piece of information has in this patient situation?
- How does this particular identified problem translate into an action?
- What are all the actions that need to result from this particular problem and why?

The reflective process involves questioning as much as it involves thought and reasoning.

Focus

Please keep in mind that a concept map may intentionally be very simple or complex, depending on the purpose and focus. A certain area of focus may be assigned to empha-size one piece of information or information links. The possibilities are truly endless and adaptable to a wide variety of circumstances and learning objectives. Using various foci to construct concept maps enables both microscopic and macroscopic analysis of thought processes, reasoning related to actions, relationship analysis, and overall critical thinking ability reflection. What this means is that detail and specificity can be added to learning. Not only does this benefit varied learning styles, but it also promotes use of and intro-spection into those styles.

This process is also integral to using and reinforcing theory related to thought pro-cessing. Taking a thought and seeing it placed on paper will always provide insight into how you look at a problem, how you determine and identify patient problems, and finally how you address problem resolution.

Focusing on various aspects of a concept map also serves to reinforce and review the nursing process. Because outcomes are part of this, use of focused concept maps stresses the importance of outcomes and problem resolution.

Of course, all of these things promote critical thinking growth, self-confidence, and readiness to fulfill the graduate nurse role. The areas of focus we consider in this section have been addressed in some fashion already. Now, however, we will take a more in-depth and detailed look into them. These areas are:

- Disease processes
- Procedures and skills
- Nursing actions
- Medications
- Laboratory and diagnostic tests
- Collaborative care
- Documentation
- Legal and ethical concerns
- Evidence-Based Practice

Keep in mind that a detailed focus is only one option for any of the areas listed. Generalized concept maps still have advantages. Both types lend themselves to use for static and living concept maps.

Disease Processes

Choosing to construct a concept map with a focus on disease processes presents many possibilities for studying and learning. Because the goal is enhanced critical thinking abilities and a greater awareness of how concepts connect and interrelate, the possibilities are truly endless. Some possible topics for more detailed, focused concept maps related to diseases are:

- Symptoms secondary to a disease process linked with the exact pathophysiology producing them
- Contrast between the systemic and localized effects of a disease
- The abnormal laboratory values resulting from a disease state and their causes

Ideas for use of a more macroscopic viewpoint could include:

- Showing the pathway of a disease process throughout the body
- Describing overall nursing actions related to nursing care of a specific disease
- Collaborative care related to a certain disease

These are just a few examples, and as we proceed, you may think of many more. Many times you will find that the current theory you are learning as well as clinical experiences will help to guide your thinking regarding the sort of concept maps that are helpful. Of course, this process is also guided by assignments you will be given as well. Looking at some examples will assist you in developing other ideas.

The map in **Figure 7-39** can be noted as a static map because it is strong on information and facts. It is true that nursing actions are implied but they are not specifically noted. It is detailed and demonstrates some baseline knowledge related to these biomarkers as they relate to acute myocardial infarction (AMI).

More detail could be added regarding specific peak times, specimen collection, frequency, and any other factors related to obtaining, monitoring, and reporting abnormal values (see **Figure 7-40**).

This concept map is much more visual than most of our other examples. Whether your learning style is strongly visual or not, memory cues of many types may be combined with concept maps to prompt you to make associations and see interrelationships for stronger critical thinking skills. Another variation would be to add notes to the side of shapes containing related concepts as a way of stimulating thought processes. *As a general rule, these notes should be incorporated into the style of the concept map; meaning they should be contained within shapes and descriptive phrases, and lines should be used to connect them to the rest of the concept map.* **Figure 7-41** demonstrates such a map.

Procedures and Skills

Outlining the steps for procedures and skills within a concept map is an effective way to think through steps and to associate rationales. At the same time, mental connections are being made between the specific procedure or skill and the equipment needed. More complex concept maps may include troubleshooting steps to follow for the particular equipment used, such as an IV pump.

Figure 7-39 **Disease processes concept map #1: Detailed and static.**

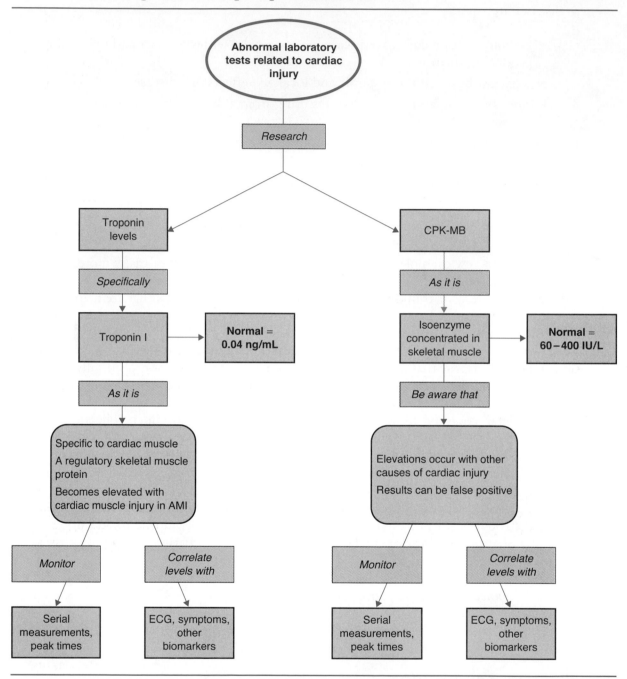

Figure 7-40 Disease processes concept map #2: Detailed static.

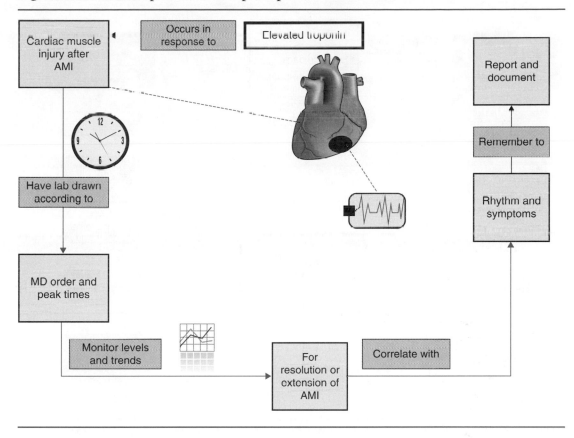

Simplified concept maps may contain only each step in the progression from beginning to completing a nursing skill. Often what is emphasized is the core skill being focused on. Although the rationale is not usually omitted, secondary related concepts often are. For example, if the focus of an assigned concept map is a wound redressing, a more simplified concept map may include the following:

- Supplies and their assembly prior to proceeding
- Specific steps to remove and dispose of the old dressing
- Necessary steps and observations in cleansing the wound
- Factors to consider prior to redressing such as wound measurement, surrounding skin assessment, and drainage type
- Specific steps for replacing and securing the new dressing
- Possible alternate steps if the traditional dressing is not able to be applied (tape allergy, anatomical challenges, etc.)

Figure 7-41 Disease processes concept map #3: Detailed static.

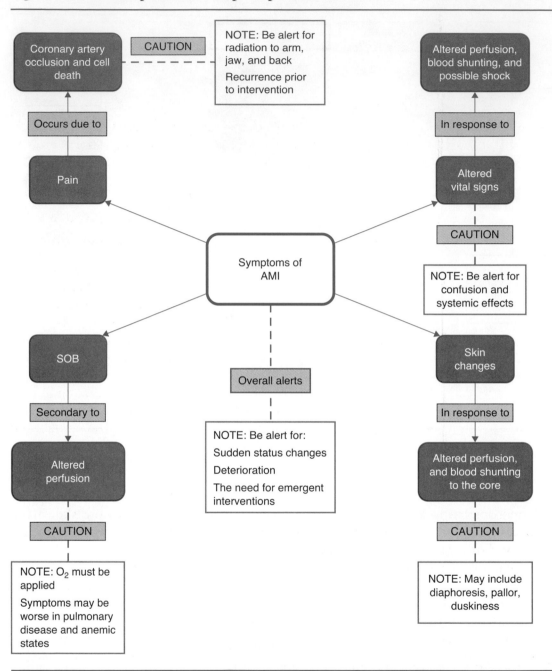

If you remember your most recent nursing skills lab, you will recall that this is how you were taught to proceed and tested according to these steps or similar ones. Normally, the progression used is from simple to complex skills and considers concepts such as readiness and scope of practice based on a learning phase within the education continuum.

In contrast, more complex concept maps can enhance the skill or procedure by asking you to include things such as:

- Defining and classifying the type of dressing to be used by purpose
- Aligning the wound type, placement, and stage with the prescribed treatment plan
- Documentation criteria
- Pre-skill or pre-procedure care considerations such as administering pain medication, checking the physician order, collaboration with the wound care team, and obtaining help to properly position the patient.

This is a wonderful feature of concept maps because they will grow along with you. You can save all of your concept maps and add to them as you progress through your nursing courses. Seeing the positive progression you have made is always stimulating and builds self-confidence!

Figure 7-42 contains a detailed, complex static concept map related to pressure ulcers. If we decided to base this concept map on an actual patient, we could easily convert it to a living concept map by adding specific patient data related to laboratory values, wound descriptions, and so on.

The concept map in **Figure 7-43** takes a simple skill and incorporates the theory and rationales behind it, including the nursing process and nursing care standards. For every skill you are approved to perform, you must know not only the proper steps and procedure to follow, and the correct equipment, but also what the expected and unexpected outcomes are. Expected outcomes are those in which the procedure or skill is completed in a timely manner, correctly and appropriately, and smoothly. Unexpected outcomes can range from inability to complete the task because of equipment failure or patient intolerance, to abnormal findings that need to be addressed before proceeding and completing the task. It becomes extremely important to include these anticipatory events into your planning. **Figure 7-44** highlights some possible unexpected occurrences along with possible solutions. Anticipating in this way not only saves time and enhances problem-solving abilities related to time management but also helps to ensure accuracy by using properly working equipment.

Any unexpected outcome, whether it is related to the procedure completion, something that occurred during the procedure to interrupt it, or an unexpected result, must be addressed immediately. Some problem-solving steps are very simple and some require several actions, including ongoing monitoring and reassessment. Anticipating these possible interruptions and considering the actions and solutions related to them contribute to managing time. This is a valuable skill to set goals for as you progress to readiness as a graduate nurse. Patients with multiple complex problems and having multiple patient assignments mean that your time management must be well honed. Time management affects safety, organization, and prioritization in terms of nursing actions and planning care. The plan of care you start your day with may change dramatically throughout the day. Anticipatory skills do not solely apply to each specific skill but also to the entire plan and all nursing actions (see Figure 7-44).

Figure 7-42 Procedures and skills concept map #1: Detailed static.

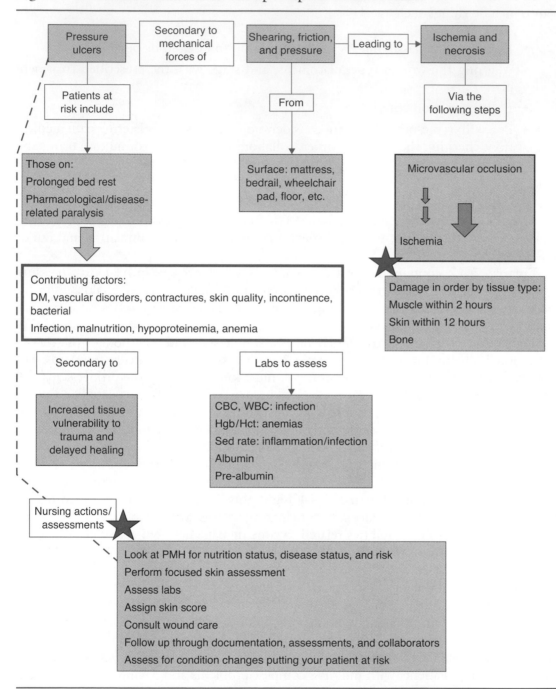

Figure 7-43 Procedures and skills concept map #2: Detailed static.

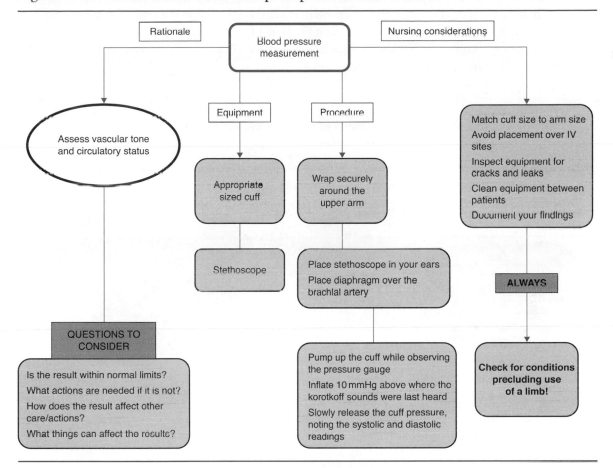

Figure 7-44 Unexpected outcomes and action to address them.

Unexpected Outcome	Possible Solutions/Interventions and Actions
Equipment Failure	Check alarm, restart the pump, replace the pump
Malfunction of IV pump	Inspect for cracks and loose connections, use another cuff
BP cuff holds no pressure	
Patient Pain Status Affects Completion	Assess and address pain prior to proceeding and offer emotional support
Patient Status Prevents Completion	Stop the procedure and assess responsiveness and ABCs
General status changes	
Mental status changes	Fully explain procedures and obtain assistance
Uncooperativeness	Reevaluate the need for the procedure and notify the co-assigned nurse
Abnormal Findings Relative to Previous Ones	Reassess, obtain new measurements, cover, and notify the co-assigned nurse
Wound is worse than previously documented	Reposition the cuff and repeat the measurement, assess for symptoms, and notify the co-assigned nurse
BP is greatly different compared to earlier readings	

Next we will take a look at a concept map generally focused on a patient assessment (see **Figure 7-45**). This concept map makes a huge statement regarding nursing care. It encompasses all we need to think about when planning care while considering the nursing process and collaboration. Again, conversion to a living concept map could be easily accomplished if an actual patient or case study was used.

Figure 7-45 **Procedures and skills concept map #3: Generalized static.**

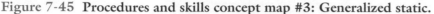

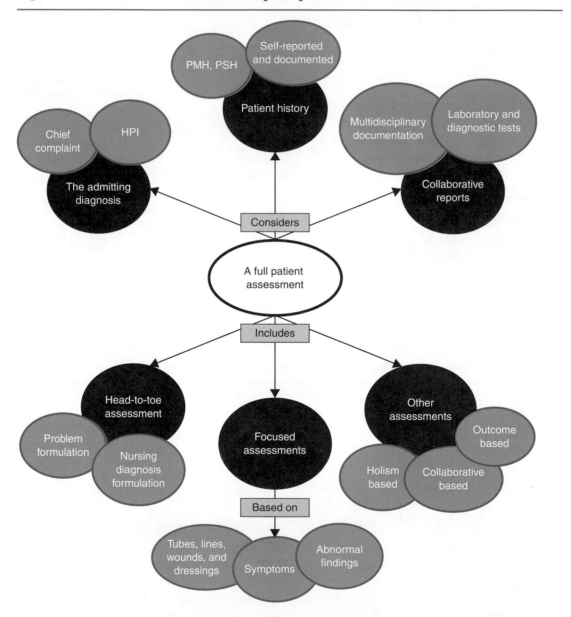

Let's do just that by using the following scenario:

You are caring for K.N., a 55-year-old female admitted with pneumonia and exacerbation of multiple sclerosis (MS). The patient had been at her baseline health level until 3 days ago when she began with upper respiratory infection symptoms that quickly progressed to her lower lungs. She was taken to see her family physician when she was no longer able to get out of bed. K.N. was immediately admitted. There is no other PMH. Data obtained from the physical assessment yield the following findings:

- Vital signs: BP 120.66, P 66, R 28, Temperature 101.8°F orally
- Generalized weakness: K.N. is barely able to move independently in bed, complains of SOB
- Mental status: alert and oriented
- Lungs: rhonchi and inspiratory wheezing auscultated throughout all lung fields
- Skin: hot and dry
- Abdomen: soft, round, and nontender; slightly hypoactive bowel sounds times 4
- Extremities within normal limits
- Slightly reddened sacrum
- Two IV sites: one as a heparin trap and one with D5 ½ NS at 100 mL/hour
- CXR results demonstrating bilateral lower lobe pneumonia
- Laboratory test results: elevated white blood cells (WBCs), decreased albumin (all other tests within normal limits)
- The patient's concerned husband states that K.N. normally needs a walker to get around, no longer drives, but is able to cook some meals and manage most ADLs, except for the past few days
- K.N. sees a specialist for her MS management and is currently taking immune modulators and steroids

Now we can take each section and add specific patient information. Any information not already provided will be added as we progress (see **Figures 7-46** through **7-50**).

Well, that was certainly quite a bit of work! Did you take note of the common threads throughout all of the concept maps? Look back over the examples and identify all of the components of concept mapping theory. Associations and critical thinking are clearly evident. When you receive a patient assignment, you never know exactly what to expect. There is a great deal of patient information that needs to be considered for formulating nursing actions and the plan of care. Monitoring for this information is an ongoing process during which much more may be discovered and will need to be addressed. While we may use the term *static* to refer to some of our concept map examples, in reality the process of caring for patients is never static.

The preceding concept map examples reinforce the need for awareness of learning styles but also show how we can break apart a concept map and still learn about the relationships we will find. We have also seen how large concept maps can become. Clarity and all of the other essential components we have previously addressed are important in every single concept map you create.

Figure 7-46 Using a step-wide approach to create a living concept map: Identifying problems.

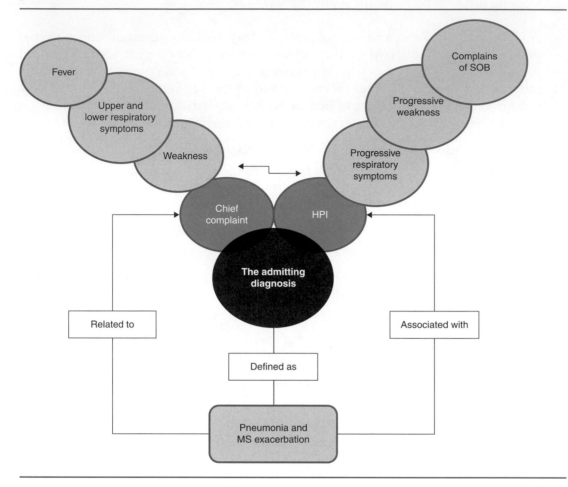

Figure 7-47 Using a step-wide approach to create a living concept map: Collecting subjective and objective information.

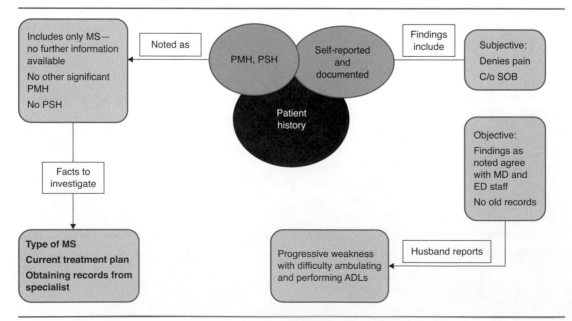

Figure 7-48 Using a step-wise approach to create a living concept map: Recongnizing collaborative concerns.

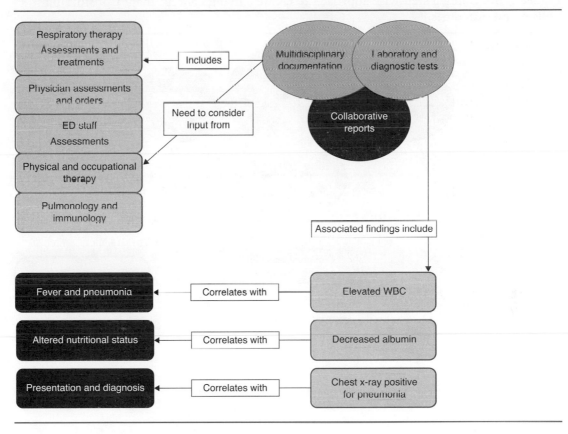

Figure 7-49 Using a step-wide approach to create a living concept map: Recognizing the need for focused assessments.

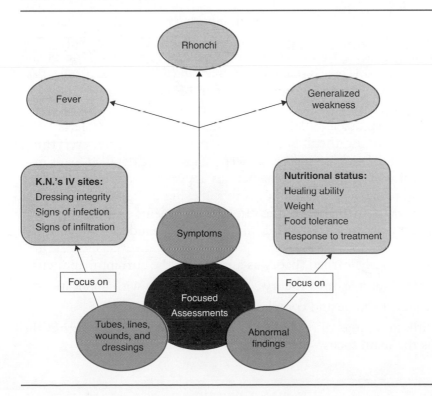

Figure 7-50 Using a step-wise approach to create a living concept map: Considering holism and outcomes.

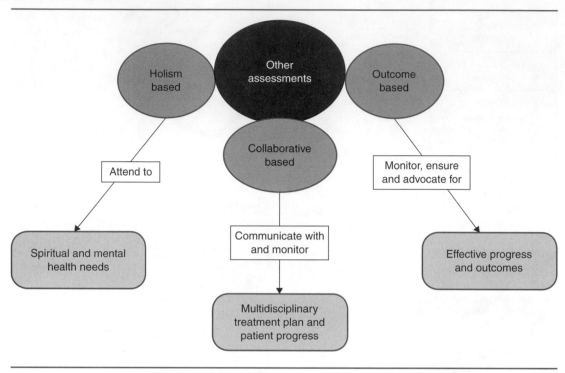

Nursing Actions

The next category used as a focus is nursing actions. We can specify a focus of nursing actions related to one problem or situation or focus on many related to a patient situation such as in the case studies used earlier. Although it is always helpful to understand all nursing actions in terms of rationales based on their linkage to theory, it is sometimes helpful within the learning process to analyze them in smaller segments. One of the points emphasized throughout this text is that concept mapping allows for self-reflection of critical thinking abilities and growth progression of those skills as your education progresses. At times, analysis and review of the smaller segments is the starting point for that reflection, because each step taken initially leads to the other nursing actions and the thought processes used in planning them. So, much like pieces of a puzzle, everything fits together to form the whole. Looking at some concept maps with a detailed focus may help you to understand this better. Also, nursing actions appear in all concept maps in some form or another and so become a prime focus in achieving competency in critical thinking abilities. As a review, remember that the various components analyzed within a completed concept map for assessment of critical thinking skills include:

- Recognition of previously learned theory as it relates to the current map focus
- Recognition of previously learned theory and its connection with application
- The ability to connect simple and complex ideas and concepts
- The ability to link groupings of related concepts to each component within the group as well as the main focus

- Recognition of how nursing care standards and the nursing process are utilized in and impact concept map content

Figure 7-51 illustrates the entire process. One other concept represented within the figure is that of cause and effect. An integral part of growth, whether in knowledge or critical thinking, is the ability to recognize how an action impacts future actions. For that to be recognized, critical thinking must be involved because relationship analysis and anticipation enable that process. The concept map examples that follow can assist you in understanding how to pull everything together.

A mini scenario for the first example in this category is as follows: Your patient has fallen and sustained a fractured right wrist. A cast is in place. Your assignment is to detail the assessment for this patient related to the main problem of the fracture site (see Figure 7-52).

This map demonstrates use of prior knowledge related to fracture care with more advanced knowledge regarding a possible complication of compartment syndrome. Theoretical knowledge of care standards is evident in recognizing the need for fasciotomy. The actions and content display critical thinking skills and relationship analysis. Simple and complex actions have been included and account for a thorough assessment that includes the nursing process, an implied ability to adjust the plan of care if necessary, and outcome consideration. Using this system for self-evaluation of concept map content, along with the checklists, will ensure that you include what is needed and at the same time reinforce learning and enhance critical thinking skills through relationship analysis.

Figure 7-51 Concept mapping summary.

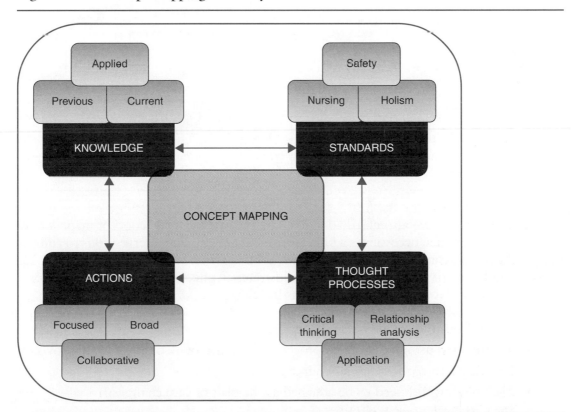

Figure 7-52 Nursing action concept map #1: Living and detailed.

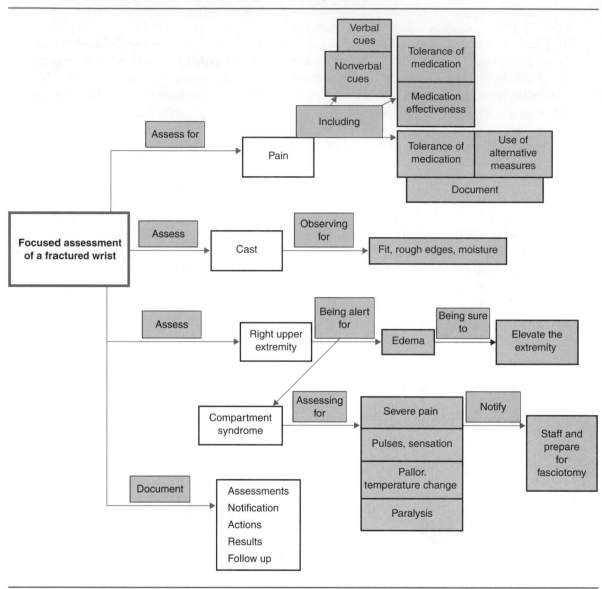

Cause and effect are also clearly demonstrated throughout the concept map. A fracture causes pain, which necessitates a pain assessment and nursing interventions to address it. In addition, outcomes have been addressed, both in terms of patient comfort as well as action completion via documentation. This illustrates an effective way to think of actions. Actions can be viewed from many angles in that they:

- Result from thought processes
- Are initiated using the nursing process to account for all phases of care provision
- Have a starting point and an endpoint
- Are ongoing and need to be adjusted as the plan of care changes
- Necessitate documentation

It is important to consider what types of things may alter the plan of care and necessitate changes in our actions and interventions. These events can occur frequently or infrequently, depending upon practice setting and patient focus. Basically you need to be constantly evaluating the plan of care as you proceed throughout your clinical day and always anticipate changes and unexpected events. A plan of care rarely remains unchanged because it is affected and impacted by so many factors. Skills such as anticipation, organization, and prioritization assist you with dealing with these changes and alterations in the plan of care.

Possible changes to the plan of care may result from:

- A complex status change resulting in the need for a rapid response or code team
- Care changes occurring post-procedure when frequent vital signs and other monitoring are required
- A less complex status change where more intense monitoring is indicated
- A patient transfer or discharge
- New care team collaborators impacting treatments and outcomes
- Patient assignment changes

All of the items listed here will lead to a deviation from the set plan of care. The first three examples can occur frequently. In these cases, possible nursing action changes include providing more focused care through frequent assessment, monitoring, and vital sign measurements; frequent documentation and notification of the physician; and refined organization to meet all of the patient's needs. In the student role, you may not be speaking with the physician personally but need to be aware of that collaboration.

Transferring a patient requires nursing actions involving education, documentation, and coordination with other staff as well as the patient's family. Usually these events occur quickly and must also be carried out quickly.

Care team collaboration may mean new physician consultants adding orders resulting in nursing actions. It may also mean other disciplines have been asked to provide care so that our actions combine with theirs. In any case, the original plan has been altered.

Patient assignment changes can occur without warning at times. Some situations warrant transferring patients off of your unit to allow room for incoming patients. So, the plan of care you thought you had ends abruptly and a new one begins. All of these things require adaptability and nursing action alteration.

Consider the following scenario:

M.M. is a 78-year-old female admitted with new possible TIA. When obtaining her vital signs this morning, you find her blood pressure to be 88/50 and her heart rate to be 162. Since admission, her other blood pressures have been 120–130/65–74 (see **Figure 7-53**).

This map is an illustration of comparing and contrasting a current event with the main diagnosis as well as the PMH. It reinforces how no occurrence is static and that one thing is always affecting or being affected by something else. With more available space, we could explore advocacy through holding any antihypertensive medications and address any other medications impacting the current event. This example also demonstrates cause and effect.

Figure 7-53 Nursing action concept map #2: Detailed living.

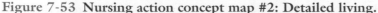

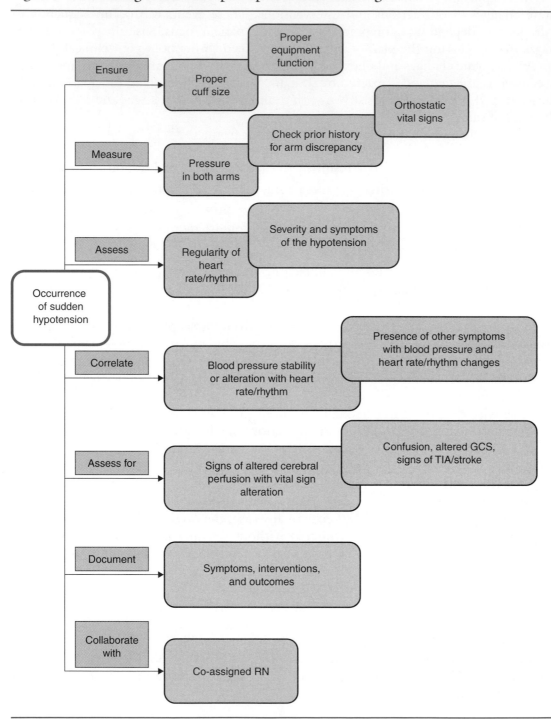

GCS = Glasgow Coma Scale

You may also notice that some of the recent concept map examples are more linear. If you prefer to "see" your mental processing in a timeline type of format, this formatting option may appeal to you. This is not to say that nonlinear formatting does not allow you to see starting and endpoints for thought processes and actions. You need to be aware of your mental processing style or method and then tailor your concept map formatting to it.

So, we have seen that concept maps with a focus on nursing actions do not solely demonstrate nursing actions. They also demonstrate the thought processes and nursing standards leading to the formulation of those actions.

Consider the following scenario for the next concept map:

J.F. is returning to your unit after receiving a PICC line in the interventional radiology department. You receive a report that J.F. has received 5 mg of midazolam (Versed) IV push during the procedure. He tolerated the procedure well and the line was inserted without problems. The dressing is dry and intact. The patient has been recovered and is now awake, alert, and oriented. When he arrives on your unit, J.F. is slightly drowsy but oriented and cooperative (see **Figure 7-54**).

This concept map incorporates safety through care of the line as well as mental status assessment. If the patient was found to be confused, additional safety measures

Figure 7-54 Nursing action concept map #3: Detailed living.

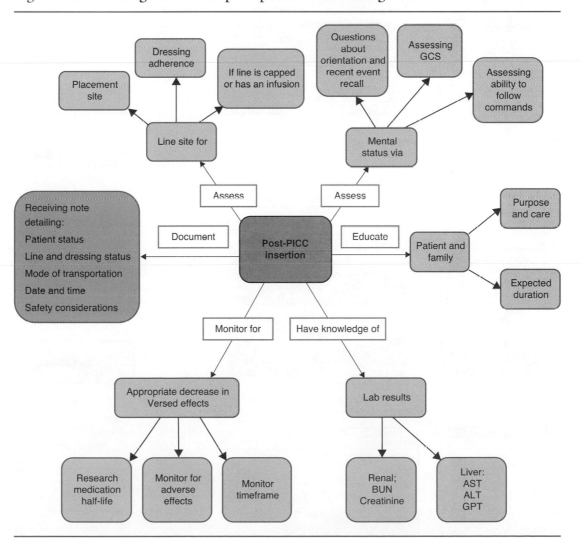

BUN = blood urea nitrogen; AST = aspartate transaminase; ALT = alanine transaminase; GST = glutamate pyruvate transaminase.

would need to be added to protect the line and ensure patient safety until the medication effects are no longer a concern. Theory related to these nursing actions originates from medication knowledge and pharmacodynamics, safe care practice standards, and PICC line–related theory. Most concept maps draw on vast amounts of integrated theory to formulate nursing actions and enact critical thinking.

The previous example is one in which prioritization can be introduced. Although you may normally think through your actions in some sort of order, chances are you have never written them down. Prioritizing steps using a concept mapping format will allow you to make associations with the order of your actions and patient needs. In this way you

Figure 7-55 Nursing action concept map #4: Detailed static.

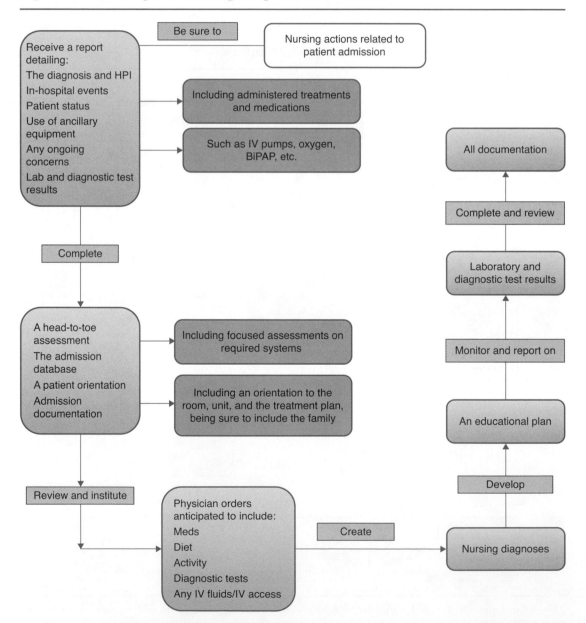

are applying nursing knowledge along with how it is best applied. Strong prioritization skills will lead to improved organizational ones, which will only serve to enhance your nursing practice. In thinking about nursing skills, it may seem fairly easy to prioritize from a general standpoint. These steps are fairly straightforward and usually include reviewing the skills, assembling the supplies, completing the skill, and then assessing patient outcomes and documenting.

When it comes to prioritizing nursing actions related to overall care, this process may seem to be more difficult because of the great number of variables and factors to consider. These considerations may include:

- Changes to the plan of care
- Unfamiliarity with the procedure or task at hand
- Inexperience plus lack of confidence
- Unexpected patient responses and problems
- Limited preparation time
- Difficulty with multitasking skills

What I am referring to here is that the picture you have in your mind of how the day should proceed may be different from what actually occurs, and this can make you feel more than a little unsettled. It does not mean you are unaware of how to proceed, but you might feel unsure of how to adjust to an uncertain situation. In some situations prioritization may seem to be very clear and simple, while in others it may appear less clear. It may help to use some guiding principles in this case.

In addition to the following guiding principles, see if you can think of some of your own:

1. **Don't forget what you already know!** As a student you may feel uncertain at times and that there is much still to learn, but isn't that the point of being a student? You are learning and it takes time to perfect and integrate skill sets related to problem solving.

2. **Stop and think!** Draw on past experiences to think through your actions and rationales required in a given situation. Odds are that you will know how to begin to proceed, even if you have difficulty with reaching the endpoint.

3. **Get help!** Rarely will you act alone as a student. Collaboration with your instructor and the co-assigned nurse is essential. Both would prefer you consult with them and explore solutions to the problem at hand, rather than follow through without having a specific rationale for and understanding of your plan.

4. **Know what resources are available and use them!** Resources related to skills, care standards, and medications abound. This refers to unit-based resources, those required by your nursing program, or those available for individual purchase. Be sure to have proper knowledge about what information they provide and have them close by.

5. **Know your patient!** The better you know your patient and the problems that may surface, both actual and potential, the better prepared you will be. If no worksheet or information collection tool is provided, use those in this book or create your own. Start a rough draft problem list on the back of it and think about relationships and actions as you provide care throughout the day.

6. **Ask reflective questions!** Ask yourself questions related to your patient and the plan of care. What is different about the plan you established and what might be changing? Why is that? What is an alternate plan for this particular situation or problem?

Let's look at a concept map that illustrates prioritization, first from a standpoint of expected actions and then from one of unexpected ones. The concept map in **Figure 7-56** has outlined the steps for this procedure, taking into consideration all aspects of the nursing actions required for its preparation. As addressed earlier, direct patient nursing actions are important, but so are all the other actions related to scope of practice. These actions also reflect the expected ones we anticipate completing for this and many other procedures.

Figure 7-56 **Nursing action concept map #5: Prioritization.**

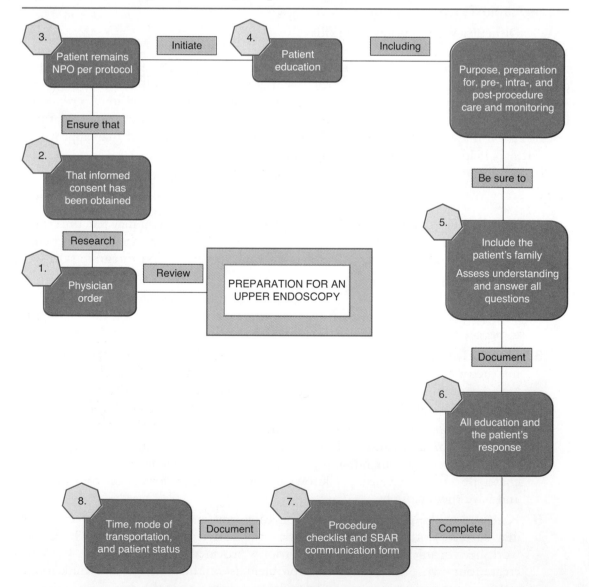

Now, let's suppose that we encounter some unexpected findings, events, or situations with this scenario. Refer back to the guiding principles and reflect on them as you review the concept map. For this portion of the concept map analysis, we will use segments from the concept map in Figure 7-56, adding callouts to indicate the unexpected components (see **Figure 7-57**).

The rationale for speaking with the patient first is that we need to clarify what is at the root of his refusal. Many patients fear receiving sedatives or anesthetics because of negative feelings related to loss of control. Often, just spending time reviewing the education and reinforcing that a registered professional will be present the entire time is enough to allay fears and obtain agreement to proceed. However, if the patient will not disclose the reason or becomes belligerent, collaboration and notification are initiated much more quickly. If the patient would agree to the procedure after the stated interventions, the original actions planned would be completed. Although the patient has agreed

Figure 7-57 Anticipating changes to the plan of care.

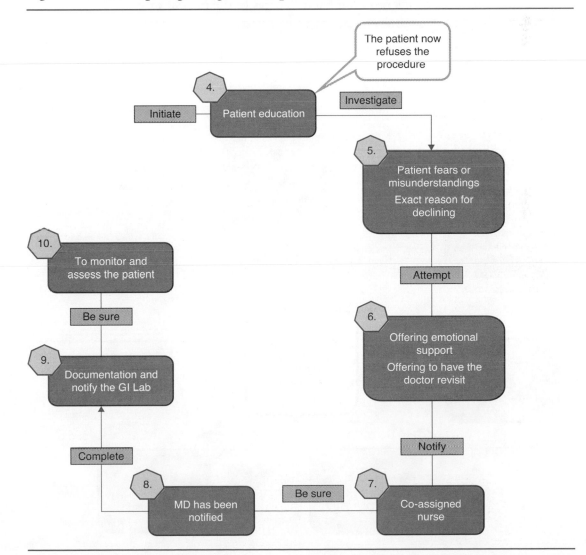

to the procedure, the initial refusal should be passed on to the gastrointestinal laboratory staff, either verbally or on the SBAR (situation, background, assessment, recommendation) form.

Now, let's suppose that we are prepared to send the patient for the procedure, but an unexpected finding occurs (see **Figure 7-58**). Because this event affects patient safety during the procedure, the procedure must be held. Another action to consider in this case is to determine why the prothrombin time (pro-time) is elevated. Is it related to a medication, liver dysfunction, or some other problem? Additionally, how prone is the patient to bleeding? What medications would you anticipate being ordered? What other precautions are needed to prevent bleeding, and what nursing actions are needed to monitor the patient for bleeding and complications? All of these considerations equate to critical thinking and knowledge application in action. While you are physically assisting the patient back to bed and answering his questions, your mind is running through all of these questions. This is what it means to function and think like a nurse.

Figure 7-58 Nursing actions resulting from changes to the plan of care.

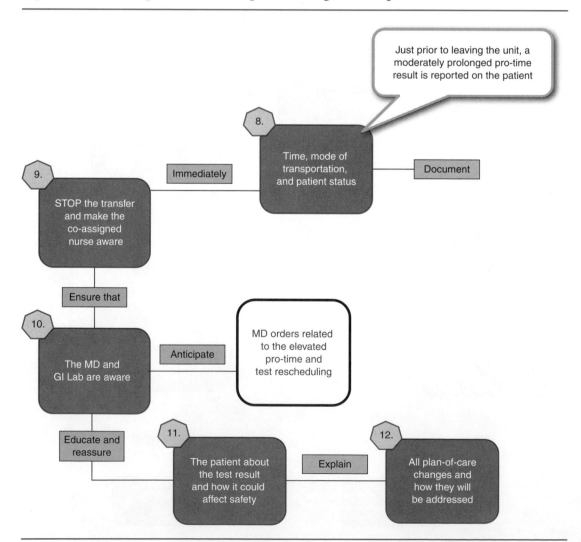

Medications

This is another focus area for concept maps. Within this category we can choose to focus on skill-related items such as the five rights and safety, the procedural aspects of medication administration, or any other aspect of medication administration, affecting our actions. This can be a great exercise as you progress in your skills and administer medications by various routes. For any possible route of administration, there are many accompanying nursing considerations. At times you may become so focused on the task that these other areas are not foremost in your thoughts. Making time to think about them and construct concept maps related to them will go a long way in increasing your critical thinking skills, not to mention your self-confidence. It is all interconnected. Concept map examples begin in **Figure 7-59**.

Obviously, this is a very simple concept map, but it is valuable in making us think about and consider the potential complications resulting from a relatively simple procedure. We could easily add rationales for each of our stated considerations.

Figure 7-59 Medication concept map #1: Simple static.

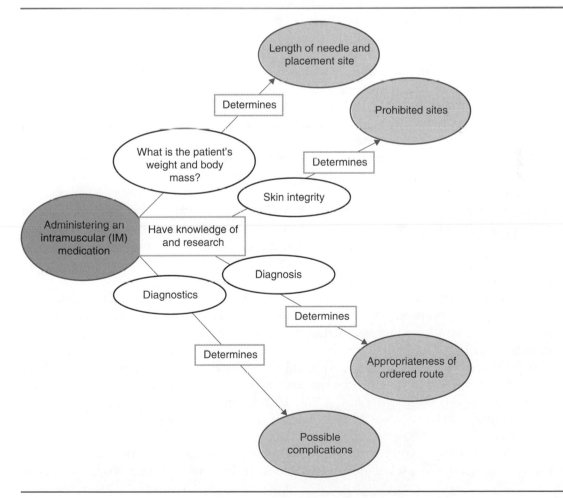

Body mass is an appropriate consideration because some patients have inadequate muscle mass. Whether this results from disease, catabolic states, or loss of muscle mass from some other cause, it may make it difficult to find a site to support the depth and volume of a given medication.

Skin integrity may not always be a strong consideration but nonetheless figures into our actions and administering an IM medication. Patients with burns or extensive breaks in the skin may not be candidates to receive a medication by this route.

Diagnosis is a strong consideration and another rationale for the statement that all things are interconnected. For instance, in a patient situation where myocardial infarction is being ruled out, placing a needle into the muscle will cause a falsely elevated creatine phosphokinase (CPK). Although troponin levels are the gold standard for evaluating myocardial damage, CPK is still used. Another diagnosis to consider is anything that affects coagulation status.

Coagulation studies are important diagnostic tests to be aware of prior to administering a medication by this route. A significantly decreased platelet count could lead to IM bleeding and hematoma formation. If this example was based on an actual patient, the map would then become a living one and we would need to include the diagnostic results and actions related to outcomes.

A concept map such as the one in **Figure 7-60** is assisting you with improving your critical thinking skills by *thinking outside the box*. Critical thinking evaluative processes in this case must be used to compare steps of a skill with specific patient information. Each skill needs to be tailored to and consider perspectives of each patient's situation.

For instance, the first several interventions under the *patient consideration* category are standard, by-the-book procedures used for all patients. However, we must never forget to match the correct MAR to the correct patient. In an age where much of this information is electronic, it has a similar appearance for each patient and is not part of a physical bedside chart; thus we need to make this step a priority.

Medication sensitivities can be as severe as patient allergies. If they are not listed in the database, on an arm bracelet, or on the MAR, you need to ask the patient about them. This step is also helpful to clarify allergy information because many patients have misconceptions about what constitutes a sensitivity, a side effect, and an allergy. This becomes a great opportunity to educate patients on the differences between these concepts.

A safety concern in medication administration is the alteration of laboratory test results. Many medications will alter laboratory results, and you must be aware of these levels prior to administering the medication.

Time-saving strategies with intravenously administered medications include assessing the IV site before you even obtain and draw up the medication. Unless a line has just been inserted or you have just assessed it, there could be a problem with patency. This especially pertains to peripheral sites in small veins that can easily rupture.

Under the *skill-related* category, compatibilities are extremely important. Although you may be flushing the line both before and after the administration, you need to be sure the medications do not mix in the line. Check compatibilities each and every time. Use a reputable resource such as Micromedex; if conflicting information is found, notify the pharmacist.

It is also essential for you to understand why you are giving this particular medication to this patient, comparing scholarly information with the physician order. In addition, the

Figure 7-60 Medication concept map #2: Complex static.

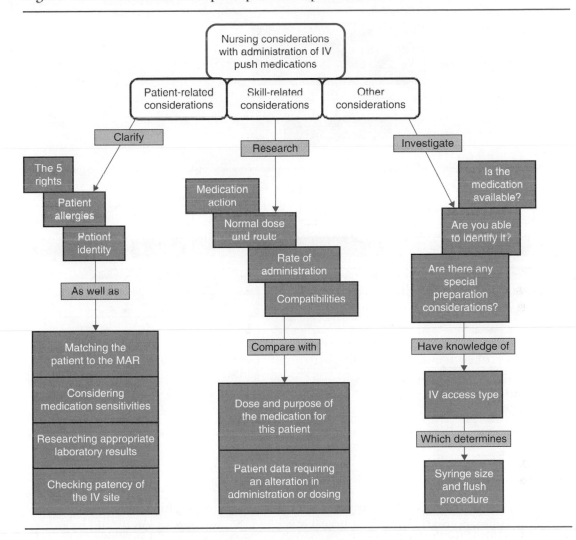

rate of administration may need alteration depending on the patient status. An example of this is slowing the rate of administration of a pain medication in the hypotensive patient.

Finally, the *other considerations* category addresses your knowledge of the medication administration system you are using, along with the unit and facility policies. Answering questions such as what the medication label looks like and how to identify packaging will help save time and ensure safety. Knowing when a medication is given via a straight push technique versus diluting it prior to administration is important to successful results. An IV medication book or other type of resource must be kept nearby at all times. Proper knowledge of the IV access devices used is a competency that must be addressed before you even attempt to administer an IV medication (see **Figure 7-61**).

You can see from the previous examples that while a concept map can have a certain focal point, related concepts can also be focused on within the concept map. Each concept map is a blend of theory, critical thinking, nursing care considerations, and nursing care

Figure 7-61 **Medication concept map #3: Complex static.**

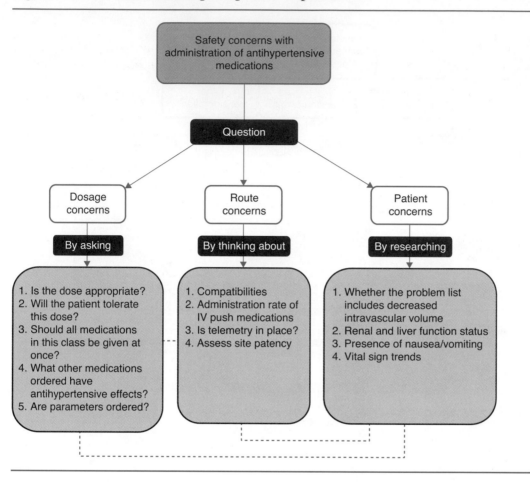

standards. All of these concepts appear in every concept map. This serves as a review of what concept mapping theory is and how it is applied. No nursing action should be carried out without knowledge of the theory and rationale behind it. In addition to rationales, the concepts of cause and effect must be considered. For every action you must ask yourself, "If I do this, what will happen?" When you think through nursing actions in this way you are making all the necessary connections between patient information and the concepts noted earlier. When we apply this principle to the concept map in Figure 7-61, the following connections emerge.

Considering and questioning dose appropriateness demonstrates an awareness of the patient's body weight and body habitus. While most medications have a recommended dose range for mg/kg of weight, this fits a wide range of individuals but may need to be adjusted for a patient outside of that range. Patient response is partly related to dosage.

Drug tolerance is in turn related to intravascular fluid status. Anything on the patient's problem list related to this may lead to potentiation in the drug's effect. This list could include:

- Dehydration
- Hypovolemia
- Anemia

- Bleeding
- Fluid shifts

Knowledge of the diagnoses each patient has is mandatory for understanding cause and effect and to properly anticipate problems and status changes. Trauma, hypernatremia, myxedema coma, and gastrointestinal bleeding are some examples.

Many patients require multiple-medication therapy to manage HTN. While they may take all of their medications at once in the home setting, many choose to separate these types of medications because of dizziness. Given that the patient may be volume depleted, it makes sense to separate the administration of this class of medications in the acute care setting to avoid complications. Obtaining knowledge of vital sign trending values and checking orthostatic vital signs would be appropriate nursing actions.

Other medications, such as loop diuretics and thiazides are used for managing HTN. Even if your patient is not receiving one of these medications for this purpose, you need to know that they will have a blood pressure lowering effect by pulling off intravascular volume.

Rate of administration connects to several concepts related to antihypertensive medication administration as seen on the concept map. As a general rule you will usually be directed to follow the recommended guidelines in whatever approved text you are using. There may be times, however, when the rate of administration is slower based on patient tolerance of the medication related to heart rate, medication sensitivities, and other factors. Use of telemetry is normally a mandate because these medications can lead to a rapid change in vital signs.

Assessing IV site patency is not only a care standard but also relates to time management nursing actions. Taking the time to obtain, prepare, and administer the medication only to find that the IV site is not viable is a waste of time. Assessing the site with the first shift assessment and prior to the medication administration time may help to avoid time mismanagement, especially with peripheral IV sites.

Nausea and vomiting would prohibit giving oral medications until that issue is resolved. However, if these symptoms are coming from the medication and are severe enough to not give it, advocacy may be needed to ask for an alternate medication.

It is very important to consider the laboratory values associated with metabolizing and excreting the medication. There are times when dosing adjustments are necessary or prohibited based upon them. It is also extremely important to look at several sets or trends of vital signs. One set does not tell you what you need to know. Suppose the cuff is not working correctly and is not tight enough. The blood pressure result would then be inaccurate. Any medication administered for vital sign parameters requires several sets of trended readings to make the best decision to give or not to give based on the ordered parameters. Once again this reinforces how all nursing care information is interdependent.

The concept map in **Figure 7-62** is basically stating the importance of safety and knowing your patient. There are so many things required for safe medication administration beyond the "five rights."

Precautions may be needed when sedatives are ordered and the patient has a change in mental status. Use of contrast media and certain antidiabetic medications can result in lactic acidosis. You must always maintain current knowledge related to medication administration. Often, facility policies related to administering medications are based on this information.

Administering a certain medication may be prohibited relative to situations, diagnoses, or routes. As discussed earlier, in any patient who is being ruled out for myocardial

Figure 7-62 Medication concept map #4: General static.

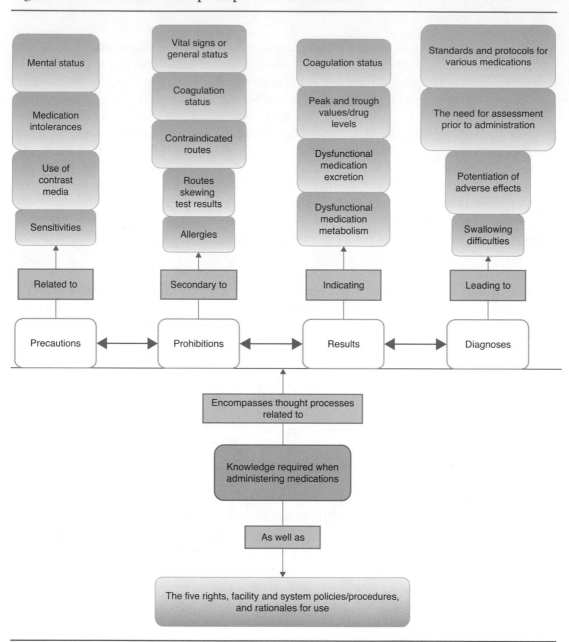

infarction, IM medications would be prohibited because they would falsely elevate the CPK results. They would also be contraindicated in patients with hypercoagulability.

Virtually all medications will have some dosage adjustment when impaired renal function is evident. Many antibiotics require peak and trough levels to dictate proper dosing. Additionally, there are many medications administered and dosed according to drug level. Researching your medications each time you use them will increase your knowledge level related to these concepts, improve medication safety, and ensure your competency with medication administration.

Knowing your medication administration system is also a key factor in safety. Each step requires you to assess your medication knowledge, check your dose, correctly identify the ordered medication and chart. Whatever system is being used, be sure to carefully follow all steps in the order directed by system and policy design, because omitting a step will most likely lead to errors.

Finally, be aware of the rationale for giving this particular medication to this particular patient. Make the connection between the diagnoses and the reason and purpose for this medication. When you have knowledge of this information, you will be able to critically think through the entire order and pick up on anything that is not appropriate. An example of this would be the following order:

- Atropine 0.4 mg PRN for heart rate less than 40 and blood pressure less than 90 systolic

Researching atropine, you will discover that it is used to increase heart rate and an appropriate order would state to use it for that purpose. Using this medication for blood pressure management is inappropriate.

Laboratory and Diagnostic Tests

Understanding laboratory and diagnostic test results and their relationship to patient diagnoses is not always an easy process. From a very large database of tests and possible results, a great many interrelationships can exist. These results assist with explaining and understanding pathophysiologic processes; their interpretation is an integral part of critical thinking as it applies to the patient problem list, anticipating new problems, and formulating nursing actions. Many times a clear pathway of cause and effect cannot be determined because many tests and their abnormal results can be applied to a number of situations and diagnoses. Concept maps are an effective method to link a specific test not only with a disease process or syndrome, but also with nursing actions. Seeing a test result as a problem or area of concern immediately spurs thoughts of possible actions. This thought draws the result into consideration in the problem list and the plan of care. This fact directs you to research and discover more about the test and its implications as well as the patient's needs in response to either the test or the result.

Possible actions resulting from a diagnostic test result include:

- Reporting the result to a physician
- Ensuring that follow-up, repeat tests are ordered if necessary (serial testing)
- Monitoring the patient for symptomatic effects
- Reporting abnormal levels to colleagues
- Educating the patient and family members about the testing and results
- Trending results

At the very least, an abnormal result, whether laboratory or diagnostic test based, may mandate doing nothing more than monitoring the patient and subsequent result or value. This would normally apply to laboratory tests but could apply to certain diagnostic tests. For instance, if your patient has a slightly low potassium level but is asymptomatic, but is receiving potassium replacement and this has been the trend or "normal" situation for this particular patient, no action is needed except to ensure that a potassium level test is ordered for the next day. The same could be said for an abnormal CXR indicating pneumonia. If the patient's status has not changed, the pneumonia is not a new diagnosis, and treatment has been instituted, you would continue to monitor the daily results and focused assessments.

Just as has been previously mentioned with vital signs, trending of both types of test results is extremely important. While it is important to note that a result was abnormal, there are a few questions you need to ask to clarify both the situation and your subsequent actions. These may include:

1. Is there a previous result to compare it to?
2. What changes have occurred?
3. Is the difference significant?
4. Are immediate actions necessary?
5. Is the patient symptomatic?

These questions reflect concept mapping theory and assist you in reasoning through the actions needed.

To foster an understanding of these tests and their results, you need to first establish some baseline knowledge of them. Become familiar with the current text used for this purpose, and read! Until you become familiar with the terminology, purpose, and normal findings, you will find it difficult to understand the abnormal and relate it to disease and nursing actions. Let's consider this in more detail for a moment.

Laboratory tests may be run on any body fluid. The knowledge you need regarding this is as follows:

- The various departments that exist within the laboratory
- The specific department that runs a particular test
- Terminology and abbreviations for the various tests
- Units of measure used for reporting
- Turnaround time
- The difference between normal and abnormal results

In addition, you need to have knowledge of the procedures for collecting and submitting a specimen for testing. All of this knowledge serves as a supplement to theory knowledge of how a specific test is used for evaluation and diagnosis as well as treatment.

Because diagnostic testing using departments other than the laboratory also impact nursing actions and patient care, you need to have knowledge of those as well. As discussed earlier in this text, there are a variety of possible diagnostic tests performed in a wide variety of departments throughout the hospital. You need a working knowledge of each department, the specific tests performed, and how and why the tests are used. Another important area to focus your research on is the normal and expected findings obtained compared with the unexpected and undesired ones. This will drive your critical thinking processes and enable you to create helpful and meaningful concept maps. The concept maps you create can be focused on:

- The purpose of the test
- Actions related to patient preparation
- Actions related to patient education
- Post-test care of patient
- Actions related to assessments and treatments

So you see, the foundational knowledge you need to cultivate is necessary for application. Everything you learn will be applied within the framework of care actions.

The concept map in **Figure 7-63** reinforces the many thought processes used in nursing care. Our nursing actions stem from a wide variety of sources. If this was your concept map, you could also use additional connecting lines to link symptom severity with the symptoms to be alert for, as well as the echocardiogram results. It is amazing

Figure 7-63 Laboratory value concept map #1: Complex static.

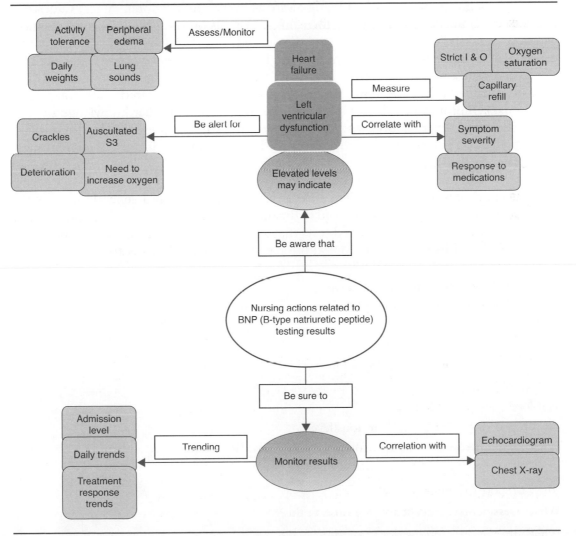

to see that so many nursing actions and our patient's status can be affected by so many different things.

This map also considers outcomes and other parts of the nursing process in that it considers the patient's response to treatment. An elevated B-type natriuretic peptide (BNP) level normally results in treatment with a diuretic. Urine output would then be expected to increase, the patient's weight and edema to decrease, and overall status to improve. Because we know that this does not always occur, this concept map also makes us think about anticipation of ineffective treatment response in the form of congestive heart failure (CHF). Overall, this type of concept map increases awareness of what a laboratory test means to the plan of care; it shows how it fits. This fact reinforces the knowledge that a laboratory test result has meaning and impact on the plan of care and our nursing actions.

Let's consider how we think about this test result. Walking through those steps and applying it to the concept map is just an enhanced way of looking at things. **Figure 7-64** provides a checklist for you to use in this evaluation process, with questions to guide your thinking. Use it as an addendum to your concept map. Both are learning tools. You begin by studying and being aware of every single laboratory test value your patient has had drawn. Because the focus in this case is on the BNP, you need to know the normal levels. When you note that it is elevated, you then have to correlate it with a cause. This is where you need to have thorough knowledge of your patient. Researching the admitting diagnosis, the PMH, PSH, and HPI should lead you to a connection. The next step is further research to make a connection between the elevated result and patient behaviors, symptoms, or possible deterioration. You then apply that knowledge to your assessments and other features within the plan of care. Part of understanding this process is to be able to see how things fit together. Either way, you need to use a concept map, a checklist, as well as a customized thought process to think all of these things through so that you can put your plan into action.

The concept map in **Figure 7-65** is static, because it is really a general listing of the types of evaluative diagnostic tests used in diagnosing renal dysfunction. It could be made more complex if we included related tests that aid diagnosis in addition to expanding on the reasons each listed test is used. Additional space would allow us to add a key. The

Figure 7-64 **Questioning and reasoning.**

Questions/Reasoning Process	Notes
What is the level?	
What unit of measure is it expressed in?	
Is it elevated?	
Is it low?	
How has it changed from the previous level?	
What symptoms are seen in my patient secondary to this?	
How do any of my patient's diagnoses fit with this?	
Must I report this immediately?	
What assessments are needed in response to this?	
What other orders/actions can I now anticipate?	

Figure 7-65 Laboratory and diagnostic testing concept map #2: Static.

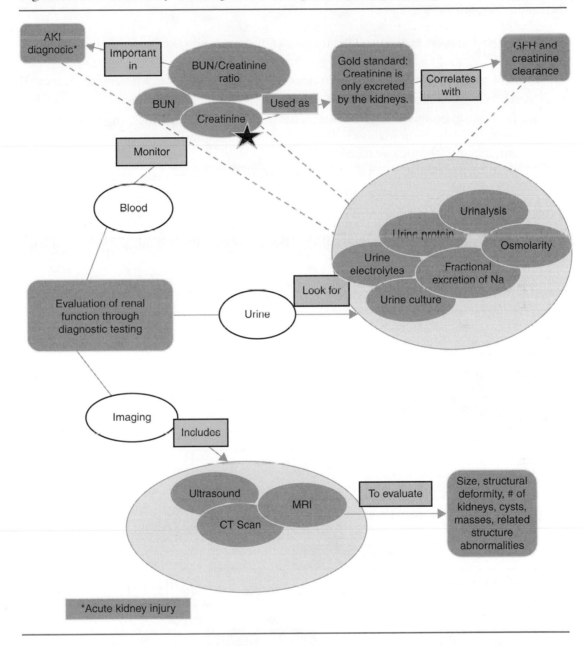

dashed lines link the various tests with the blood-based testing results as well as to the glomerular filtration rate (GFR) and creatinine clearance.

Although this concept map is static, it is still based on the theoretical knowledge necessary for understanding the purpose and diagnostic value of each test. It also serves to promote more critical thinking related to subsequent nursing actions and some perspectives related to result interpretation. The formatting of this concept map also pulls the various sources for renal dysfunction diagnosis together. This reinforces the valuable resources needed for research and application of the plan of care.

When considering the various meaning of diagnostic tests, remember to think about four main categories:

1. **Blood-based testing:** This includes any test result taken directly from a blood sample.
2. **Urine-based testing:** This refers to any urine sample, whether it is a small amount collected or a 24-hour specimen.
3. **Imaging-based diagnostics:** This area of testing includes any type of diagnostic visualization such as radiology, ultrasonography, fluoroscopy, and scanning enhanced with nuclear medicines.
4. **Procedural testing:** This normally refers to invasive instrumentation and could include biopsy, arteriography. or visualization with an endoscope.

Considering all of this provides another awareness of the overall connection between testing and our nursing actions. Anything ordered for or affecting our patients will have an impact on the plan of care.

Figure 7-66 Laboratory and diagnostic testing concept map #3: Static.

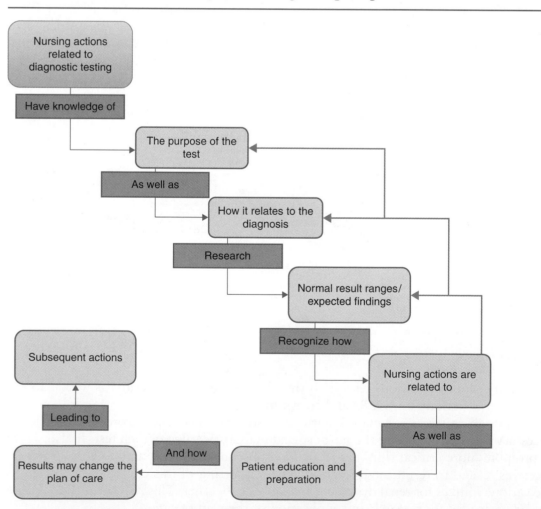

Concept Map 3 (**Figure 7-66**) demonstrates relationship analysis and a prioritized thought process in a very thorough way. The map is easy to follow, and its meaning is clear. This is a very general map yet still it addresses outcomes and includes the nursing process. This is the type of concept map that could be used for studying and could be added to as your knowledge level increases. Have you noticed that every concept map example reinforces the importance and indicates the presence of concept mapping theory? No matter how simple or complex a concept map is meant to be, the basic components and theoretical bases are present. Reinforcement and connections are two of the strongest building blocks of learning for comprehension and application.

The concept map in **Figure 7-67** delineates a starting point with a heavily weighted arrow. In this way actions can be prioritized. Checking the physician order is always the first step. This ensures that we are collecting the proper specimen for the correct patient. Similar to the "five rights" of medication administration, you can use the "six Ps" as actions when sending off laboratory tests. They will serve as a procedural type of checklist and are found in **Figure 7-68**.

Collaborative Care

As a student in today's world of nursing practice, you will work alongside many collaborators. Although each will have his or her own responsibilities in ensuring fulfillment of patient care standards, it is the responsibility of nurses to coordinate and oversee this process. This means that you must develop an understanding of each collaborative specialty, the purpose of it, and the role it plays in the plan of care, how it affects nursing actions, and how it impacts patient outcomes. As a nurse you will always wear many hats but must also be aware of the hats others wear. It may help to think of these collaborators

Figure 7-67 Laboratory and diagnostic testing concept map #4: Static.

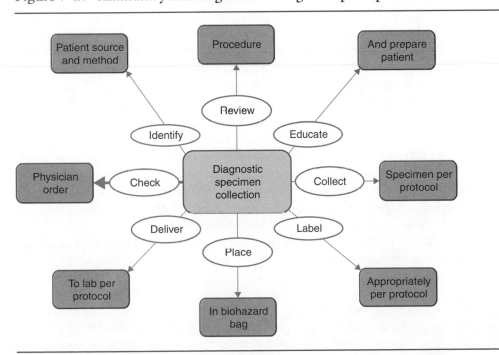

Figure 7-68 The six Ps.

Physician:	Most specimens are collected in response to a physician's order. Check that you have matched the correct patient to the correct test and that an order has been written.
Protocol:	There are times when unit or facility protocols are the stimulus for a specimen being sent. Check that a protocol covers you to do this if you do not see a physician order.
Patient:	Be sure to identify the patient using at least two identifiers.
Procedure:	Research the procedure and be sure that you are following all the steps correctly and according to standards.
Proper Label:	Label the specimen appropriately with the patient's information along with your initials, the date, and the time. Enclose the proper paperwork as well.
Proper Send-off:	Always place the specimen in a biohazard bag. Check institutional policies on how to deliver the specimen to the laboratory.

as anyone the patient comes into contact with regularly. **Figure 7-69** highlights some of these collaborators.

Care collaborators can also be defined as colleagues on the healthcare team who have a responsibility in providing patient care. Their roles assist with and enhance nursing care to meet patient goals and outcomes. Collaboration is teamwork in action; for it to be effective, each party must know the roles of the others and ongoing communication must take place so that everyone remains on the same page, keeping the patient as the main focus. Some common methods used to accomplish this are interdisciplinary patient rounds and/or meetings, documentation using interdisciplinary progress notes, and face-to-face updates as needed. As mentioned previously, nursing is the main coordinator of all collaborative care. Meetings and updates must also be provided to family members.

One thing to mention here is that an integral role for nurses concerning collaborative care is that of educator. A patient may feel overwhelmed at all the faces appearing at the bedside and have difficulty understanding what each person is assigned to do. While we as professionals know that collaborative care is effective, it may be difficult for patients to accept and develop a rapport with so many caregivers.

Let's take a brief glimpse at the collaborators listed in Figure 7-69. The attending physician admits a patient, writes admission orders, and generally oversees all medical care. Shifting trends in the acute medical care setting have led to hospitalists taking over this role as opposed to the patient's own personal physician. Patients may need time to adjust to someone they are unfamiliar with managing their care.

Consulting physicians are called in when the attending physician feels that specialty care is warranted. The number of consultants depends on the patient problem list and the specific care needed.

Physical therapists, as well as occupational therapists, have a role in assessing and providing a plan for patient mobility and management of the ADLs. Whether this is in response to an alteration in ambulation, an active problem with pain, disability, or prolonged bed rest, this discipline will develop a plan to address these specific needs.

Figure 7-69 **Interdisciplinary patient care collaborators.**

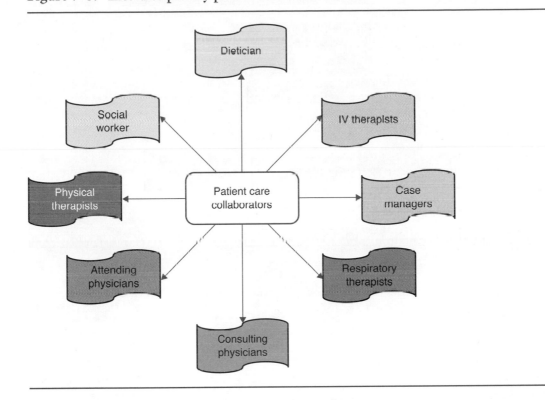

Social workers and case managers ensure that all patient needs are being met with respect to services in the outpatient setting. This may include procuring financial assistance or durable medical equipment. Both disciplines also play major roles in discharge planning; either by investigating placement options or homecare services.

Because nutrition plays such an important role in healing and lowering mortality and readmission rates, the registered dietician has become a main care collaborator. The dictician assists with planning adequate nutritional care through providing education and sample meal plans, arranging for outpatient education related to meal planning, and monitoring laboratory results relative to nutrition, such as albumin and pre-albumin levels.

IV therapists assist with maintenance and insertion of IV access sites such as peripheral angiographic catheters (angiocaths) and PICC lines. Having this discipline manage access devices provides for consistency and has been shown to lower infection rates secondary to IV therapy.

Respiratory therapists focus on respiratory care. Normally they will administer inhalers and aerosol treatments, coordinate and manage ventilator care, and participate in ventilator-weaning protocols.

The concept map in **Figure 7-70** accomplishes several things. First, it promotes an awareness of what a dietician's role in patient care is and allows you to compare his or her role to yours. Many of the pieces of information you obtain will also be used by the dietician to complete a thorough nutritional assessment. Secondly, the map establishes a pathway of nursing actions correlating to those of the dietician that demonstrates how communication and collaboration will take place. In addition, it reinforces collaboration

Figure 7-70 Collaborator concept map #1: Static.

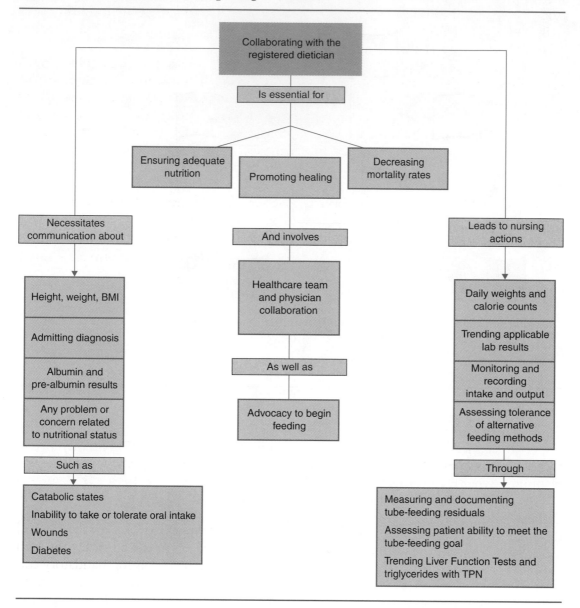

among the entire healthcare team so that all team members should have knowledge of patient problems just as you do. Finally, the concept map is establishing a relationship between nursing actions necessary to both nutritional assessment and collaborative nutritional care.

Getting to know your collaborators allows a rapport to be established, opens up communication, and allows for multidisciplinary goals to be set. Within this process and integral to it is the promotion of multidisciplinary advocacy. True collaboration leads to an exchange of ideas, integration of multidisciplinary EBP applications, and hopefully better patient outcomes.

Always be aware of all collaborators' roles and responsibilities as well as what is being documented. Have knowledge of where documentation is completed on the medical record and how to access it. Read the daily notes and communicate patient needs in relation to those notes to other collaborators. Make every attempt to meet with collaborators daily and update the plan of care as needed. Build these actions into your time management portion of nursing care.

Figure 7-71 assumes that we would also be collaborating with the physician if needed but recognizes the need for collaboration with the respiratory therapist at this time. Again, note the reinforcement of both disciplines needing to have knowledge of the patient status, problem list, the impact of the PMH on the current situation, and available interventions. In modern healthcare, it is the respiratory therapist who administers both scheduled and PRN aerosol therapies. Both disciplines should document assessments, when a PRN aerosol is needed, the patient response to the treatment, and any subsequent actions.

Common themes used when working collaboratively include the following:

- Each discipline needs to have knowledge of the other's roles and responsibilities
- Each discipline provides supportive documentation of its own assessment findings
- Each discipline must have in-depth knowledge of the patient's diagnosis, history, and problem list
- Communication must be daily, shift-to-shift, and ongoing
- Current standards of care must be followed by all disciplines

Every action related to collaboration in the previous example also relates to safety (see **Figure 7-72**). This is a great example of cause and effect. If there was no communication between the nurse and physical therapy personnel, an adverse event could occur. The patient may have had a great deal of blood loss resulting in a subnormal hemoglobin and hematocrit. This would lead to volume depletion and orthostasis, which could precipitate a fall. Collaborative communication would reinforce the need for at least two to three assistants to maintain safe transfer or ambulation. Other factors to consider as potential fall-risk contributors in the postoperative patient are pain medication administration, the pain itself, and generalized weakness or grogginess.

The impact of all of this is that the patient should not be ambulated until the physical therapist has been given a report by the nurse. The nurse can initiate advocacy through establishing a rapport with the physical therapist, initiating protocols for mandatory collaboration prior to getting a postoperative patient out of bed, promoting use of a written SBAR form to communicate patient information, and by using multidisciplinary rounding to communicate these policies and protocols. This is an example of nursing's role in overseeing the function of all collaborators. This is what nursing leadership is about.

Documentation

Many pages and examples within this text have emphasized documentation. That is because our documentation serves as proof of actions we have taken and validates those actions. Documentation via flow sheets, medication administration notes, and narrative notes is an essential part of nursing practice. Documentation techniques must be competent, adequate, professional, and thorough. As part of the permanent chart and legal medical documents, these notations become a timeline of patient problems and our actions and responses to them.

Figure 7-71 Collaborator concept map #1: Static.

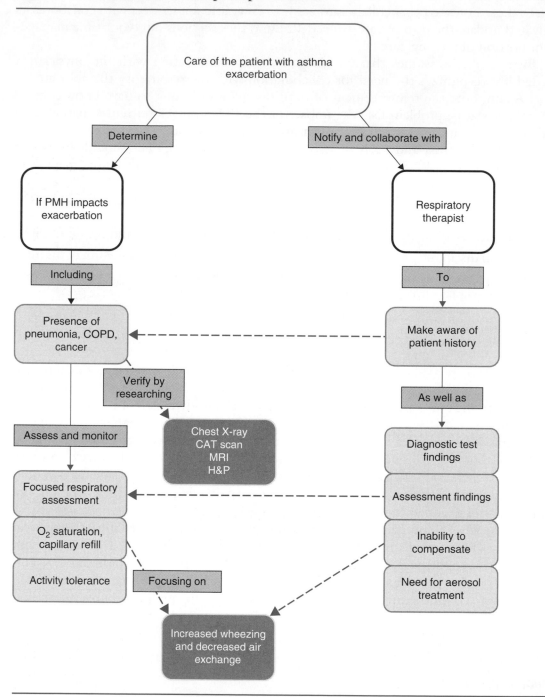

Figure 7-72 Collaborator concept map #3: Static complex.

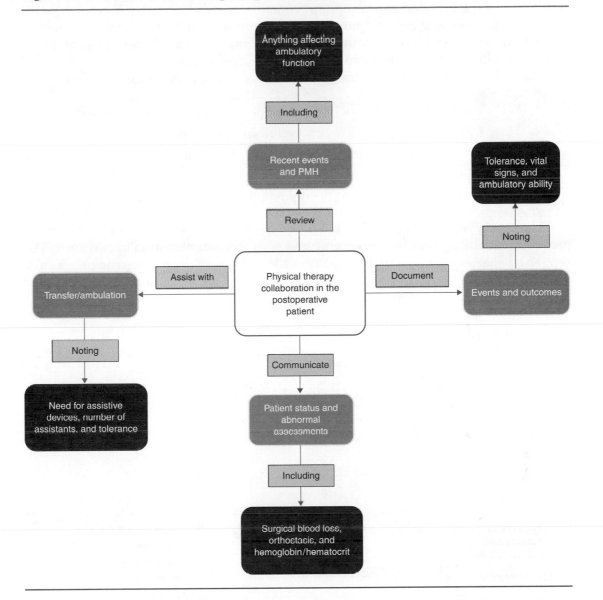

Assessment documentation is normally fairly straightforward and follows a head-to-toe assessment pattern. In today's nursing care environment, this usually entails charting by exception. Within this format abnormal findings are charted while any normal findings are indicated through checking a box labeled WNL (within normal limits). *Whether you record an abnormal assessment finding or the WNL box, you are stating that you are aware of the difference between the normal and abnormal assessment findings pertaining to that system.* This assumption can have legal ramifications if a case ever goes to court, so this fact adds responsibility to all nursing documentation. Simple notations and checking boxes should never be completed without critical thinking and complete knowledge related to whatever you are charting.

A narrative note is a required addition to further explain the assessment documentation. Although many electronic programs contain preloaded narrative notes, there will always be situations that demand more specific documentation. You will need to maintain current knowledge of charting formats and the information that needs to be included in each note. While it is recommended that the note be concise, more charting is preferred to none at all. Some questions to use as a checklist for how to chart can include:

1. What can I document that will best explain the event, situation, or action?
2. Have I addressed the problem, intervention, and outcome?
3. If another colleague is reading this note, are the situation and any actions taken clearly stated?
4. Have I shown that I followed up and followed through on a patient concern?

The concept map in **Figure 7-73** outlines the expected documentation for the stated procedure. It also stresses the importance and need for documentation in two areas. The flow sheet charting is necessary to document the addition of the nasogastric tube as well as the standards related to its care and management. This ensures that the tube is assessed and maintained per set protocols.

Figure 7-73 **Documentation concept map #1: Static.**

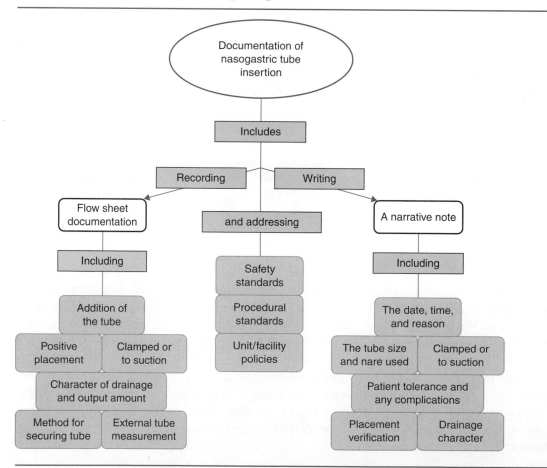

The narrative note is necessary to explain procedural steps and patient tolerance of the procedure as well as the reason for its insertion. The reason and rationale for insertion, other than that related to the physician order, will link with and determine the need for other actions. Let's suppose the tube was placed secondary to gastric distention and possible ileus. A subsequent note and accompanying nursing actions would include reporting any x-ray results, improvement or change in abdominal assessment, and patient status updates. Many times the first recorded narrative note serves as a baseline for others throughout the shift.

Other reasons for nasogastric tube insertion, each requiring a specific narrative note tailored to the situation include:

- Surgical decompression
- Bowel obstruction
- Upper GI bleeding
- To administer enteral feedings

Each time an event occurs, a note is needed to explain the event and any actions taken. Each note must be timed and should be written as needed. One long note recorded at shift's end does not allow for adequate follow up and monitoring of a concern or problem.

For the next map, let's suppose a patient has a CXR showing a pneumothorax. The patient is symptomatic and requires the intervention of chest tube placement (see **Figure 7-74**).

This concept map example is focused on a specific situation relative to an abnormal finding requiring intervention. Please remember that the chest tube would also be added to the flow sheet as well. It is clear to see that this situation requires multiple notes. Not only is this done to accurately time events as they occurred, but it also is done to show ongoing assessment and monitoring—that the nurse remained with the patient and assisted with the procedure. In addition, it indicates that ongoing follow-up care has been and will continue to be provided. There are so many things to think about and recall when writing a narrative note. This is why you must practice and reflect on your skills related to narrative note writing. As you learn and practice, a core group of common components will surface that should be included in each note, as we have discussed.

Legal and Ethical Concerns

Everything we have discussed thus far has a connection to legalities and ethics within nursing practice. In fact, ethical and legal standards are always part of nursing education. This is because standards of care are based on the premise of doing no harm to patients. Professional standards ensure that legalities are respected within nursing care. The two concepts go hand in hand with each other. The American Nurses Association has created a code of ethics to guide nursing practice. It is each nurse's responsibility to have knowledge of and practice according to this code. Other professional standards for nursing practice are set by the individual state boards of nursing, The Joint Commission, and individual care facilities. It is important to realize that these standards begin at the national level and affect all practice in all settings. Satisfying and maintaining all practice standards are conditions of nursing licensure. Legal and ethical concerns affect our practice, and our actions have implications in respect to both. While you are a student, you

Figure 7-74 Documentation concept map #2: Complex living.

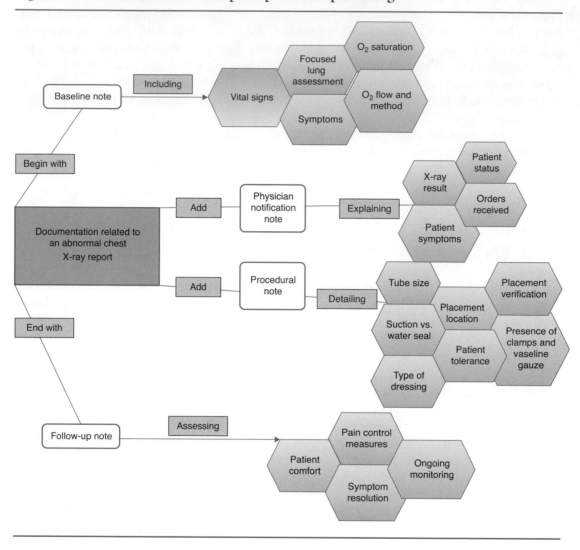

must learn as much as possible about these implications and the huge impact they have on nursing practice. Almost any nursing action will touch on some aspect of ethics and legalities within care. Recognition of this will enable you to add ethical and legal nursing action implications to the plan of care. In addition, as with any other patient problem, legal and ethical problems and concerns have the ability to alter the plan of care. Some examples of this are:

- A change in a patient's code status
- A patient's refusal of medication
- A patient's refusal of any prescribed treatment, medication, or diagnostic testing

Many times for students, this knowledge is accumulated gradually and can seem very confusing. It is also an area that is somewhat abstract, and the interventions employed may be somewhat different with every patient.

There will be helpful links at the chapter's end to assist you in educating yourself. Some additional examples of the impact of ethical/legal implications on nursing actions are listed in **Figure** 7-75. These are only a few examples but occur often in the acute care setting. Once you have reviewed the sample concept maps, review the others in the text to look for legal and ethical implications.

To fully understand the meaning of the example in **Figure** 7-76, let's consider it in the format used for documenting the main concern—the narrative note format.

Problem/Concern

The patient has refused a medically recommended procedure. Although we have not used a case study per se, we could assume that the patient agreed previously and now has had second thoughts. However, a patient could refuse at any point along the care continuum. So the main problem is that this patient has refused and now we need to determine why so that we can understand what action is needed next.

Nursing Action(s)

In many instances, a patient's fears and misunderstandings may make them more likely to refuse procedures. Exploring the root of that fear may help the patient to express it so that

Figure 7-75 Examples of the impact of ethical/legal implications on nursing actions.

Example	Legal Implication	Ethical Implication	Rationale
A patient refuses further treatments and "wants to be left to die."	X	X	Further collaboration and advocacy are needed to determine if the patient is alert, oriented, and in sound mind.
A patient's family states they are unhappy with the physician's care and wish the patient to be transferred to another facility.	X		The family may decide to take legal action.
A nurse administers a medication against a patient's wishes.	X	X	This violates the code of ethics and has legal implications as well.
The nurse institutes palliative care after the patient and her family agree with this plan.		X	This has no legal concerns because the patient and family agree.
A patient is asked to consent for a surgical procedure but the procedure and risks have not been explained.	X	X	If the procedure is carried out, the patient could claim coercion.

Figure 7-76 Legal and ethical concerns concept map #1: Static

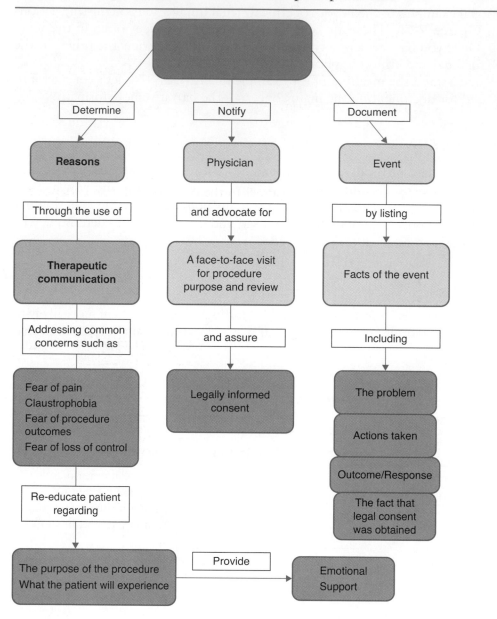

you can help deal with it. Many patients will verbalize that they fear pain as well as a loss of control. In some cases, re-education and empathetic listening will calm the patient's fears. Subsequently, they will agree to the procedure. So, the first step in addressing the problem is to speak with and re-educate the patient.

The next step would be to notify the physician. Whether the patient agrees to undergo the procedure or not, the physician should still be aware of the concern. As a patient advocate, you would request that the physician speak with the patient to further allay fears.

Response/Outcomes

You need to document specific patient and physician responses as well as the fact that the patient made an independent decision to proceed. Legally and ethically, a patient must never be coerced into submitting to a procedure.

Concept maps can assist you in understanding legal/ethical perspectives in nursing care and how nursing actions are impacted by them. They also reinforce use of the nursing process in decision making. In addition, they are a great tool for assisting you with thinking through how to document these types of instances, allowing you to better apply the basic ethical/legal principles you have learned to practice (see **Figure** 7-77).

Although you may feel intimidated and out of your element when adverse events occur, it is important for you to keep focused. You will not have to handle the situation, concern, or problem alone, so notifying colleagues in the chain of command is a positive thing. These colleagues will support you and assist you in dealing with the issue at hand

Figure 7-77 **Legal and ethical concerns concept map #2: Static.**

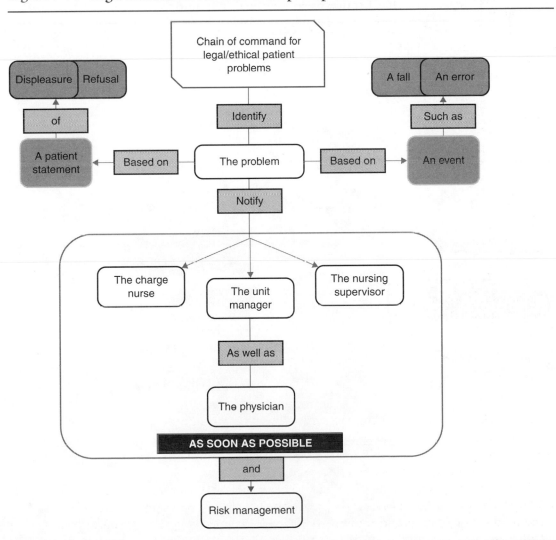

as well as how to proceed with documentation, patient or family communication, and follow up. All of this is necessary should legal action be instituted. The physician will also want to be made aware of any patient problems so that the patient can be examined, if that is what is required, or to speak with the patient or family.

Risk management personnel are often called in when there is a possibility of legal action. They will also review charts and determine if hospital lawyers should be involved. This is why documentation is so crucial. The last example for this topic addresses this concern (see **Figure 7-78**).

Be aware that this map example provides a general guideline. Each facility will have its own specific decision tree or some other document describing the appropriate procedural pathway. This concept map example could be made more detailed by adding specific information. For example, subjective data would include exact quotes made by the patient and/or family. This clarifies the concern at hand and helps to justify future actions and notifications. Objective data would include specific observations you made

Figure 7-78 Legal and ethical concerns concept map #3: Static.

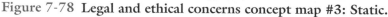
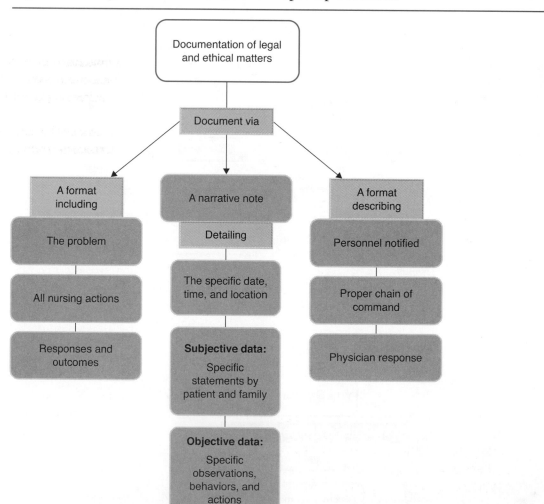

in terms of behaviors, nonverbal cues, and actions. Again, this completely and clearly describes what occurred and whether or not correct procedures and protocols were followed. Any charting or other documentation is part of the legal patient record. On one hand you are explaining how you cared for and advocated for a patient, and on the other hand you are justifying your actions.

You will learn a great deal about legal and ethical concerns in nursing care throughout your career. Set a goal to learn as much as you can. Many continuing education programs contain current and relative information on this topic.

Evidence-Based Practice

EBP stems from nursing research and guides all care that, in turn, affects all nursing actions within the set plan of care. When you began to learn about rationales accompanying skills and nursing actions, did you ever wonder where that rationale originated? Rationales do not exist because of one person's thoughts and ideas. They exist because research has shown that particular action reflects the best practice for the best patient outcomes. Often, this research is a combination of medical and nursing research as physician orders impact nursing actions. Research leads to nursing policy and protocol institution; in other words, it directly affects nursing actions during patient care at the bedside.

It is important to recognize that the process of nursing research is ongoing. As new research results concerning best practices are accepted, nursing care and nursing actions are adjusted to the new practices. Once the newly recommended practices are implemented, research continues to monitor effectiveness of those practices. You then become a direct participant in nursing research by documenting findings relative to policies, procedures, and actions.

The concept map in **Figure 7-79** is a very basic static map showing recommended nursing actions and rationales for the actions. It could easily be expanded to include actual research sources and comprehensive information on the procedures for mouth care and oral gastric tube care. Learning about and recognizing rationales are other ways to view relationship analysis and the concept of cause and effect. Both concepts reinforce education through making connections. In this case those connections are made between rationales and actions. The connections justify how nursing research is applied to practice. Anytime this link is made and understood, meaningful learning has taken place—moving past simple knowledge or awareness to true comprehension and recognition of how it can then be applied. Use of concept mapping in nursing education allows and promotes all of this. What a powerful tool!

Summary

This chapter has delved more deeply into nursing applications for concept mapping than any other. We have revisited concept mapping theory and demonstrated how it is applied through various purposes, processes, and focus areas within nursing care. The section related to purpose reinforced not only why we use concept maps in nursing education but also how purpose is applied. That application takes place by using concept mapping theory and then employing it within a concept map.

Figure 7-79 EBP concept map: Static.

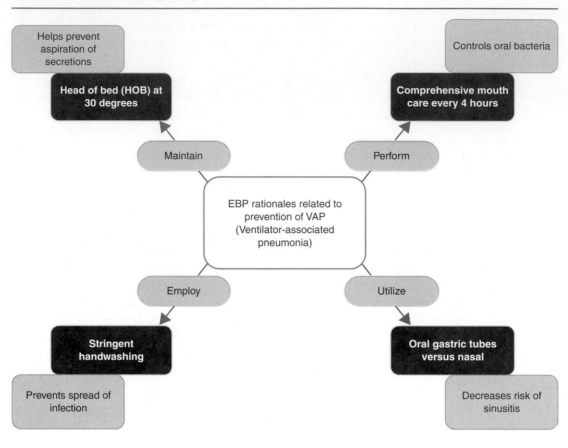

The next section focused on various processes through which nursing care and our nursing actions are applied. Even though concept mapping theory is what guides concept map creation, it is the nursing process and holism that guide nursing practice; therefore, this must also be demonstrated within any concept map. The many and varied sample concept maps reinforce this and make an important statement that concept maps are a tool. They cannot and do not replace the nursing practice processes that serve as the foundation of nursing care.

The last section demonstrated the use of specific focus areas to address critical thinking, relationship analysis, and theory application. This section also strongly emphasized rationales. Rationales tell us when we are performing along recommended guidelines. They tell us what makes sense and explain the purpose of our actions. They also link patient outcomes to nursing actions.

All of these components are reflected within the current National League for Nursing (NLN) curriculum guidelines and program outcomes. They are also components of the National Council Licensure Examination (NCLEX) and the Quality & Safety Education's (QSEN) graduate competencies. You have also probably recognized by now that they are part of your clinical competencies as well. This should provide great motivation to actively pursue strong critical thinking skills—skills that cross over clinical performance boundaries to blend with theory for the best application of what is learned. Rationales are a huge part of successful critical thinking application. Concept maps assist with learning, processing, recognizing relationships, and mapping out a pathway of how you think. Once you truly understand that, you will know yourself more deeply, your learning will become more meaningful, and you will be able to grow professionally

Critical Thinking Questions and Activities

1. Reflect on and discuss three ways in which you have seen your critical thinking skills improve since beginning to read this text. Supply specific examples.

2. Explain how the nursing process is demonstrated and correlates with the nursing-based plan of care when creating a concept map from the time the problem list is created until the completion of the map.

3. Discuss and share stories of patients you have cared for in the past. What components of holism were part of the care you provided?

4. Create a static concept map demonstrating how holism is applied to nursing care. (To use a Concept Map Creator, see the Student Companion Website at http://go.jblearning.com/schmehl.)

5. List at least five ways that safety is reinforced within a completed concept map. (To use a Concept Map Creator, see the Student Companion Website at http://go.jblearning.com/schmehl.)

6. Explain how nursing actions result from patient information that has been identified as a problem or concern.

Case Studies

Directions: Read through each case study and answer the questions using the chapter material provided.

1. Elaine is trying to make connections between her patient's symptoms and what she has learned about the pathophysiology responsible for them. Some of them seem to make sense but others do not seem to have a rationale associated with the disease process. She has started to ask questions but is unsure of how to proceed.

   a. How can Elaine begin to ask critical thinking questions related to her assessment findings?

   b. What part of concept mapping theory will guide her questions?

   c. How will comparing and contrasting information help her to find the correct answers?

   d. What types of resources would contain the best information for Elaine to use to make connections and provide answers?

2. Andy is thinking through the steps to create a concept map about his patient's main problems of HTN and anxiety/depression. Although he has been trying for about an hour, he does not seem to be any further along than when he first started. He has written the main concept and one associated one but cannot seem to come up with nursing actions and descriptive phrases for dealing with them.

    a. In addition to writing some of his thoughts on paper, what other suggestions can you think of that would help Andy complete his concept map?

    b. What steps should he follow to get the best results?

    c. What might be the cause of Andy's feelings of frustration?

    d. How will formulating nursing diagnoses for these problems assist Andy in making connections?

3. Maria is caring for a patient who has just had a PICC placed. Her patient was admitted with chest pain and has been ruled out for myocardial infarction. He is stable with the exception of atrial fibrillation. The patient had no prior history of this and has now been started on warfarin (Coumadin). The PICC line was started for long-term antibiotic therapy because the patient has developed hospital-acquired pneumonia (HAP) during this admission. It will likely remain in place for 3 weeks or so, according to the collaborative note recorded by the case manager.

    Maria's instructor has asked that she create a concept map focused on PICC line care. This is Maria's problem list:

- Presence of an invasive line
- Mild discomfort
- A need for dressing changes
- Risk for infection because of invasive line

    a. Which is the main concept?

    b. Does the related problem list contain everything from every available resource?

    c. What other sources contain information that correlates to the main problem?

    d. How does that information link with classroom theory *and* nursing actions?

    e. How will that information alter Maria's nursing actions?

4. John is caring for a patient who is confused and is at high risk for falls. Use the nursing process and the additional information provided to answer questions for this case study. L.H. is an 80-year-old male admitted with urinary retention and urosepsis. L.H. resides in an assisted living facility and normally cares for himself. While his history states he has an enlarged prostate and does have difficulty emptying his bladder at times, this is the first time L.H. has been unable to empty his bladder at all. At this time, his sepsis is resolving with the administration of IV antibiotics, and an indwelling Foley catheter is in place. The sepsis has led to generalized weakness and interferes with L.H.'s ability to ambulate. L.H. has had one episode of nighttime confusion thought to be secondary to zolpidem (Ambien), which has been discontinued. This patient is allowed out of bed only with assistance and generally requires two people to assist him.

    a. Assessment

        1. What specific physical assessment findings correlate with an increased risk for falls?

        2. What other types of assessment findings may contribute to an increased fall risk?

b. Diagnosis
1. What nursing diagnoses can be developed that correlate to this patient as well as the fall risk?

c. Planning
1. What ideas do you have for planning overall collaborative care for L.H.?
2. Who else must this planning phase involve?

d. Implementation
1. What nursing actions are specific to the assessment findings?
2. What nursing actions are specific to tubes, lines, and medications?
3. What nursing actions stem directly from holistic care?

e. Evaluation
1. Explain what it means to follow up on a patient problem.
2. Why is there a need for multiple nursing actions and multiple phases of follow up at times?
3. In what ways are actions used to follow up? What form do the necessary actions take?
4. What are some of this patient's collaborative and holistic needs that must be followed up on?

5. Amanda is caring for a patient admitted with new-onset DM. Review this patient's information and then answer the questions. T.K. is a 50-year-old male admitted after he saw his physician for complaints of fatigue, frequent and excessive thirst, and frequent urination. A fingerstick glucose performed in the office was greater than 400. T.K. was immediately admitted. The rest of his information is as follows:

PMH:
- Mild depression
- HTN
- Family history of CAD—father had myocardial infarction at the age of 50

PSH:
- Left inguinal herniorrhaphy 20 years ago
- Tonsillectomy as a child

Medications:
- ASA 81 mg chewable daily
- Lisinopril 10 mg daily
  Current vital signs:
- BP 166/74
- HR 88
- Resp. 20
- O_2 saturation on room air 99%

Abnormal laboratory test results:

- Glucose 430 mg/dL
- Creatinine 1.6 mg/dL
- Potassium 5.6 mEq/L
- Urine ketones positive

On assessment, Amanda finds that T.K. is anxious. He states, "I don't feel that bad and do not know why I'm here. My doctor told me I have diabetes. Will I have to take insulin forever? I don't understand any of this." He states that he feels no pain but does have a slight frontal headache and his vision is blurry. He also feels fatigued and just wants to sleep. Additional assessment findings are:

- Patient is alert and oriented.
- Lungs are clear to auscultation bilaterally.
- No open skin areas are noted.
- An IV angiocath is in place and normal saline infuses at 125 mL/hour.
- Abdomen is soft and nontender with normoactive bowel sounds times four.
- Both feet are slightly cool to touch.
- Bilateral pedal pulses are palpable but weak.

   a. Create a problem list for this patient.
   b. What are at least three nursing diagnoses for this patient?
   c. How will they lead to nursing care actions?
   d. What are T.K.'s needs that should take priority in the short term?
   e. What needs are more long term?
   f. Review the concept map in **Figure 7-80** dealing with T.K.'s anxiety. Complete the concept map, adding the appropriate descriptive phrases and shapes as needed to address all problems/concerns. A few entries have been inserted to get you started. Add as many shapes as needed to complete the concept map so that all needs are addressed.

6. Steve is reviewing his patient's chart prior to the start of his clinical day. His goal is to identify and differentiate between this patient's actual and potential problems. Read through the patient information and help Steve to identify them.

   L.R. has been admitted with a fractured left ankle. She awakened during the night to use the bathroom but became dizzy making her way there. She held onto the wall for support and felt better after 1–2 minutes. On her return to bed, she tripped over a rug in the hallway, twisting her ankle on the way down. L.R. was unable to stand back up and, because she lives alone, had to crawl and find her way to the phone in the dark to call 911. Ambulance personnel had to break in to attend to her and found L.R. to be alert and oriented with stable vital signs. Her left ankle was edematous and extremely sensitive to touch. An x-ray in the emergency room showed a fracture. L.R. is NPO for an open reduction and internal fixation later today.

   L.R.'s PMH includes: HTN, hypothyroidism, and three previous falls within the past year requiring admission. Past workups for the dizziness were

Figure 7-80 **Completing a concept map with a specific focus.**

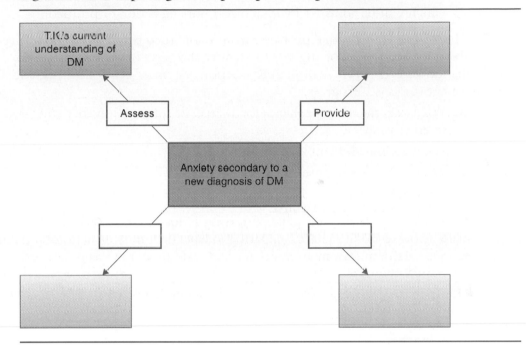

inconclusive. Her medications include metoprolol (Lopressor) 50 mg twice daily and levothyroxine (Synthroid) 50 mcg daily.

a. Use the chart below to make a problem list for L.R. Begin with each problem and add a rationale for why you have identified it as a problem or concern. You may need to add rows.

Patient Problem/Concern	Rationale

b. Now you need to compare and contrast the items on the list to differentiate between the actual and potential problems. Make a second chart for this purpose and include your rationales for placing them in either category.

c. Identify which problems will be addressed through a physician order and which will be addressed with a direct nursing action or protocol.

7. Choose one of the actual problems from Case Study 6 and write a narrative note about it. Use the following key to identify the parts of your note: **I/E** = information or event; **A** = action; **AR** = action response; **F** = follow up; and **PR** = patient response/progress.

   a. What was the main problem, focus area, or information that your note centered around?

   b. What actions did you take to address it?

   c. What was the response to those actions?

   d. How did you or would you plan to follow up on the patient's progress?

8. Using Case Study 6, make a list of nursing actions for this patient. Use the template below to make a chart comparing independent nursing actions and nursing actions originating from a physician order. Add more rows as necessary.

Independent Nursing Action	Action Secondary to Physician Order

9. Eugenia has constructed a concept map on nursing actions related to her patient's diagnosis of peripheral vascular disease (PVD). The example is in **Figure 7-81**.

   a. Reflect on this concept map. Does it demonstrate a link between theory and applied knowledge?

   b. What depth of critical thinking does it demonstrate?

   c. Does this concept map adequately reflect the nursing process? Why or why not?

   d. How does this map reflect and demonstrate the process of relationship analysis?

   e. Does this concept map demonstrate adequate knowledge about PVD?

Figure 7-81 Using reflection to evaluate critical thinking.

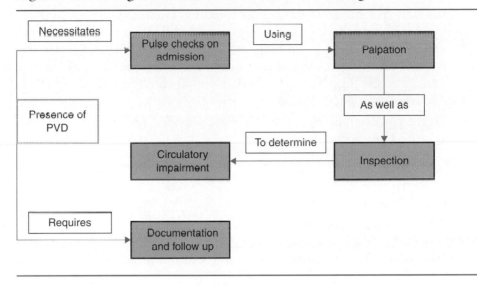

10. You have admitted a 60-year-old male with a diagnosis of upper GI bleed. He reported to the ED after experiencing two episodes of vomiting bright red blood. He states he felt "woozy" after the second time he vomited. He drove himself to the ED. His assessment findings and medical history are as follows:

Assessment
- Alert and oriented
- Odor of alcohol on the patient's breath
- Cooperative but slightly restless
- Lung sounds slightly coarse in both bases posteriorly
- Moves all extremities with slight tremor noted
- Abdomen soft and nontender, but slightly distended
- Bowel sounds are normal in all four quadrants
- Skin is intact without open areas
- Vital signs are stable except his blood pressure which is 188/98

Social History
- Divorced and lives alone but has a girlfriend
- Drinks 1.5 cases of beer daily
- Unemployed—is on medical disability for "a back problem"
- Smokes 1 pack of cigarettes per day
- States he does not have a physician and practices no health maintenance
- States he has never been to a detox center

Additional Information

Currently the patient is not having any bleeding. He denies any abdominal pain or cramping. He states he is only slightly nauseated. He remains restless with slight tremors in his extremities and keeps asking where his girlfriend is. He is ordered to have two units of packed red cells infused for a hemoglobin of 7 and a hematocrit of 28%. His liver function studies are all elevated and his CXR indicates possible aspiration pneumonia.

a. Create a problem list using the template provided and the following categories of related problems:
  - Actual problems
  - Anticipated problems
  - Collaborative problems
  - Psychosocial problems

Actual	Anticipated	Collaborative	Psychosocial

b. Use lines to draw problems that are linked across various categories.

c. List all the nursing actions required for the patient's main diagnosis of GI bleed and the other abnormal physical findings.

d. Create five nursing diagnoses for this patient.

e. How will the use of differential diagnoses factor into this patient's care?

WWW   For a full suite of assignments and additional learning activities, use the access code located in the front of your book to visit this exclusive website: **http://go.jblearning.com/schmehl.** If you do not have an access code, you can obtain one at the site.

References

Albanese, M. P., Evans, D. A., Schantz, C. A., Bowen, M., Disbot, M., Moffa, J. S., . . . Polomano, R. C. (2010). Engaging clinical nurses in quality and performance improvement activities. *Nursing Administration Quarterly, 34*(3), 226–245.

Amerson, R. (2010). The impact of service-learning on cultural competence. *Nursing Education Perspectives, 31*(1), 18–22.

Brown, R., Feller, L., & Benedict, L. (2010). Reframing nursing education: The Quality and Safety Education for Nurses Initiative. *Teaching & Learning in Nursing, 5*(3), 115–118.

Carlson, E., Catrambone, C., Oder, K., Nauseda, S., Fogg, L., Garcia, B., . . . Llewellyn, J. (2010). Point-of-care technology supports bedside documentation. *The Journal of Nursing Administration, 40*(9), 360–365.

Chan, E. A., Chi, S. P. M., Ching, S., & Lam, S. K. S. (2010). Interprofessional education: The interface of nursing and social work. *Journal of Clinical Nursing, 19*(1–2), 168–176.

Cornell, P., Herrin-Griffith, D., Keim, C., Petschonek, S., Sanders, A. M., D'Mello, S., . . . Shepherd, G. (2010). Transforming nursing workflow, part 1: The chaotic nature of nurse activities. *The Journal of Nursing Administration, 40*(9), 366–373.

Cornell, P., Riordan, M., & Herrin-Griffith, D. (2010). Transforming nursing workflow, part 2: The impact of technology on nurse activities. *The Journal of Nursing Administration, 40*(10), 432–439.

Gilliss, C. L. (2010). On interdisciplinarity and why it matters . . . A lesson from primary care. *Nursing Outlook, 58*(3), 119–121.

Jarzemsky, P., McCarthy, J., & Ellis, N. (2010). Incorporating quality and safety education for nurses competencies in simulation scenario design. *Nurse Educator, 35*(2), 90–92.

Johansson, B., Fogelberg-Dahm, M., & Wadensten, B. (2010). Evidence-based practice: The importance of education and leadership. *Journal of Nursing Management, 18*(1), 70–77.

Macdonald, M. B., Bally, J. M., Ferguson, L. M., Lee Murray, B., Fowler-Kerry, S. E., & Anonson, J. M. (2010). Knowledge of the professional role of others: A key interprofessional competency. *Nurse Education in Practice, 10*(4), 238–242.

Melnyk, B. M., Fineout-Overholt, E., Stillwell, S. B., & Williamson, K. M. (2010). Evidence-based practice: Step by step. The seven steps of evidence-based practice: Following this progressive, sequential approach will lead to improved health care and patient outcomes. *American Journal of Nursing, 110*(1), 51–53.

Nemeth, L. S., & Wessell, A. M. (2010). Improving medication safety in primary care using electronic health records. *Journal of Patient Safety, 6*(4), 238–243.

Sullivan, D. T. (2010). Connecting nursing education and practice: A focus on shared goals for quality and safety. *Creative Nursing, 16*(1), 37–43.

8

Other Educational Uses for Concept Maps

Learning Objectives

- Explore additional options to utilize concept maps in nursing education for more comprehensive, meaningful learning.
- Create specific concept maps as learning tools within the clinical setting.
- Consider methods for concept map utilization as an adjunct to theory.

Introduction

As you have read through this text and viewed the sample maps, you may have questioned how it would be best to use them for more meaningful learning. The purpose of this chapter is to discuss that question in more depth.

I have frequently mentioned throughout this text that concept maps are easily adapted and tailored to each patient and situation. Remember that they can also be tailored and individualized to each student as well. Whether for use in note taking or studying, adapting each concept map to your learning style, mental processing, and way of viewing information will make a concept map one of the most valuable tools you have. The secret is that not only are you reinforcing knowledge, but you are also creating associations. This aspect alone takes a learning tool such as a concept map a step beyond simple note taking. The act of creating links and associations while taking notes is an important component to later application of that theory. You are not just writing something down, but thinking about how it relates to other things you have learned and what it means to take that piece of information to the bedside and incorporate it into the plan of care.

As we proceed, you will see that the possibilities for use of concept maps are virtually endless. Use of concept mapping has recently been recognized by the National League for Nursing (NLN) as one of several effective educational strategies used to prepare nursing students for the graduate role. This chapter is dedicated to you, the future graduate nurse.

Key Terms and Definitions

- **Nursing performance competencies:** goals set to be accomplished and achieved satisfactorily for successful course and program completion
- **Clinical performance competencies:** course and program competencies to be demonstrated, accomplished, and achieved through patient care in the clinical setting
- **Academic performance competencies:** course and program competencies to be demonstrated, accomplished, and achieved through written assignments and examinations
- **Theory Rationale (related to nursing theory):** a statement explaining causation of a disease, symptom, or treatment

Nursing Performance Competencies

Placing an emphasis on enhanced critical thinking skills means that learning must be proactive. If you expect that everything you will need to know as either a student or a graduate nurse will be prepared and served to you as a gourmet meal, you will surely be disappointed. For learning to be meaningful and successful in terms of critical thinking and ultimately, applicable, you need to dig in, investigate, and question (see **Figure 8-1**).

Proactive learning means many things. Among them is a desire to learn all you can. This is sometimes known as inquisitiveness—one of the characteristics of critical thinking. Proactivity is closely related to critical thinking in that it is an active form of seeking knowledge. Other characteristics of proactive learning include:

- *Active initiation.* This phrase refers to you being instrumental in your own learning. You need to employ active initiation in all learning situations. There are several reasons for this. First, you are in charge of your learning. What you make of each learning experience is up to you. Seeking out opportunities to learn helps you to better prepare for your role as a graduate nurse. Secondly, taking control of learning will build self-confidence. The more you know, the more comfortable you feel, and the easier necessary information in a given situation is to recall.
- *Preparation.* This is one of the most essential actions to take in your quest to make learning meaningful. Where theory is concerned, preparing prior to class is a must. Coming into a class without preparing wastes everyone's time. Think about it. If you are trying to take notes and follow the lecture without having prepared, how effective is any learning that just might happen to take place? While

Figure 8-1 **Proactive learning.**

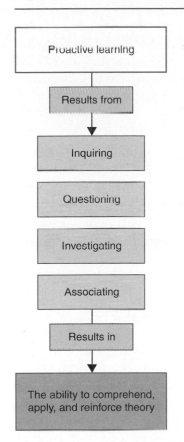

it is true that multitasking has its time and place, the classroom is not usually one of them. If you are focused on what is being said, you cannot take effective notes. If you try to write down everything that is said, you will be too distracted to truly learn anything or ask helpful questions. The same goes clinically. Preparing by reviewing and practicing commonly used skills and assessments not only means you will feel more confident and competent, but you also will actually perform satisfactorily.

- *Researching and investigating.* These characteristics go hand in hand with the first two. Because each of us has a different learning style and way of thinking, we each need to prepare differently. So, once you have taken a look at required lecture readings for class, you can research and investigate the best method for reviewing that material. Repeated exposure and reinforcement is integral to learning for comprehension and application. Using a variety of methods and sources effectively accomplishes this. The same is true for clinical experiences. To become familiar with skills you need to practice, know what the equipment is, how it works, how it feels in your hands, and how it can be manipulated. Doing so will improve your comfort level to troubleshoot and recognize what actions are required when unexpected events occur during a procedure or skill. I often tell students that although practicing skills on a mannequin is not the same as completing them with a patient, with each practice session comes familiarity in handling the equipment, reinforcing sterile technique, and increasing knowledge of what to do and how to do it. All of this is being integrated into your thought processes and foundational knowledge. When you have to complete the skill or procedure on or with an actual patient, the only part you will feel uncertain about is how to approach the patient, which you can easily work through. The rest is a piece of cake!

- *Active reasoning.* This is the process of thinking through not only what you know, but also what you need to know more about. This is where critical thinking and relationship analysis fit into the picture. It is about taking what you have learned and thinking about it in different ways. Compare it to past knowledge. Think about how that knowledge is used in nursing care; what makes it work? What is the rationale? It is about asking questions that lead to other questions and putting a new spin on things. The point is that you should always feel as if you are growing professionally. In your entire career, you will have never learned enough or applied enough, because the process is ongoing.

- *Reviewing and reflecting.* Both of these characteristics need to be integrated into all phases and cycles of learning. Another way to think about this is that on the learning continuum, from a starting point of first exposure to an endpoint of application, a great deal of review and reflection have to occur (see **Figure 8-2**). Reviewing occurs when you reread articles or chapters and when you study lecture notes. Reflection occurs during the active-reasoning process and also when you assess how well you feel you know the material—the depth to which you comprehend it. It is very much a self-evaluative process. But use it positively. Negative thinking is not a stimulus to learn. Instead of thinking things like, "I am good at skills but terrible when it comes to understanding theory," say, "I am competent with my skills. Now, I need to set goals for better understanding theory." Positive reinforcement works.

Figure 8-2 The learning continuum.

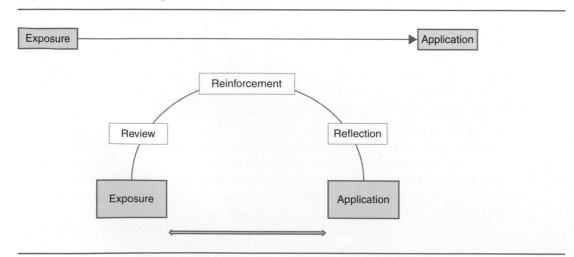

All of these characteristics blend together to some extent and are interdependent. They become a continuous process—not only with brand-new knowledge, but also with knowledge that is being reintroduced in a new way but is built on previously learned material. Much of what is learned in nursing education is progressive. Setting goals for studying, reinforcement, and application according to these characteristics and your learning style will help you to achieve success. It should be easy to spot the link between all of this and concept mapping theory. Using personalized learning styles, proactive learning, and concept mapping theory to learn for comprehension and application is the greatest recipe for success. Concept mapping can integrate all of these concepts and be applied to the following student uses:

1. Theory-based competencies
   - Note taking
   - Studying
   - Test taking/Case studies
2. Clinical-based competency
   - Procedural skills
   - Overall clinical performance
   - Organization
   - Prioritization

Theory-Based Competencies

Note Taking

Note taking is a must. Preliminary notes taken during preparation for class are a step beyond a first exposure or introduction to theory and begin reinforcing the material. This would be an ideal starting point. This is also a great time to add in the research and investigation. Depending on your learning style, this could entail web-based resources such as animations and videos or additional reading of articles and text chapters.

The note-taking format you choose should be aligned with your learning style. In addition, be sure to include space for the following:

- Rationales
- Explanations
- Connections
- Questions

Rationales accompanying theory learning, much like those accompanying skills learning, help to lend meaning to what is being studied as well as to reinforce what is learned. A theory rationale is a statement about why something is occurring. For example, a rationale for a lung disease would be what has led to its occurrence. Where theory on disease pathophysiology is concerned, you could add rationales for the disease or syndrome, the symptoms, treatments, and nursing actions. Including rationales for all of this is an effective critical thinking strategy. Rationales affect each piece of information as well as the whole. *HINT: Review the class lecture outline provided as you prepare. Format your notes from that and add a rationale section for each area covered.*

Making space for this in your notes serves as a reminder to think about theory rationales every time you study. Although not often formally included in notes, rationales are part of making links and relationship analysis. Be creative and use your learning style to add rationale sections. Once you develop a format that works, make open-copy concept map notes to use. This method is especially helpful as you receive more in-depth theory that has been built on previous information. Including rationales helps you recall past information and how it fits into what you are currently learning—a double bonus!

Explanations are a bit different from rationales. Explanations may be in the form of examples or mini case studies. They are normally a bit more involved and elaborate on the rationale. For instance, if the rationale for a lung disease such as chronic obstructive pulmonary disease (COPD) is nicotine abuse, the explanation states how that occurs. Each cause of a disease or syndrome may have its own rationale and explanation. Explanations may also be thought of as the pathophysiology behind a disease, but you do not have to focus on rewriting what the text is saying. Use this for putting things into terms you can understand and that will help you comprehend the topic. *HINT: If you are taping the lecture, use this section to note where on the tape the explanation can be found. You can also list correlating text pages as well.*

Connections fit in with both rationales and explanations. However, choosing to put them into a separate section may help to emphasize them, thus reinforcing them at the same time. It is also much less time consuming during studying when key pieces of information are easier to find. Connections can link rationales with more elaborate explanations.

Questions will surely pop up as you prepare. Ideally, any questions you have should be answered in class, either during the lecture or in any accompanying discussion. Lecture is meant to clarify material with which you are already familiar. There may be times when you still have questions, though, so dedicating a section to them ensures they will be answered. *HINT: Questions should be geared toward rationales, the concept of cause and effect, and relationship analysis because that will serve as the best reinforcement of the theory leading to application.*

All of these things are so valuable for effective learning. Learning for comprehension and application demands multiple exposures to theory sources. Considering only one source is equivalent to seeing that theory in only one way. It also minimizes exposure and negates the use of learning styles. The first exposure should occur prior to class as you prepare. The second occurs either in class or during additional reviews and reflections prior to class. Subsequent exposure occurs during review, research, and investigation. Exposure equals reinforcement. Employing these actions helps to enhance critical thinking skills.

All of this also brings out how involved notes need to be. Once you develop a preferred format and make open copies, you can record some preliminary facts during preparation so that lecture time can be spent on listening. Minimal time would then be required for writing.

I would highly recommend focusing on concept mapping theory in order to use a concept map format for note taking—it is a highly effective format for including the concepts we've been discussing. If it truly does not appeal to you, and your learning style could benefit from use of another format, there are hybrid formats you can create.

Let's look at some examples. We can use the following sample lecture outline to work from:

I. Allergic Asthma
   A. Definition
   B. Causes/predisposing factors
   C. Pathophysiology/symptoms
   D. Acute versus chronic development
   E. Common allergens
      1. In home
      2. Environmental
      3. Work related
   F. Diagnosis
      1. Skin testing
      2. Pulmonary function testing
   G. Treatment recommendations
   H. Nursing actions related to:
      1. Education
      2. Compliance
      3. Medications
      4. The home environment
      5. Culture and beliefs

The formatting of **Figure 8-3** is very simple and not only organizes the notes but also allows your mind to organize thought processes. This takes place in the cyan shaded areas, first by linking pathophysiology and symptoms with acuteness and chronicity. Immediately your mind is making a connection that enhances and accelerates learning. Relationship analysis is promoted through use of side-by-side blocks and a specified area to compare and contrast acuteness and chronicity. The formatting also helps prioritize your thoughts—you need to know the preliminary information before you can understand pathophysiology and symptoms.

The light gray shaded areas link common allergen sources and assist with considering commonalities among the allergen groupings. This can help in planning care because all areas of a patient's life may be affected by allergens, exacerbating their condition.

Finally, the side-by-side, dark gray shaded areas will allow for cause-and-effect comparison between diagnosis and treatment recommendations. Nursing actions then stem from this as part of the plan of care development. The nursing action section can easily be tailored to include holism, safety, and cultural and other standards of care. Include the framework used by your program, whether it is Gordon's Functional Health Patterns or some other framework. It may also be helpful to include the nursing process (see **Figure 8-4**). You can also include an area for care collaborators.

This type of note taking can expand the way you are able to think about planning care. All areas are included, and it is simple to create and implement. You may need to use larger paper or multiple pages for notes so that arrows and lines can be used to integrate the *rationales*, *explanations*, *connections*, and *questions*. More space allows this, and you are reinforcing the connections as you take notes. You can also make use of balloons and callouts for information you want to emphasize. Please remember to use formatting that works best for you and your learning style. You may need to experiment until you find the most comfortable format. This will be the one that matches with your learning style and your approach to learning.

Figure 8-3 Example #1: Concept map format.

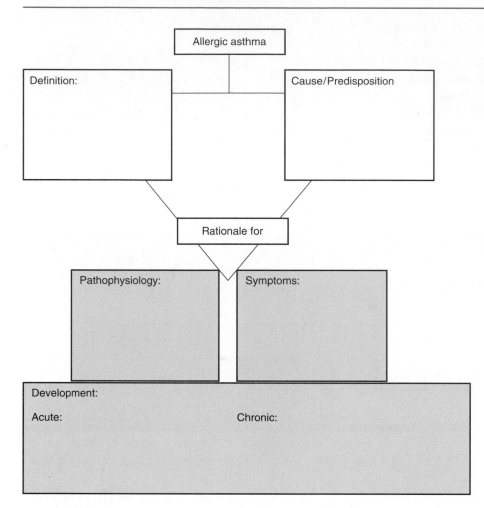

Figure 8-3 (*Continued*)

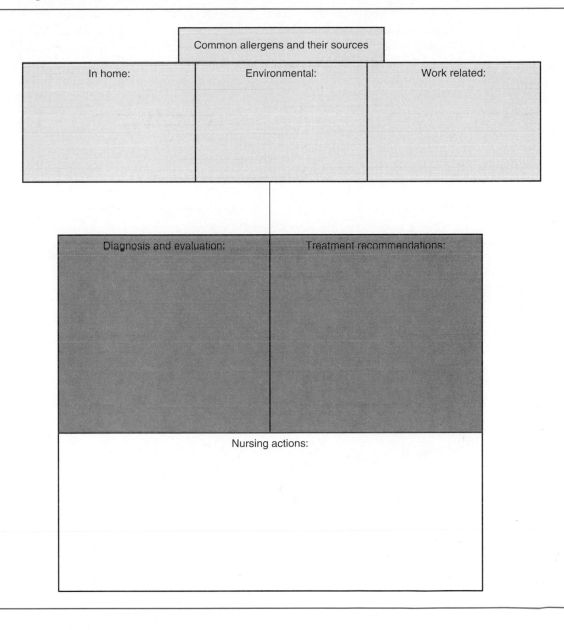

Figure 8-4 **Nursing actions and nursing process.**

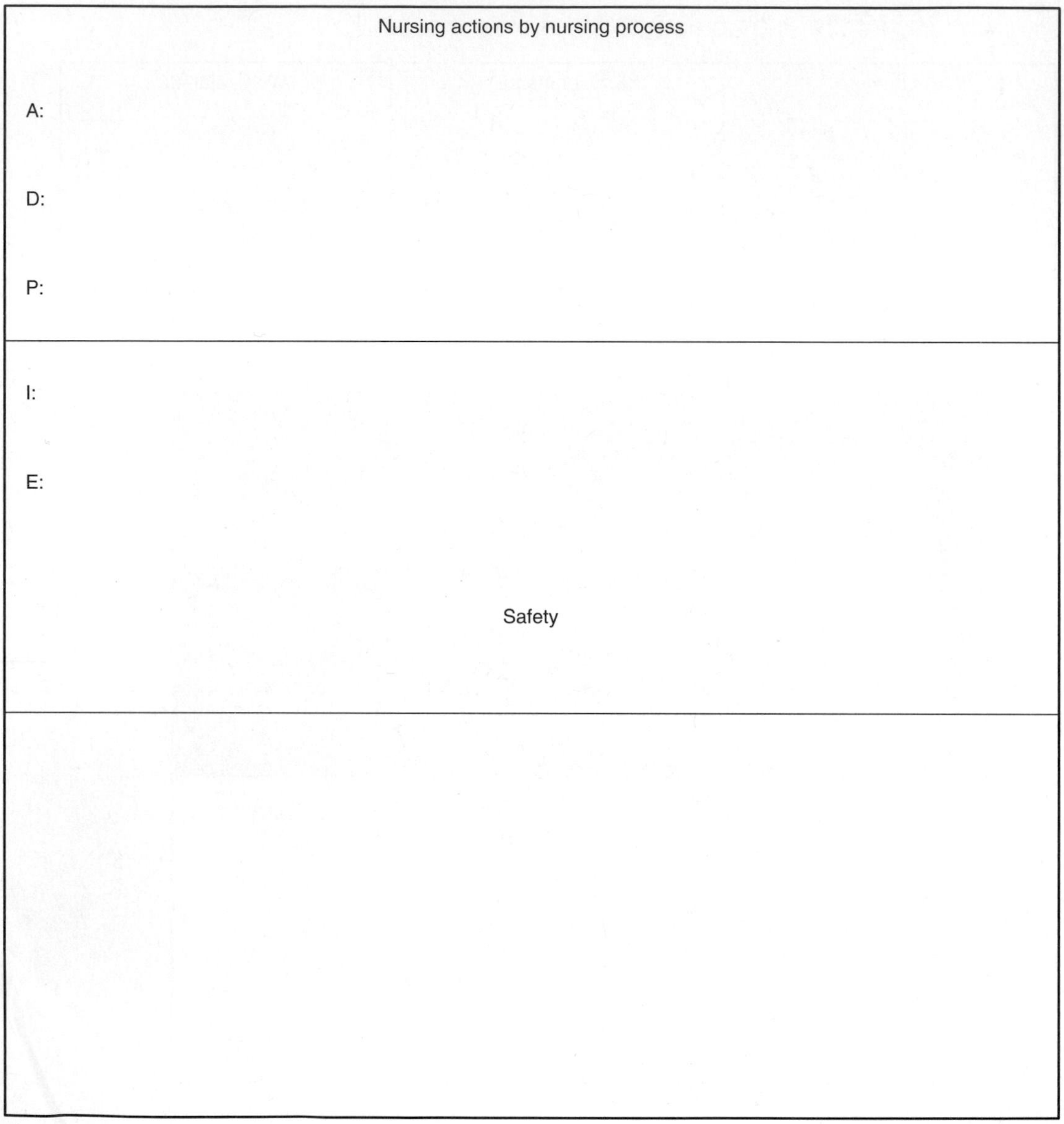

Nursing actions by nursing process
A:
D:
P:
I:
E:
Safety

Figure 8-4 (*Continued*)

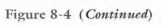

Health maintenance/compliance

Cultural

Spiritual

Condition acceptance

You can also choose to use a concept map–like format for pre-lecture note taking and then using standard notepaper to add in information presented in class. You are only limited by your creativity.

Verbal learners may prefer an outline format. **Figure 8-5** presents a hybrid sample where the outline note-taking format has been accentuated by the addition of sections including the *rationales, explanations, connections,* and *questions.* The section on questions can be incorporated into any format or left as a separate, free-standing section at the end or off to the side. For this option, use of larger paper adds more available space. In addition, you could use a separate piece of paper with a blank copy of this outline and fill in the notes you want under the corresponding heading.

Figure 8-5 **Example #2: Outline format.**

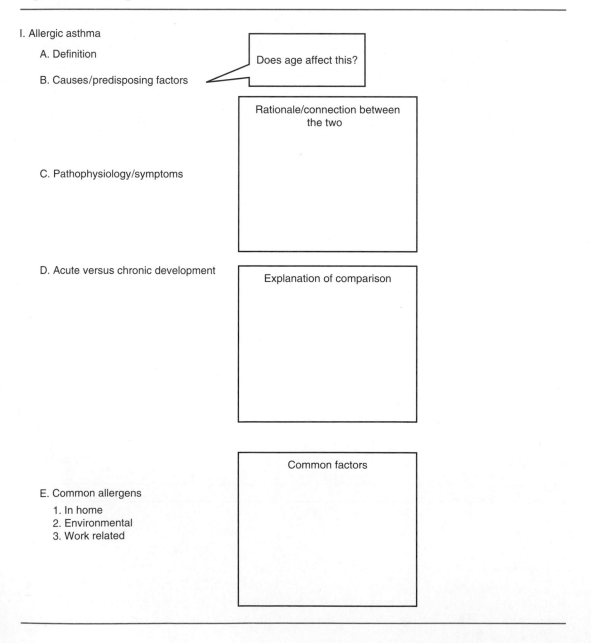

The example in **Figure 8-6** uses the least visual format. The notes section adds more room for additional information but keeps it lined up with the original outline. Another idea would be to double-space the outline to allow more room.

So note taking can and should be much more than following a simple outline. It should be an act of creativity that stimulates your thirst for knowledge and works to quench it. I highly recommend the use of larger paper so that your thought processes can flow and you have enough space to add all the notes you need without cramming. Creative note taking means nothing if the final copy is illegible.

Example 3 (see Figure 8-6) makes different use of the coded key you learned about earlier in the text. To save time when writing notes, use the key to emphasize the category. This way, more time can be spent recording your notes. The following chart could also be used as an alternative format.

Outline component	R	E	C	Q

The important point is that you think outside the box. Reflect on the way you learn and process and what note-taking format best fits. This creativity may feel foreign at first. Many students have a preconceived idea about what note taking is and how it is accomplished. It takes additional time to creatively format note-taking strategies. However, one size does not fit all, so it is time well spent. Using a note-taking format that is congruent with your learning style will make studying easier and accomplish meaningful learning more quickly. Every part of learning should be geared toward correlating critical thinking and learning for ultimate application. This is the basis of nursing education.

Studying

Successful studying can more easily occur with organized notes. Any time you have to spend trying to read illegible notes or organizing material cuts into valuable study time. But studying is more than viewing notes. Concept maps can be used to contain and clarify information such as charts, graphs, lists, and pictures. These sources may come from

Figure 8-6 Example #3: Side-by-side outline.

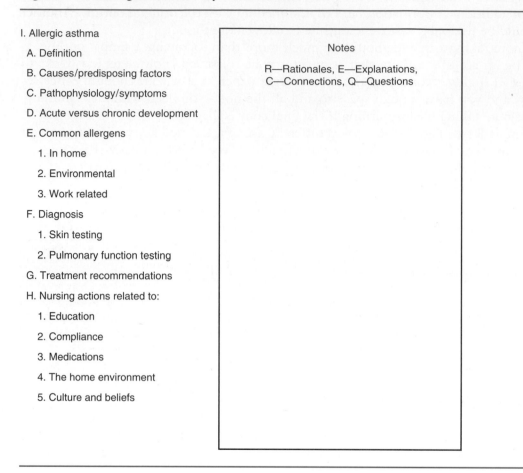

I. Allergic asthma

  A. Definition

  B. Causes/predisposing factors

  C. Pathophysiology/symptoms

  D. Acute versus chronic development

  E. Common allergens

    1. In home

    2. Environmental

    3. Work related

  F. Diagnosis

    1. Skin testing

    2. Pulmonary function testing

  G. Treatment recommendations

  H. Nursing actions related to:

    1. Education

    2. Compliance

    3. Medications

    4. The home environment

    5. Culture and beliefs

Notes

R—Rationales, E—Explanations, C—Connections, Q—Questions

handouts in class, pictures form articles, or charts from your textbooks. Placing them into concept map format may help to better explain the source itself, reinforce explanations, or connect it back to the lecture notes.

Effective and meaningful studying must come from multiple sources. This is true no matter what your learning style is. Remember that mental processing is the accompanying component to learning style. Using various sources satisfies aspects of both components. Additionally, each source may offer a different method of presenting the information, so there is layering of information for the best comprehension of it. This allows you to consider the information from many different angles. Have you ever studied something and after finishing, you did not feel sure how much you really learned? If you did not review and use other sources, you never really learned or comprehended that information. Nursing knowledge is too valuable to waste time on ineffective study methods and habits. For every bit of theory you study, multiple resources should be included. Some examples are:

- *Nursing texts.* These are often the primary resources and are listed in course guides as required reading. Fortunately, many of today's texts contain information addressing the various ways of learning. This methodology can be included within the book or as external links.

- *Nursing-based articles.* Articles can be research-, theory-, or skill-based and assist with clarifying, emphasizing, and applying theory. Articles are available in both hard copy and electronic forms.
- *Streaming video.* The Internet provides instant access to video learning, and can be accessed through a variety of devices. Video content can address all types of learning styles, not just visual ones.
- *Electronic resources.* These include websites and Internet-based programs. Many approved nursing/medical sites offer choices including case studies, animations, quizzes, flash cards, and other critical thinking exercises.

Effective and meaningful studying also includes the characteristics listed in **Figure 8-7**. These are time, exposure, reinforcement, and methodology. Time refers to the amount of study time employed per week. Currently, leading nursing educators recommend 3 hours per course credit per week. A 9- or 10-hour nursing course would translate into 27–30 hours of studying weekly.

Exposure includes review, using multiple sources and reflection on what was learned. These things serve as a checklist of sorts so that you are evaluating your learning accomplishments as you go. Every time you study, be sure you are moving through the learning domains and reaching comprehension. If you are not, it is time to try a different approach.

Reinforcement occurs when you have reached comprehension and are now studying with a goal for application. Effective studying methods must be in place to achieve this

Figure 8-7 **Effective studying.**

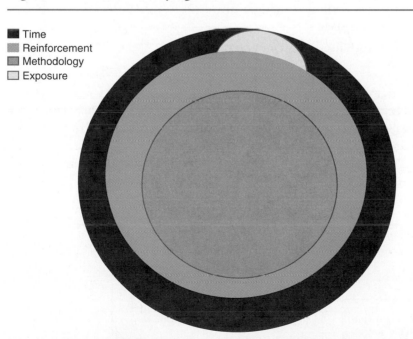

Time
Reinforcement
Methodology
Exposure

You can see that time invested applies to all studying and even includes the first exposure to the material. Time also encompasses reinforcement and the methodologies used to achieve goals of comprehension and application.

goal. Using the appropriate methodology according to learning style and mental processing ability will assist you in achieving this.

Using concept maps for studying, besides those used for note taking, can be accomplished in several ways. Other than creating checklist and question-type concept maps, you can create separate maps for various study resources to emphasize and clarify information. Let's look at some examples.

The example in **Figure 8-8** provides a starting point for analyzing your current study habits. It also allows you to reflect on study habits and take another look at your learning style. Correlating study resources with personal learning style will result in easier, more effective studying so that you spend less time but comprehend much more.

Aligning resource content with the lecture objectives and outlines assists you in setting goals for organization and prioritization. Knowledge of what is going to be covered sets the stage for planning study sessions prior to lecture. It also provides another opportunity for review and reinforcement.

Although you may be provided with recommended or required learning resources, some of these may be self-chosen. I am sure you have already found that various resources approach and present theory differently. In order to avoid confusion, use the provided outline and objectives for your lecture to assist with resource choice. This streamlines the research process and assists you in choosing those resources that best align themselves with what will be taught and addressed in class.

Satisfying the RECQs (rationales, explanations, connections, and questions) is an ongoing process in effective studying and learning for comprehension and application. The example in **Figure 8-9** can be tailored any way you choose and used as an open copy. Advantages to its use are as follows:

- Resource information is compiled using a universal format agreeing and correlating with your learning style
- Key information for studying is kept in one place

Figure 8-8 **Example #1.**

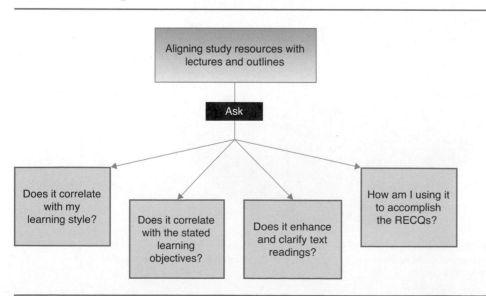

- Summarizing it means you will not have to search through resources to remember where you found specific information when you are spending valuable time studying
- Increases knowledge of your learning objectives and outline content
- Simplifies studying

As with any concept map, keep your mind open to the type of paper and format used to employ this. Larger paper provides more space for note taking. Any size paper can then be folded to fit into a folder for ease in carrying it. Do not be put off from using alternate styles of paper. A web resource can be printed out and stapled to this form if you desire.

Figure 8-9 **Example #2.**

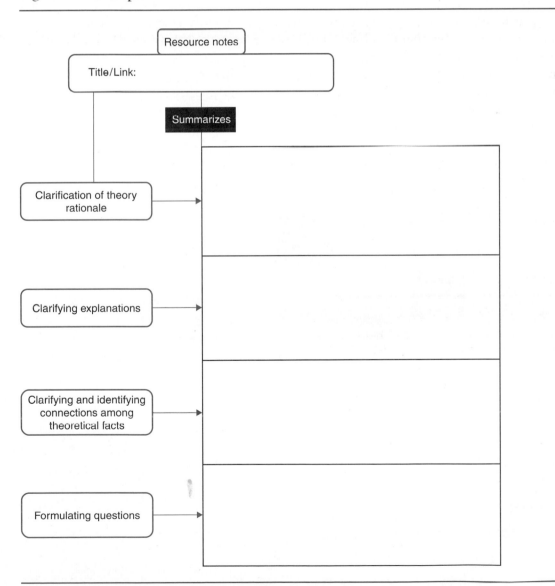

This format could also be used for web-based animations. Use it to emphasize the main points you have learned from such a visual resource. Remember, the point is to maximize learning for comprehension and application. This is the ultimate goal of anything you are learning and studying. Also keep in mind that a concept map for resources can be formatted in many different ways. Use what works for you.

The example in **Figure 8-10** reinforces the fact that all theory eventually has an impact on nursing actions and patient-centered care. Adding this consideration into your studying should help you to understand the theory and its meaning more effectively. Thought processes in this vein also assist with clinical reasoning during nonclinical activities such as case studies and reviewing National Council Licensure Examination (NCLEX) style questions.

Overall, studying should encompass learning for comprehension and application. This is ensured through using critical thinking to ask questions regarding relationship analysis. Analyzing relationships and connections assists with answering questions surrounding concepts such as cause and effect, initiating nursing actions, and creating a patient-based problem list. So, none of what has been mentioned is truly taken in isolation. As you study and prepare for testing, some helpful questions to consider include:

- Do I understand the link between lecture objectives and what I am studying?
- Can I identify the rationale for symptoms of a disease based on its pathophysiology?
- Do I understand what I am seeing and why?

Figure 8-10 Example #3.

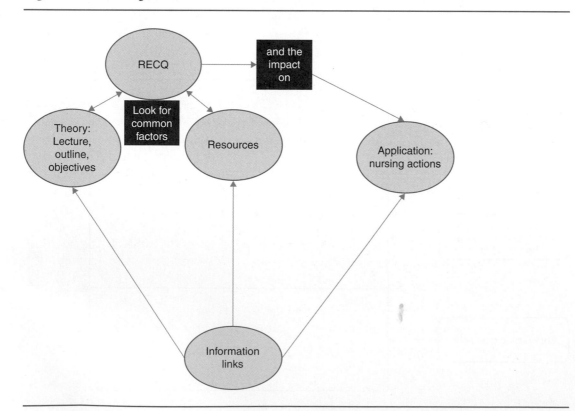

- Does this enable understanding of diagnostic tests and the treatment plan?
- Does this clarify nursing actions?
- Am I able to anticipate necessary actions?

These questions are progressive and may assist thought processes to take individual pieces of information and give them meaning in a larger sense, where application is included. You may be able to think of many more questions, or ask them differently depending on how you best learn. Each is another way to think about and view concept mapping theory and how to apply it. Progressive questioning may lead you to further thoughts regarding test success strategies, which are addressed next.

Test Taking/Case Studies

Concept mapping theory and use of concept maps in nursing education satisfy not only clinical aspects and clinical competencies of that education, but are also integral to achieving academic competencies. **Academic performance competency** is assessed through testing, and concept mapping lends itself well to use in test success planning. Leading experts in the field of nursing education agree that evaluating competency in critical thinking means assessing cognitive abilities with higher level cognitive questions. This is not only to prepare for the NCLEX examination but also to prepare students for successful practice in the graduate role. Therefore, meaningful note taking and studying lead to successful testing. Studying for application and critical thinking must be done with the learning domains in mind. A higher level question means that you can expect a more detailed question where multiple facts are presented and you will need to use application and analysis to arrive at the correct answer.

Many books are available on successful testing strategies. Although most are geared toward the NCLEX examination, these methods and thought strategies can also be used in studying for program examinations. Most address the concepts discussed in this chapter through reinforcing how to take a question apart and analyze its portions to be able to determine exactly what that question is asking. Each question has a stem, facts and information about the stem that could include distractors, and a segment forming the end of the question. This could be thought of as a beginning portion forming the basis of the question, a middle portion providing additional information, which may or may not be correlated, and finally an ending portion to complete the question. An example question follows:

A patient has been admitted with congestive heart failure (CHF) and anemia. The nurse recognizes that the most important information from the patient's past medical history impacting nursing actions and care outcomes would be:

    a. A remote history of anxiety and depression

    b. A history of stage 4 chronic kidney disease (CKD)

    c. A past admission for venous stasis ulcers of the lower extremities

    d. A history of gastroesophageal reflux disease (GERD)

In this case the stem or beginning portion is the patient's case. The middle portion is the section on the patient's past medical history relevancy, and the end portion asking the question is the section addressing the part of the statement on *important information* and *nursing actions*. The question contains a fair amount of information, but what is it really asking? From a critical thinking and higher cognitive level perspective, it is asking several things.

First, what is the pathophysiology of CHF? Before you can competently answer this question, you need to have the answer to that. This leads you to recall what CHF is, how it presents, and what nursing actions are employed in response.

The next question to answer is regarding the anemia. What is anemia, and what is its connection to CHF? Is there one? So, in addition to answering the same questions about anemia that were asked about CHF, you need to look for any possible connections between the two.

Finally, the question itself is asking you which part of the patient's past medical history has the most impact on the patient's status and nursing action at this point in time. This means that you need to have knowledge of each of the possible answers provided to choose the correct one. This would lead you to answer "b." The rationale is that CHF manifests as fluid overload. CKD can also lead to the same problem. In addition, if the kidneys are not working properly, the usual treatment of furosemide (Lasix) may be ineffective, leaving the patient at high risk for compromise. Compromise in this case could be respiratory failure leading to mechanical ventilation and an inability to diurese, leading to emergent hemodialysis. Current textbook information on anemia will tell you it is common in renal disease and exacerbates CHF.

Answer "a" is incorrect because these conditions are listed as remote. This would lead you to think they have been resolved. If that is not true, they will impact the patient's care but are not life threatening or primary problems at this time.

Answer "c" would make you question the presence of peripheral vascular disease and lead to a thorough skin assessment, but there is no information stating this is a current problem at all.

Choice "d" is something to be aware of but does not have the impact that CKD does on this situation.

To arrive at the correct answer mandates a great deal of knowledge, critical thinking, and analytical ability. This is the same type of thinking and reasoning used in case studies and clinical situations. Reviewing chapter questions, along with case studies and NCLEX questions from separate sources, helps to reinforce theory as well as the review processes used to study and prepare for comprehension, application, and test-taking competency. This is concept mapping theory in action. To solve this question and choose the correct answer, relationship analysis must be used to make connections—drawing on prior knowledge and employing concepts such as cause and effect. Overall, studying for successful academic grades must follow this format. It allows you to see the multiple factors to be considered and that from a single question, many more must be answered to arrive at the correct answer. This situation mirrors that of the clinical situation where many factors must be sorted through to choose the correct and most appropriate nursing action.

The examples in **Figure 8-11** and **Figure 8-12** are another way of looking at how to consider question analysis and evaluation. They also serve as reinforcement of the fact that the deductive reasoning processes used to arrive at the correct answer include critical thinking and concept mapping theory. Within those processes are the rationales, explanations, connections, and questions you have used during studying theory that allow you to apply critical thinking.

Figure 8-11 Example #1.

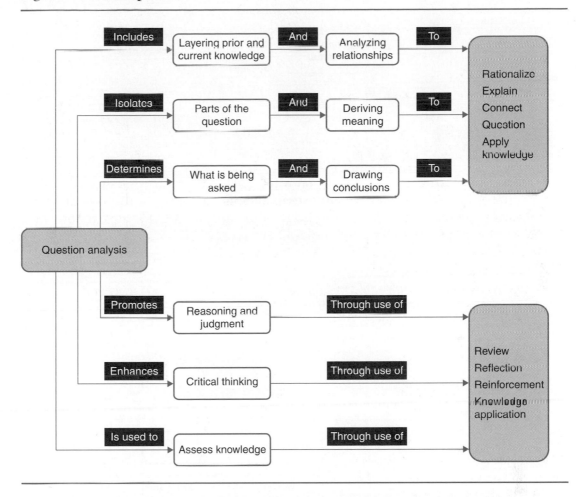

The first example is broader and provides a starting point for question analysis. Questions of a higher cognitive level are asking you to analyze and apply what you have learned. This is actually no different from your nursing actions during bedside care. Each patient situation is like a mini case scenario because of these types of questions. Past knowledge is blended with current knowledge to reason through what is happening or being asked and what nursing actions are needed. This reinforces how critical thinking and judgment skills apply to the academic as well as the clinical setting. In many ways, academic study, preparation, and testing set the stage for clinical performance and practice. Both are strongly dependent on your commitment to and your proactive participation in your own learning.

Example 2 (Figure 8-12) is more detailed. If you examine it closely, you will see that it is asking you to read through the entire question—slowly and thoroughly. This is the fact-finding step. You cannot come to any sound conclusions if you hastily skim the question. Although each examination has a set time limit, you still need to follow all the steps to choose an answer that makes sense. Prioritization is also important. Performing the analysis in order will save time, because you will know what to look for each step of the way. Strong baseline knowledge along with strong critical thinking skills cultivated

Figure 8-12 Example #2.

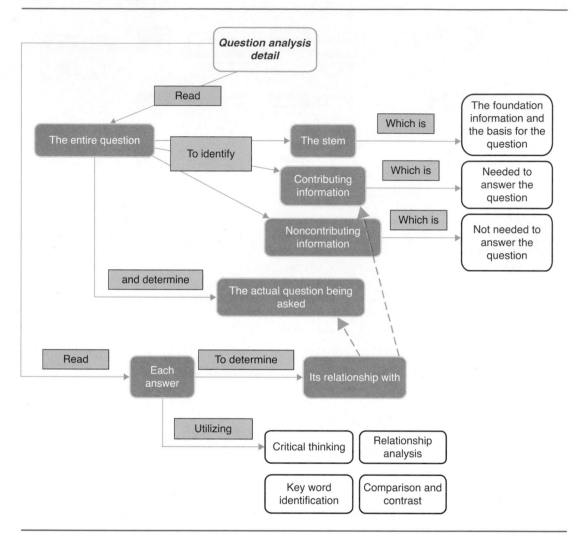

through note taking and studying will strengthen reasoning abilities and the likelihood of choosing the correct answer quickly yet accurately.

As stated earlier, use of concept maps to analyze test questions for academic success can also be used for improving critical thinking related to clinical situations because the two are similar. The only real difference is that instead of a mini case study on paper, there is a real-time, patient-related situation or event taking place. You still use the same critical thinking and reasoning processes featured in the previous examples to evaluate the situation and your response to it.

Let's look at another example (see **Figure 8-13**). This third example signifies and emphasizes the link between theory and practice. Knowledge must be paired with critical thinking and other concept mapping theoretical processes to apply it in academic and clinical situations. Although the main concern must be identified, you must have knowledge of all patient-related information so that you are able to isolate what is important in

Figure 8-13 Example #3.

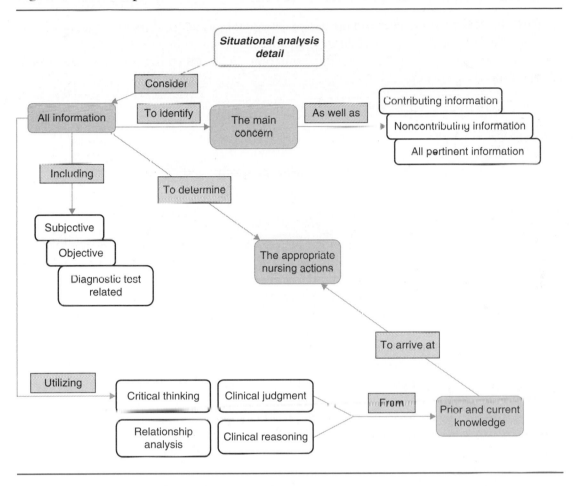

the given situation. This is where concept mapping is so valuable. Formulating a problem list identifies all areas of concern; this will help you to prioritize what is important and address it using appropriate nursing actions.

Each example we have used can be employed in both academic and clinical situations. Ideas for use include:

- Making static concept maps for use in studying
- Individualizing more complex or living concept maps for clinical use
- Laminating concept maps for ease of use in multiple situations
- Using individualized open maps as learning and reflection tools to accompany clinical experiences

Most photocopiers can shrink documents, making it easier to transport and/or laminate them. Individualized open copies can be used either during or after a clinical situation to fill in specific information. This maximizes learning and theory application.

Clinical Competency Satisfaction

In 2010 the NLN formulated and presented a national model for nursing education. The comprehensive model applies to all nursing program types and includes educational core values, integrating concepts and program outcomes. Central to the theme of the model are the following concepts:

- Safety in care across the entire healthcare continuum for all populations
- Holism
- Patient advocacy
- Maintaining practice standards in legalities, ethics, and professionalism
- Maintaining continuous professional growth and competency
- Maintaining a practice guided by the most current evidence-based research

Stemming from the central theme are three main categories including core values, integrating concepts, and program outcomes. They are summarized in the **Figure 8-14** and have been the basis of the care standards this book has addressed.

Each nursing program has stated outcomes from which all curricula originate. Within each course of the program skills, performance objectives and competencies are in place to achieve those outcomes and are normally included in a syllabus and/or handbook. In addition there is normally some type of clinical evaluation document. This document is used to record your clinical performance progress through the clinical portions of each course in the entire program. In order to be successful, you need to have a thorough knowledge of what each competency means, how it is evaluated, and how you apply it to clinical practice.

A typical evaluation form may contain broad headings emphasizing the main or core competencies. Beneath each competency would be the ways they might be achieved. See **Figure 8-15** for a sample. No matter the format, the important thing is to have full awareness of what the competency is asking for and how it is to be achieved. You also need to know how it will be determined, whether you have achieved the competency or not. Normally, a key or rubric is included to explain this process.

This would be an example of one singular performance competency focused on safety. The types of actions evaluated are merged from both learned theory and skills that are applied to patient care. As each clinical day progresses, you need to reflect on what this competency is asking you to achieve and then be sure to meet all components in the care you provide. Although it may be tempting to think you are performing only for evaluation purposes, do not fall into this way of thinking. Everything you apply to care is a nursing

Figure 8-14 Core values, integrating concepts, and program outcomes.

Core Values	Caring, Diversity, Ethics, Excellence, Holism, Integrity, Patient-Centeredness
Integrating Concepts	Context & Environment, Knowledge & Science, Personal/ Professional Development, Quality & Safety, Relationship-Centered Care, Teamwork
Program Outcomes	Human Flourishing, Nursing Judgment, Professional Identity, Spirit of Inquiry

Figure 8-15 **Competency evaluation.**

Competency A: The student will adhere to and follow appropriate safety standards in all aspects of care.			

Performance competency objective	Achieved	Partially achieved	Not achieved
1. The student will properly identify each patient prior to administering medications or performing procedures.			
2. The student will demonstrate an awareness of situations, symptoms, and assessments that could affect patient safety.			
3. The student will monitor the patient for safety risks through documentation of behaviors and recording the fall risk score.			
4. Proper procedural and sterile technique will be followed for all treatments and procedures.			
5. The student will verbalize and demonstrate nursing actions related to safety and the plan of care.			
Comments:			

care standard that you will need to maintain as you travel the pathway from novice to expert, wherever your career may take you. So, competencies play an important role in honing skills related to professional practice.

Normally, an overall statement on the competency to be achieved is included on the evaluation form. Under that are included the specific performance objectives that a student must satisfy to successfully attain competency.

Take some time to study your program's evaluation criteria. If you look closely, you can see that being able to satisfy competencies translates into having a sound knowledge base and using learning for application processes—critical thinking and relationship analysis—just as we have been discussing. Concept maps lend themselves well to reinforcement of theoretical information carried over into clinical practice. You can consider each competency, look at them from different angles, and come up with a wide variety of concept maps to use. Possible competency headings, based on the NLN information provided earlier, include:

- Safety in care
- Professionalism/professional behavior
- Critical thinking
- Holism
- Organization/prioritization
- Collaborative care

Of course, there are many others. They may also be worded differently depending on specific program and course competencies. Although we have seen examples of these throughout the text, let's consider a few of them from a different perspective. The examples you choose to create will be based on your learning and mental processing style. This will influence whether you start thinking about the whole concept and then break it into specific sections or the other way around. To satisfy competencies, it is necessary to know what each is asking of you. Basic concepts that can be applied to any competency are:

1. Planning
2. Preparing
3. Reflection
4. Evaluation
5. Confidence

These five things are very much correlated and interdependent. *Preparing* signifies feeling secure in your nursing knowledge base. You will be caring for a patient without the benefit of a great deal of preparation. Having a sound educational base allows for the critical thinking processes necessary to provide safe, effective, quality care. It allows for improved problem-solving and clinical judgment skills.

Planning refers not only to knowledge review but also to organization and prioritization. Each program will provide information on clinical expectations. This tells you what your role will be. First-year students may complete fewer skills and be much less independent than upper level students. As you proceed through your nursing education, more will be expected of you. Planning also involves thinking through a question prior to posing it. While this will help to build your problem-solving and critical-thinking skills, it also shows professionalism and initiation on your part—to improve and be proactive in learning. Questions you need to ask yourself prior to the clinical experience are:

1. Am I aware of my exact role expectations?
2. What skills might I have to complete?
3. Am I prepared to fulfill my role?
4. What resources are needed for the clinical site?
5. What type of tool would best help me to be organized and prepared?

It is all about planning, thinking ahead, and anticipating.

Reflection and evaluation have been addressed a great deal in this text. Reflecting on past clinical performances helps you to evaluate your performance. Introspection follows this and eases you into an honest self-appraisal of areas where you feel competent and those areas needing improvement. This leads to goal setting and ongoing reflection and evaluation. If you are a beginning student and have had few clinical experiences, reflection is more about knowledge and skill review.

Confidence speaks for itself. Confidence comes from many things. For you as a nursing student, confidence should grow as you progress through your nursing education. Experience and performing a wide variety of skills will build confidence. Critical thinking, relationship analysis, and problem-solving skills also build confidence. Use of concept mapping and its theory is another way of accomplishing this. Confidence is then manifested through self-assurance, independent practice, and initiation of actions. Everything we have been discussing is linked and connected.

The example in **Figure 8-16** is associated with diagnoses and situations affecting safety outcomes. You could just as easily create a concept map directed toward the following:

- Medication safety
- All safety problems you have identified in an actual patient
- Safety in communication
- Safety in consideration of care provision where collaboration and advocacy are the focus
- Safety concerns related to shift report
- Safety concerns with increasing leadership roles and multiple patient assignments

The key is knowing what objectives define the specific competency. What exactly are you being asked to achieve and how will you achieve it? The answers to these questions come from a variety of sources and situations. Program-level and course orientations provide a primary introduction regarding expectations, requirements, and competencies. Skills labs or other activities focused on clinical performance preparation normally continually reinforce and expand upon care standards and protocols. Any rubric, set of performance objectives, or evaluative tool will explain all of this as well. It is your responsibility to read through and understand each one.

Finally, theory and other classroom work are often used to address performance competencies in some way. Nursing actions outlined in texts and lectures directly reflect current care standards and use of the nursing process.

The example in **Figure 8-17** is broad in one way because it encompasses many aspects of what professionalism is and how it is defined. From another perspective, it also indicates what specific objectives might be used for achievement of this competency. It may be difficult to teach some of these aspects of professionalism, but you will see them modeled by faculty and clinical-based nursing staff. Often, networking that occurs from watching, interacting with, and listening to others provides great examples of desirable professional behaviors. As you study this example, it should be apparent that concept mapping theory contributes to development and growth of professionalism, as do other concepts: reflection, self-evaluation, preparedness, and learning styles. Everything is connected.

The example in **Figure 8-18** is another perspective of critical thinking competencies and their origins. This concept map reinforces that critical thinking is part of all aspects of patient care. The roots of critical thinking stem from the nursing process and all nursing theory. Other key points brought forth by this concept map are:

- Knowledge application in patient care and critical thinking
- Having a complete and thorough knowledge of each patient's diagnoses and history
- The standards and protocols to be applied to all patients in all care settings
- How the nursing process is used as a pathway to guide care
- The importance of individualizing the plan of care
- The fact that all nursing actions lead to effectiveness, compliance, and outcomes

The fact that one concept map can say so much is a great demonstration of the value of using concept maps within nursing education—what wonderful benefits are gained.

Figure 8-16 Example #1.

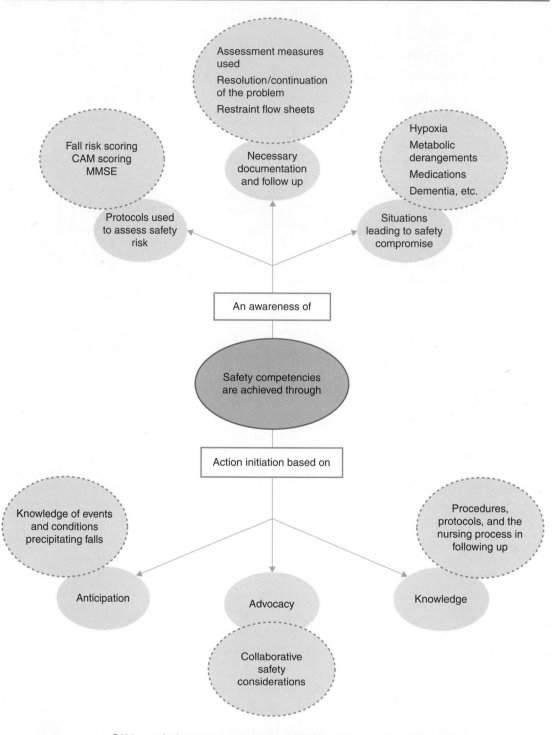

CAM = confusion assessment method; MMSE = mini mental state exam

Figure 8-17 Example #2.

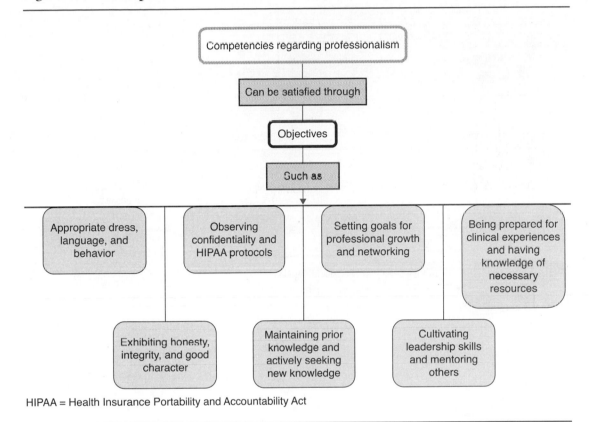

HIPAA = Health Insurance Portability and Accountability Act

Figure 8-18 Example #3.

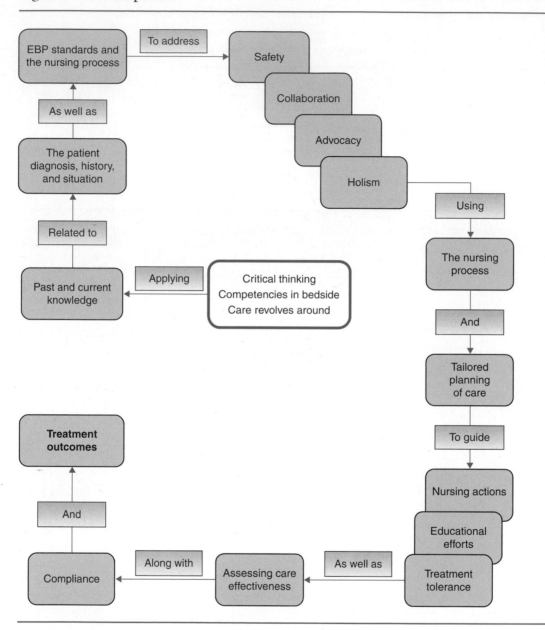

Nursing Skills Lab

The nursing skills lab provides numerous and varied opportunities for concept map use. Although the step-by-step process of a skill is straightforward, as we have seen, there is so much more to consider related to a particular skill. Nursing actions, rationales, and considerations related to skills can be applied to the timeframe immediately prior to, during, and after the skill is completed. Let's examine this area in a bit more detail.

Creating a simple, static skill-based concept map where the focus is on just the skill is quite easy. Creating these, laminating them, and keeping them with you on the clinical site can serve as a quick review prior to performing a skill. They can also be used for studying prior to any required skills lab testing you may have to complete. These could even be formatted electronically and placed on a smart phone or other electronic device as a resource. This is a wonderful idea for quick review, whether the skill is one you perform frequently or infrequently. Clinical situations may require you to perform a skill on a moment's notice. Having review resources on hand that you have tailored to your learning style will help to decrease some of the anxiety you will undoubtedly feel at this time. In an effort to lessen the anxiety in these situations, I have students follow this procedure:

1. Review the procedure either in a textbook or by using an electronic resource.
2. Think about the patient situation and ask questions related to completing the procedure such as:
   - Is there anything about this patient situation that may mean I will have to prepare an alternate plan to complete the skill?
   - Will I need assistance in any way?
   - What could happen to complicate the situation and prevent completion of the skill?
   - What is my backup plan for any unexpected findings, events, or situations?
3. Discuss the procedural steps and patient situation with the instructor prior to gathering the equipment and entering the room.

This method uses concept mapping theory in that a student must recall past learning and then use critical thinking about the particular patient situation to apply it. It also reinforces and promotes the use of relationship analysis. To answer the questions and be fully prepared to proceed, the student must make repeated connections between the patient and the procedure or skill.

So, what types of things have the potential to affect completing a skill or procedure? The following section includes some situations that necessitate forming an alternate plan for carrying out a particular skill. Basically, categories of situations requiring an altered plan can include: *patient factors*, *equipment-related factors*, and a *miscellaneous* category.

Patient factors include:

- *Body habitus.* For some skills, this factor can affect positioning and safety not only for the patient, but for staff as well. Examples would be Foley catheter insertion and wound care. Patients with an extremely thin body habitus present a concern when they are to receive an intramuscular (IM) injection.
- *Respiratory status.* Patients in respiratory distress will have difficulty lying flat for certain procedures. In addition, if oxygenation is a concern or main patient problem, any anxiety-provoking procedures mean increased oxygen demand, which may lead to rapid decompensation.
- *Confusion and combativeness.* Obviously, this situation requires a bit of extra consideration and care. The patient may have difficulty understanding what you are going to do.
- *Sensory deficits.* This could include any deficit affecting information processing. Examples are hardness of hearing, macular degeneration, legal blindness and other visual deficits, receptive and expressive aphasias, mental retardation, and

anything else leading to delayed or incomplete processing/understanding. This category could also include psychiatric disorders affecting response such as severe depression and catatonic states.

- *Cultural beliefs.* This may mean that a patient would refuse a procedure.

Necessary action and approaches in this category would include knowing all you can about your patient prior to proceeding. This will prevent delays and hopefully avert any safety concerns. Holism is a necessary action where emotional support and patient preparation play integral roles. Procedures and skills will be ordered and expected to be carried out despite these considerations, so you need to figure out ways for dealing with them. Using concept mapping theory and the nursing process, along with creativity and consideration for safe, holistic care will be key factors in your success.

Equipment

Equipment-related factors include:

- *Equipment availability.* This normally translates into timing and organizational factors because you must reorganize your schedule to perform a skill or procedure once the needed equipment is brought to your unit. Examples of this can also refer to inadequate stock inventory, not just those items that are not normally stocked on the unit.

- *Equipment malfunction.* This can happen at any time, although equipment is inspected regularly by biomedical personnel. Rest assured that this will always happen when you least expect it and when the equipment is needed rapidly. This can occur with machinery as well as "kit" equipment such as Foley catheters and nasogastric (NG) tubes.

- *Unfamiliarity with equipment troubleshooting.* Lab practice time is more about this than learning to perform the procedure. This may seem like a contradictory statement, because you may practice on a mannequin and complete a procedure step by step. However, we all know this is not the same as having to perform it on a real patient. I believe that the hands-on time with the equipment—feeling it, handling it, getting used to it—is just as valuable as actually walking through the skill itself.

Necessary action and approaches in this category include having full knowledge of what each piece of equipment is, how it works, and how to troubleshoot it. In addition, know where it is stored on your unit or elsewhere, and plan ahead for problems. Collaboration with other departments and personnel who work with or repair the equipment is helpful as well. This represents well-rounded, knowledge, which helps to make your work easier.

Miscellaneous factors usually refer to those factors affecting your role in performing and completing the procedure and can include:

- *Your knowledge of the skill or procedure steps.* Familiarity breeds comfort and confidence. Setting goals coinciding with these concepts goes a long way in improving your critical thinking, care provision, and confidence level.

- *Being familiar with procedural protocols.* This area necessitates that you ask some questions about why you are going to perform this skill or procedure. Is there a physician order? Is this procedure covered through some type of protocol? Is that protocol unit based or facility wide?
- *Knowing when to ask for assistance.* Many procedures cannot and should not be performed alone. Most go more smoothly when you have help. Taking time to request assistance also indicates advocacy by preserving the safety and standard of care required. Lack of assistance for inserting a Foley catheter, for example, can compromise sterile technique and lead to urinary tract infections.
- *Having a backup plan.* Being prepared for the unexpected and having a plan in place to deal with it is both recommended and expected.

Necessary action and approaches in this category include frequently practicing with and handling equipment and studying about and preparing for equipment and procedural troubleshooting. Any recommended approaches relate to those in the other categories. Every thought and action is interrelated and interconnected.

A simple, basic static concept map for a skill/procedure should include:

1. The skill
2. Its purpose and rationale
3. Necessary equipment
4. A stepwise procedural pathway
5. Finishing steps
6. Documentation criteria

A simple approach can be used at any level of nursing education but may be most helpful to newer students learning new skills. Higher level students may find them especially helpful if it has been a while since last performing a certain skill, as well as for new skills. Any type of action that could be defined as "skill related" would fall into this category.

It is important to mention here that throughout your nursing education, the term *skill* can also be aligned with skill sets. This transfers the term to other areas and roles you may encounter such as skills related to patient education, leadership and delegation, medication administration, communication, and so forth.

Any competency you have to fulfill will have certain specific skills and skill sets. The first example (see **Figure 8-19**) is a simple depiction of all the steps and considerations that are related to the skill. Subsequent examples will show how you can use a concept map for creating a "Plan B" or backup plan for procedures that may not follow the expected plan or flow smoothly. There are so many variations for creating these associated concept maps. It is fun to use creativity in learning. The creativity itself helps with making connections and reinforcing what is learned. As you know by now, comprehension and the ability to apply knowledge quickly follow these steps. No matter what type of concept map you create, or for what purpose, never forget the associated considerations. This is like creating a mental problem list, including the main problem, primary related problems, and secondary related problems. See how everything fits together?

Figure 8-19 **Example #1.**

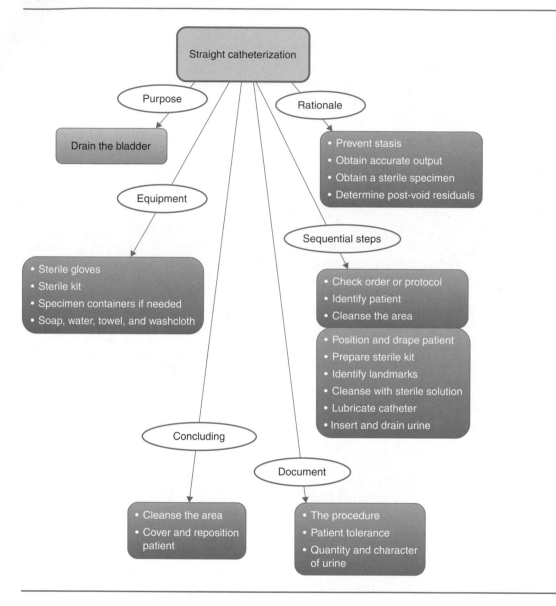

Our next step is to create examples based on the things discussed earlier; namely, those influential factors affecting our ability to complete a skill, task, or procedure. These are examples of more complex concept maps. Parts of these types of concept maps can then be blended into living maps based on actual patients and bedside care situations.

Situations such as the one in example 2 (see **Figure 8-20**) are encountered frequently in nursing practice. Any skill or procedure carried out must be approached from a holistic standpoint as far as the patient is concerned. This ensures that each plan of care regarding that skill or procedure is tailored and personalized based on patient need as well as the current standards of care. Safety and comfort should always be prime considerations. In many instances, this safety aspect is related to that of nursing staff as well. Basic concepts such as lifting mechanics and lifting techniques must be applied to avoid injury—either to the patient or to the nurse.

Figure 8-20 **Example #2.**

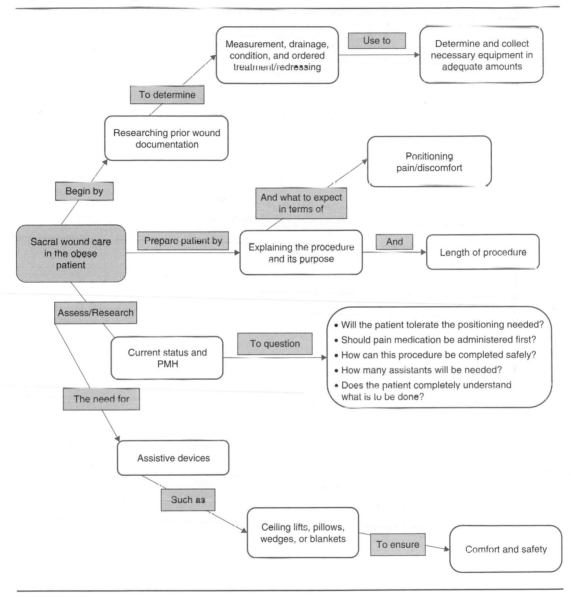

This is how critical thinking and relationship analysis are applied in nursing care. Each aspect of care, as well as the entire plan of care is carried out using critical thinking. Relationship analysis and continued questions accompany this process. Concept maps assist you with how to think through what you know—to review and reflect as well as to process and reason through that knowledge for the best ways of applying it. This is critical thinking in action.

Another reason this is so important to nursing practice is that based on individual patient situations you will need to alter how you perform or complete a skill. Knowledge of how to alter the plan of care while maintaining safety and comfort is not an ability that always comes easily. Experience and exposure help, but what happens before you have those? The answer is to have strong critical thinking skills in order to reason through any given situation. You accomplish this through using concept mapping and all we have spoken about. You have the solutions; you just have to be able to develop them. Concept mapping will allow you to do that by showing you how your mind takes in information and eventually how that information is expressed via application.

All of this shows how unexpected situations force an alteration in skill or procedure completion. That does not mean we deviate from the standards we learned, only that we have to approach and apply them differently based on patient need. This concept sometimes causes distress among students because it may be very different from what was learned. Altered approaches do not mean unsafe approaches. They simply become another method to use.

The examples in **Figures 8-21** and **8-22** demonstrate how specific aspects of as well as the entire plan of care must be considered when using critical thinking and concept

Figure 8-21 Example #3.

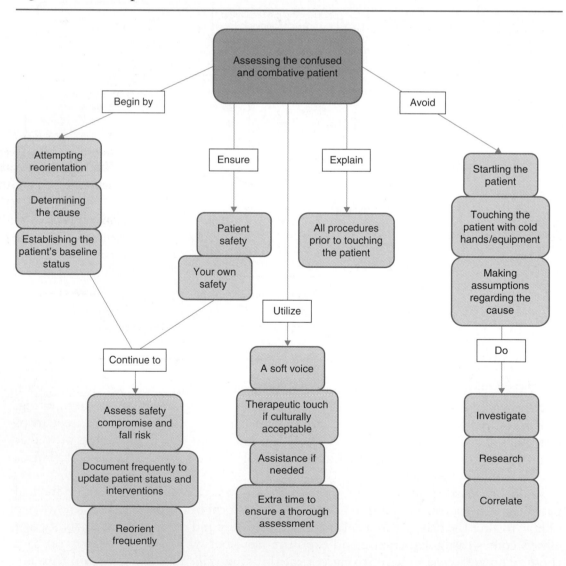

Figure 8-22 Example #4.

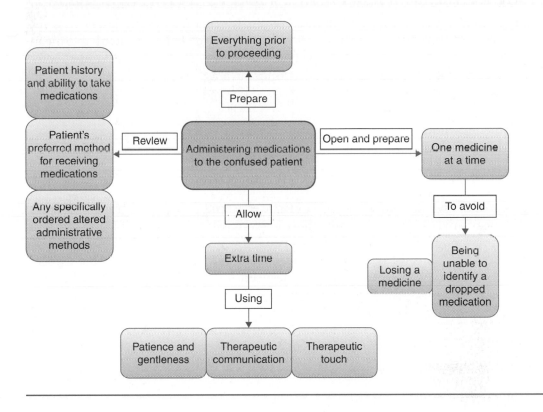

mapping theory. Many more concept maps could be created for these example patients within the patient consideration category. Some questions to ask yourself in these situations include:

1. Why does this situation dictate a different approach?
2. Which part(s) of the skill or procedure must be altered?
3. What is the best way to accomplish this without compromising safety and standards?
4. What are the basic pieces of knowledge I need to utilize?
5. What are the newer pieces I have to apply?
6. Who are my resources if I have questions?

Over time you can create more of your own questions. But what about the answers? Realize that as you continue traveling the pathway of nursing knowledge you will continually be formulating your own answers. Sometimes this happens without your own realization of it. Your brain is always working—observing and learning, processing and categorizing.

As we have seen from our examples, the first two questions have been answered in part. Altered approaches are necessary in response to patient-, equipment-, and staff-related concerns. The altered aspects or parts of a skill or procedure are dependent on things such as patient response, sensory deficits, and mental status.

Safety and other care standards dictate that no shortcuts are taken. In other words, do not omit the accepted, evidence-based standards and methods, and just utilize a different way to implement them, as is indicated in our concept map examples.

As emphasized throughout this text, all nursing knowledge has a useful and meaningful place in application. Prior knowledge blends with new to provide safe and effective care. Basic pieces of knowledge may include things such as:

- Proper body mechanics
- Sterile technique
- Therapeutic communication
- Accepted procedures

Newer pieces of knowledge are those you continue to learn or are just beginning to apply. This could mean anything from learning more about telemetry monitoring and interpretation to caring for a patient with a diagnosis you know very little about to using experimental medications. This list is endless and can occur any time in your nursing career.

Equipment-related problems requiring the need for troubleshooting can be huge organizational and time management roadblocks. Hopefully, all equipment will have not only necessary information attached to it, but also a manual on the unit if needed. Attached information could be in the form of laminated cards outlining basic operations and troubleshooting or even information printed directly on the equipment itself, which is often the case with modern intravenous (IV) pumps (see **Figure 8-23**). You will need to familiarize yourself with all pieces of information necessary to use equipment safely and for the purpose it was intended.

The second example (see **Figure 8-24**) refers to a situation that may occur frequently. Depending on the exact equipment, use may be hospitalwide or unit specific. At times there may be a lag between when the in-services are held and when the use of the equipment begins. If the company supplying the equipment changes, keeping updated on how to use it is more urgent than when the issue is just an equipment upgrade. Some examples of new equipment purchases include:

- Chest tubes
- Glucose meters
- Electronic thermometers
- IV pumps
- Medication carts

This situation may also include the use of:

- New protocols
- New orders and order sets
- New software for charting or other procedures

Unit-based educators or company representatives will normally hold the in-services and may even be present on each shift to assist staff with orientation. Another option would be to orient staff as so-called "super users" to assist in the orientation process.

Figure 8-23 Example #5: Equipment-related factors.

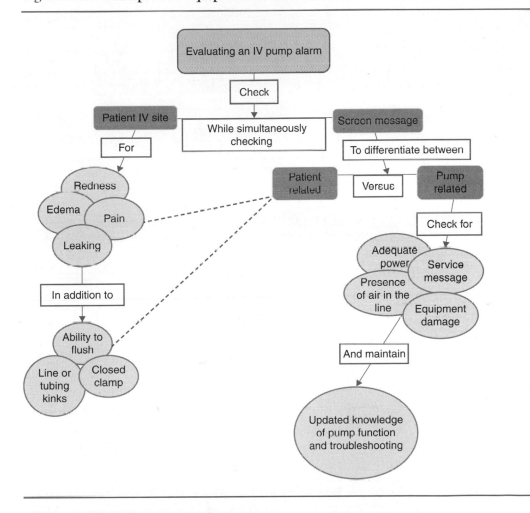

Even with all of this, you may have to use this equipment for the first time unexpectedly, so a proactive plan would be very helpful.

I encountered several examples of this on nursing units with students. In one case, one of the nursing units we were assigned to specialized in cardiac diagnoses and often received post-open heart surgery patients. During our rotation there, staff members were being in-serviced by the company representative on a new chest tube setup with electronic readouts. Apparently, a decision had been made by the cardiothoracic surgeons to use this with any lung surgeries as well as coronary artery bypass patients because it allowed for a more accurate assessment of air leaks—crucial to assess prior to chest tube discontinuation.

In another example, a student was caring for a patient with a pericardial effusion who needed to have a cardiac echocardiogram done to evaluate for tamponade. The student was busy preparing the patient for the test and hanging magnesium as well. Everything was going fine until the transporter arrived for the patient. At this time, the IV pump alarmed continuously and displayed a message saying that service was needed. The student was lucky to find another channel for the pump in the room that would work. She had to literally run after the transporter to stay with the patient until the medication was

Figure 8-24 Example #6.

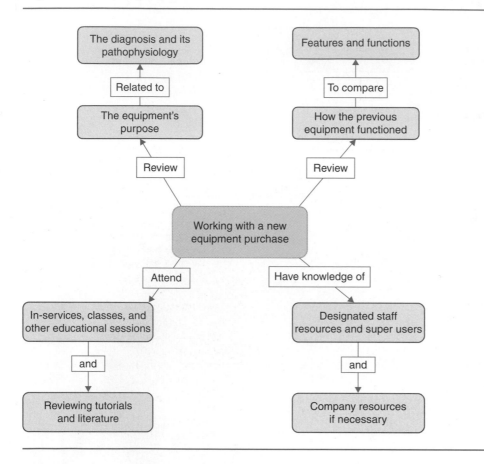

safely hung. Needless to say, the student was a bit rattled but had handled the situation well. Things may have been perceived differently had she had a large assignment. These situations and examples show that the need for a nurse's critical thinking abilities extends far beyond patient care. Anything related to patient care affects the patient and in this always necessitates critical thinking. Honing these important skills will ensure that you have a very successful journey in nursing.

Plans and Backup Plans

The examples in **Figure 8-25** and **Figure 8-26** essentially sum up the purpose of this text and how you can apply concept mapping theory in specific situations as well as in a broader fashion. Critical thinking is indicated in every patient care situation, from the simplest nursing action to the more complex ones. Setting a plan helps you to build very effective habits and practices, enabling you to be the best nurse you can possibly be. This should be your ultimate goal.

You will find that although I have spoken of applying critical thinking to all patient care situations—whether simple or complex—it is not always possible to isolate each situation in clinical practice. Often, you will need to be thinking about smaller details while simultaneously planning and executing more complex nursing actions. Take some

Figure 8-25 **Example #7: Miscellaneous factors.**

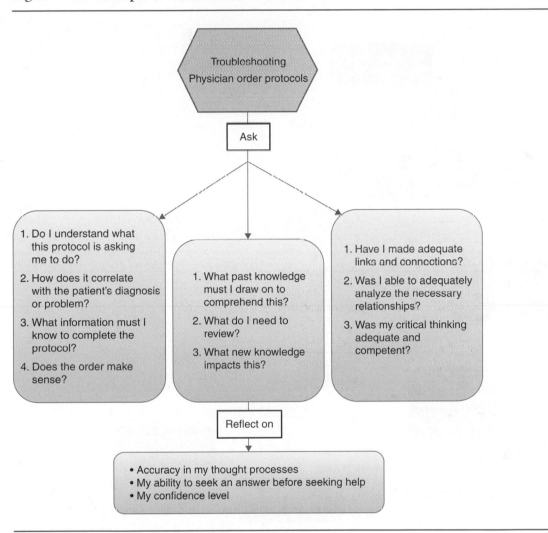

time now to review some of the concept map examples throughout the text and you will see that this is the case. That is why it is so crucial for you to work hard on your critical thinking skills. To better illustrate this point, let's consider some examples.

Suppose your patient is complaining of nausea. This seems like a simple and straight-forward problem—easily remedied with an as-needed (PRN) medication. However, you need to put the complaint in context and correlate it with what else is going on. So, you will need to ask some questions such as:

- Is the nausea occurring because of the main diagnosis or some other problem?
- Is this symptom/complaint new or has it occurred before?
- What has either exacerbated or relieved it?
- Has the patient vomited? If so, what were the quality, character, and quantity?
- What are the differential diagnoses?
- Is the physician aware?
- Are any laboratory results affected by the nausea/vomiting?

Figure 8-26 Example #8: Miscellaneous factors.

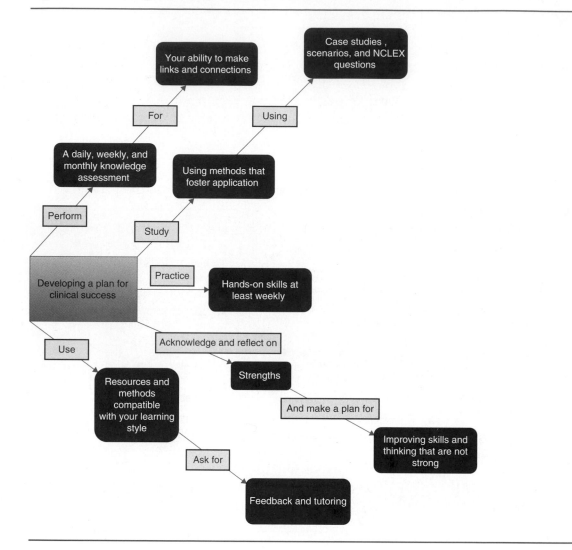

These questions directly reflect concept mapping theory and critical thinking. Some nursing actions would possibly be:

- Providing emotional support to the patient
- Providing mouth-care supplies
- Recording accurate intake and output
- Assessing for signs of dehydration
- Reporting and documenting this complaint
- Relieving the patient's discomfort
- Ensuring oral hydration
- Assessing and reassessing the patient's response to any interventions

So, from one seemingly simple problem/concern/complaint, many thinking and reasoning processes have been applied to and stemmed from it. During any 8-hour shift, these processes and actions are carried out numerous times. Such is the breadth and depth of a nurse's critical thinking. We think this way not because we are supposed to, but because we have the responsibility of lives to care for.

Let's look at another example. Let's suppose that the patient you are caring for has not responded well to treatment and is taking a turn for the worse. This change in status has necessitated calling in the rapid-response team. Now, in addition to completing focused assessments, you have to delegate to other staff members, report to the rapid-response team, and try to figure out what is happening to your patient. Examples of some questions to ask in this situation include:

- Why has this happened?
- Was the event sudden or have there been subtle clues that the patient was in trouble?
- What changes have occurred in the patient's vital signs, blood glucose, and oxygen saturation?
- What must be done now and what can wait until later?
- Who will notify and speak with the patient's family?
- What new orders and nursing actions can you anticipate?

Accompanying and correlated nursing actions would be things such as:

- Ongoing overall status assessments
- Ongoing focused assessments
- Frequent vital sign and oxygen saturation measurements
- Providing communication to the patient's family
- Providing emotional support to the patient and family
- Reviewing the physician orders
- Administering stat medications

Recognize that the thought processes you have just used for this scenario are the same ones used with creating a concept map. This is your critical thinking in action. Using concept maps reinforces this type and depth of thinking, allowing you to more easily transfer it to bedside care.

Within this scenario you see cause and effect, comparison and contrast, and critical thinking. So, depending on your learning style, this process can also be reinforced through verbally sounding out actions and reasoning using cause-and-effect statements (see **Figure 8-27**). Some examples of this from the previous scenario include:

- How do my patient's symptoms compare with a normal response?
- How do these symptoms relate back to the main diagnosis?
- How do the abnormal assessment findings relate and compare to what is happening?
- What assessment should be performed first and why?
- What communications take priority?
- How have my patient's needs and the plan of care changed?

Figure 8-27 **Types of reasoning used in critical thinking.**

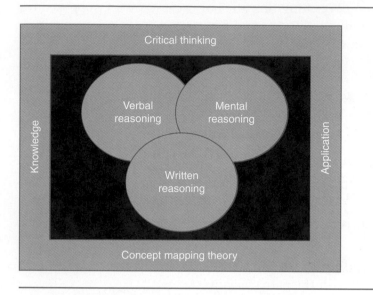

Setting Goals

It is so important to realize that critical thinking and reasoning skills are a blend of many varied processes. Using several in various ways is the most effective application with the most effective benefits. Using thinking and reasoning processes in concert with critical thinking in creating concept maps will help you to more easily apply what you have learned. Use this to set goals for yourself. Goal setting can be accomplished in several ways:

1. *Set goals for increased comprehension:* You now know that comprehension is the starting point on your journey to applying what is learned. Create concept maps focused on small bits and large bits of information you want to better comprehend. Remember that in order to apply theory, you must pass beyond learning it for the first time. Reflecting on the theory and how it translates into nursing actions will help you to more effectively comprehend it for future application. Some goals related to this might be focused on:

   • Realizing how normal physiology differs from pathophysiology
   • Realizing how symptoms are assessed and evaluated
   • Making connections between altered assessment findings and your nursing actions

2. *Set goals for putting your thoughts into action:* You have learned that nursing actions take many forms. Goals can be set focused on each of these forms. Think of goal setting as a form of reflection on your practice and thought processes. An ongoing pattern of setting and resetting goals is what you should be focused on. This correlates with your changing knowledge and skill levels. Goals focused on actions may take the following form:

   • I will use reflection after each clinical experience to evaluate my performance and thought processes.

- I will analyze and compare each concept map I create to reflect on and evaluate my progress.
- I will align my studying with my learning style for maximum success.
- Each time I study I will think about nursing actions related to the theory.
- I will use NCLEX questions to reinforce knowledge and application.

3. *Set goals for evaluating knowledge related to both a narrow and broad focus area:* You now know that critical thinking skills entail seeing both the whole picture plus smaller pieces of it simultaneously. While this may seem more than a bit challenging at first, in time you will be able to use blended methods within your learning style to accomplish this. This is an extremely important and necessary part of critical thinking because patient conditions may change rapidly. You need to be able to respond and make decisions just as rapidly. Goals in this area would contain main concepts such as:

   - Completing case studies and critical thinking exercises to compare each patient problem with the bigger picture of what is occurring (This is what a problem list is used for.)
   - Taking current theory and being sure to study it as a complete entity as well as the smaller pieces of it
   - Comparing the effects of pathophysiology of one body system to that of the entire body functioning
   - Isolating localized symptoms and comparing them to systemic ones.

You will be able to formulate more overarching goals as well as more specific ones based on your program, learning style, and clinical experiences. Concept mapping allows you to tailor your learning needs to all of these things.

Differential Diagnoses

Part of the critical thinking and reasoning process involves formulating nursing diagnoses. These are then used for specific and overall problems. In addition to this, *differential diagnoses* can also be used. Think of this process as an addendum to nursing diagnoses. While official diagnoses do lead to nursing actions and are part of the nursing process, they are normally placed into a plan of care. In contrast, differential diagnoses may be formulated more quickly and used in more rapid judgment and decision making taking place at the bedside. To better illustrate this concept, let's look at the following scenario:

You are caring for a patient admitted with fever. She has a history of chronic pain secondary to osteoarthritis. Suddenly, she calls you into the room and is holding her lower abdomen and crying. She states she has severe pain in her lower abdomen, rated 10 on a scale of 0–10. There is no information from her past medical history (PMH) or past surgical history (PSH) suggesting a cause for this pain.

In this situation the nursing diagnosis related to the patient's status change is:

- Acute pain related to undetermined etiology as manifested by patient complaint of severe pain while crying and holding her abdomen.

Because the patient was not admitted for this newly occurring problem, differential diagnoses can assist with the critical thinking and reasoning processes necessary in formulating nursing actions. Obviously, the first step is to perform a focused assessment quickly and call the physician. The focused assessment will reveal specifics of the problem as well as possible patterns that assist the physician in making the formal medical diagnosis. For instance, guarding and rebound pain may point to perforation while pain concentrated on a specific side of the abdomen may indicate possible appendicitis. So, in essence, these differential diagnoses are possible causes for symptoms. Focused assessments can lead to differential diagnoses, but this is also a two-way street. A differential diagnosis, or suspected cause, can lead to a specific type of focused assessment, leading to even more clues. Differential diagnoses have a place in all clinical situations and in fact are incorporated into code blue situations via advanced cardiac life support (ACLS) protocol. The point of this is that they can be utilized when an "unknown" occurs—whether it is a symptom, verbal complaint, or a behavior. Correlated facts used to formulate differential diagnoses can include:

- Laboratory values
- Diagnostic test results
- Behaviors and responses
- Recent events
- The patient's diagnosis and history
- Recent procedures
- Recently administered medications

For this patient's problems, you would want to have knowledge of laboratory results such as the white blood cell (WBC) count, diagnostic test results such as abdominal x-rays or an abdominal computed tomography (CT) scan, and whether or not any recent invasive gastrointestinal (GI) procedures were performed. These results are paired with the assessment findings as well as ongoing patient behaviors to provide the best clues as to what might be happening.

Differential diagnoses formed with patient condition changes also teach you to anticipate what might come next. Some of these anticipated events might include:

- Receiving orders for stat x-ray or CT scan
- A physician order for a surgical consult
- An order for pain medication
- An order for stat laboratory work to aid in physician diagnosis
- A visit from the physician to examine the patient
- The need for an IV site for fluids and IV contrast dye administration
- Frequent vital sign measurement and trending
- Using situation background assessment recommendation (SBAR) communication to report these abnormal findings to the physician

There are most likely many more things happening simultaneously as you continue to critically think and question, linking relationships and anticipating even more actions.

Actual nursing diagnoses and differential diagnoses blend together to form the plan of care and to serve as contributors to our decision making. As you think through a situation and formulate these differential diagnoses, you are following concept mapping theory by asking questions and making associations. Then, as you create nursing actions based on this process, you integrate the nursing process to complete and follow up on all care decisions and nursing actions. Everything really does tie together. This entire process is ongoing as the plan of care changes. Our actions and decision making adapt to any changes our patient is experiencing to fit the patient's needs. This pulls together everything we have been discussing. The next two concept maps are based on this concept (see **Figures 8 28** and **8 29**).

Each of these examples shows a different way to consider what is happening when a patient's status or condition changes. Differential diagnoses are formulated simultaneously with assessments, current and anticipated nursing actions, and reporting the

Figure 8-28 Example #1: Differential diagnoses.

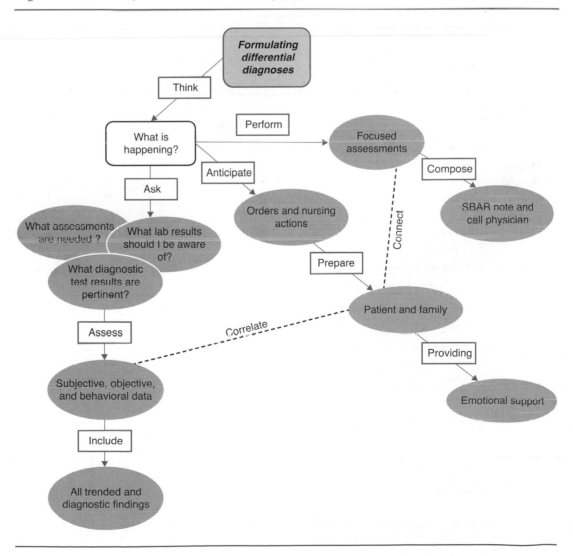

Figure 8-29 Example #2: Differential diagnoses.

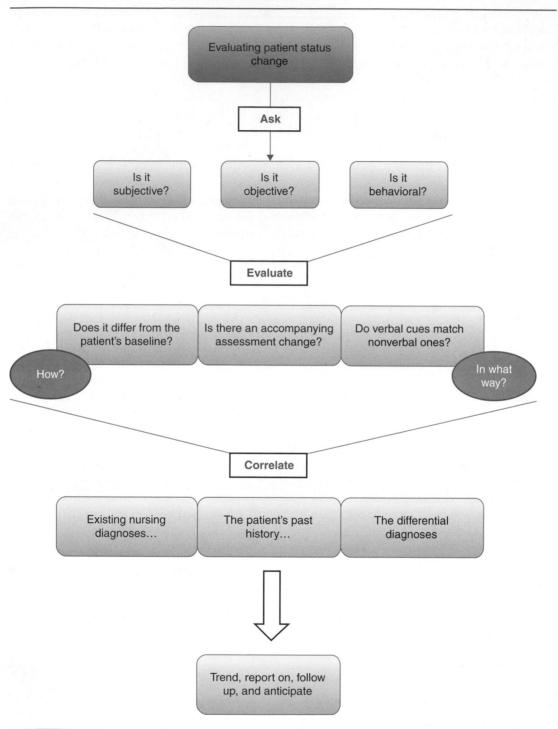

changes. Of course, along with critical thinking, relationship analysis and application are evidenced as well.

Use of differential diagnoses does not have to play a role only during patient status changes that are acute and decompensating. You use them each time you perform small tasks too. Some examples of this are as follows:

- Assessing a patient's complaint of pain at the IV site
- Evaluating subjective complaints such as pain
- Evaluating and assessing a patient to determine why he or she is now confused
- Determining how to complete a focused assessment to evaluate a new finding

In short, anytime you are comparing and contrasting, making links and correlations, and evaluating findings, all types of differential diagnoses play a role. It is simply an act of questioning and reasoning why something is happening. If we add in the concept of anticipation, we can then consider use of them as information is noted, researched, and trended. Everything we do is connected.

Anticipation

Anticipation is a part of critical thinking. In time, this skill becomes sort of like a sixth sense. In other words, there are times when anticipation is easy and relatively concrete, based on what the patient or the patient's information is indicating. In other situations, changes, cues, and clues are more subtle and more findings must be researched until we are able to recognize that a problem might occur.

A concrete example is (referred to earlier) the patient develops an acute pain and obvious assessment changes. A more abstract and subtle example is the patient in the very first stage of shock, where all changes are metabolic—occurring beneath the surface. In that case we need to link the diagnoses or clustered symptoms to anticipate undesired changes. Then we can direct data collection, assessments, and trending toward what we anticipate happening and where and how it would first appear. So, anticipation is very much an integral part of the nursing process, our nursing actions, and use of concept mapping theory and differential diagnoses. It plays a key role in completing assessments, where you are comparing expected with unexpected findings as well as in your nursing actions. In the case of nursing actions, you are comparing actions you may take with those you have learned and observed others making.

Organization and Prioritization

Anticipation also plays a role in organization and prioritization. You have seen this concept in action throughout this text, but now is a great time to address it in more detail. These two concepts play such an important role in your nursing education and a successful nursing practice. This is not only for the purpose of establishing patterns and effective ways to complete assessments and collect information. Practicing and employing adequate organizational and prioritization standards assists with the best time management practices. This becomes truly valuable and meaningful when you care for multiple patients—whether as an advanced student or a new graduate.

These two concepts can and are frequently applied to situational patient problems and the entire plan of care. You can organize and prioritize morning care as well as your patient's care post-procedure, which is a narrow focus, or plan a collaborative discharge, which is a broader focus. While we could easily separate these two concepts, normally they are considered together. Think of them in this way: When you organize, prioritization becomes a large part of how you organize. From another perspective, it is difficult to prioritize completely without having some type of organization. Let's say you are planning to change a patient's sacral wound. In assembling the necessary supplies, you mentally talk yourself through it using statements similar to these:

1. I need this many of this type of dressing, because first I need to cleanse the wound to better assess it.

2. In order to complete this skill, I need to arrange my dressings in the order I will use them.

3. First I will cleanse the area and then I will dress it.

All of these statements speak to how you will organize the supplies and the completion of the task. This demonstrates that it is very difficult to have organization without prioritization. One cannot really be applied without the other.

The concept map in **Figure 8-30** demonstrates and summarizes how critical thinking and concept mapping theory can be directly applied to organizing and prioritizing. Critical links, connections, and associations are made continually between our thought-based actions and how they are to be implemented. So, the types of thought processes we have been speaking of do not solely apply to the plan of care, patient assessments, and the problem list. They also apply to any action we carry out. Since thought processes lead to actions and implementation, the theory applies to those as well. This is where anticipation and planning play key roles. Just as we form the problem list and then anticipate important nursing actions, we can use anticipation to visualize and plan how all actions can be carried out from thoughts through to completion. Suppose you are caring for a patient in contact isolation. If you gown up and enter the room to complete an assessment and find there are no wound care supplies present, you then have to remove the gown, leave the room to gather necessary supplies, and start all over again. Pre-planning and anticipation mean adding those supplies and necessary pieces of equipment to the problem list as well. Recall that "problems" are synonymous with concerns or anything that affects the patient and the plan of care. Everything just addressed would fall into this category. Thorough anticipatory planning allows you to focus on what needs to be done. The whole process is similar to completing a pre-procedure checklist. So, before entering the patient's room, ask yourself:

- What tools and supplies will I need to complete the overall assessment?
- Are any special items needed to complete any of the required focused assessments?
- Are there adequate supplies of linen?
- Will I need incontinent care items?
- Is every piece of equipment I need in working order?
- Have I done all I can to organize?
- Have I done all I can to prioritize?

Figure 8-30 Example #1: Organization/prioritization.

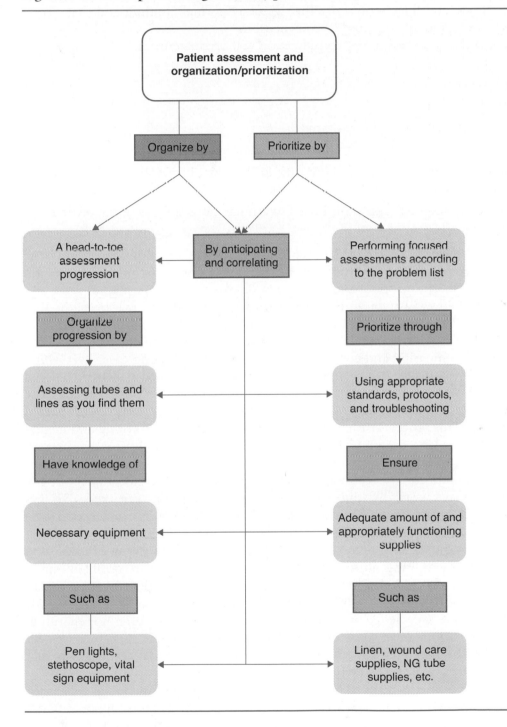

When thinking through this list, include everything related to the patient's assessment, procedures, tubes, and lines—anything that is not a "normal" finding and that would require assessment, monitoring, and documentation.

Answers to the questions under consideration will originate from:

- Shift report
- The plan of care
- The patient's status and condition
- New findings and changes to the current plan of care
- Physician orders
- Subjective statements
- The medical record

In other words: *Know your patient!* In-depth knowledge of anything concerning the patient enables complete and holistic care. Research and obtain as much information as possible. Use concept mapping and an open or blank copy concept map to serve as a data-collection tool to assist you in this process of research and information gathering. This streamlines the process, contributing to overall organization and prioritization so that you can then use a narrower focus on individual patient problems. There is that reference again—comparing and contrasting areas of focus in nursing care. Everything contributing to the patient's care becomes part of the whole but can also be broken down into smaller parts for more intense focus. This is, again, critical thinking in action. The ability to see each and every patient concern plus address it adequately is a necessary part of critical thinking. This process is affected by many things including: learning and mental processing styles, the large amounts of patient information and the ability to sort through it, and the constant flow of information that comes at you from the patient, physician orders, and other sources. Concept mapping theory and the use of concept maps are the tools needed to focus, critically think, and put a plan into motion. **Figure 8-31** lists some examples of what we have been addressing. Organization and prioritization have nursing care applications via anticipation and nursing actions.

Figure 8-31 is simply an example of some of patient-related concerns and how you might respond to them using nursing actions. Glucose fingersticks are normally timed per hospitalwide protocols, yet meal times may differ per unit. While it is great to plan for set times, be aware that the test should be performed within an hour of the meal. It is also helpful to have knowledge of the equipment used, where it is stored for charging, and how to troubleshoot any displayed messages or alarms. Many care agencies have a kit containing all needed supplies. Part of your anticipation would be to investigate whether supplies are adequate as well as to replace those you use.

A patient with a chest tube must be assessed for adequate lung function as well as for proper tube function. You want to know that the tube is doing what it is supposed to do. This involves checking the orders related to its use as well as having knowledge of what actions to implement when this does not occur. You also need to consider what other diagnostic tests impact the use of chest tubes and anticipate when they might be removed. Chest x-ray results and physician progress notes can assist you with providing that information.

One way organization is used to assess a hemodialysis graft is to plan for its assessment during the first shift assessment. This is standard procedure. Other valuable pieces

Figure 8-31 **Examples of organizing, prioritizing, and anticipating nursing actions.**

Problem/Concern/Focus	Organization	Prioritization	Anticipation
Fingersticks for glucose	Plan timing	Correlate to meal times	Check that unit is charged and kit has adequate supplies Have knowledge of protocol if results are abnormal
Chest tube placement	Check applicable orders for suction versus water seal, etc.	Follow up and reassess per protocol	Have clamp and vaseline gauze with unit
Hemodialysis access site	Assess with first shift assessment	Check for bruit and thrill before and after access Reassess and follow up as needed	Be aware of signs/symptoms of site compromise
Amputation	Have knowledge of limb affected, when it was performed	Correlate with plans for ambulation	Check if prosthesis as well as other assistive ambulatory devices are needed
Capped IV	Prepare for flushing and site assessment during shift assessment	Flush before site is needed for meds to avoid time delays	Research insertion date to anticipate site change
Isolation status	Plan and cluster care	Maintain isolation protocols	Assess need for supplies before entering room

of knowledge to have are when the access was placed and if there have been any known difficulties with it. Some patients experience repeated difficulties necessitating replacement. Knowing this normally leads to more frequent assessments as well as allowing for patient education sessions focused on detecting decreased flow through the graft.

Consider a patient with an amputated limb (I chose this example because many patients have this history). You will need to anticipate how this affects ambulatory status because ambulation to prevent the complications of bed rest is a prime preventive measure employed in today's nursing care. Ask yourself questions. Does the patient have a prosthesis? Has it been brought into the hospital? Is the patient able to ambulate without it by using a walker and having assistance? How does all of this affect the fall risk score?

A capped IV site is relatively easy to deal with but can easily become displaced. Assessing the site with the first shift assessment alerts you to any actual or potential problems and allows for alternate planning to occur.

There are many types of isolations a patient could need. Some of those can be hazardous to staff, so time of exposure must be limited. For other types, cleaning equipment that is taken into the room becomes part of your actions.

All of this sums up the statement that everything is connected and has a relationship to patient care as well as your actions. You need to put your critical thinking to work and think of every possible connection. This directly ties into safety standards and other care standards as well.

These examples provide you with more perspectives and ways to consider, review, and understand concept mapping theory and how it assists with knowledge comprehension and application.

The next concept map example is based on the following scenario:

J.S. is a 70-year-old male admitted with right upper quadrant pain (RUQ) later determined to be secondary to gallstones. He is scheduled for a laparoscopic chole- cystectomy tomorrow in the early morning. At this point his pain is fairly well con- trolled with morphine sulfate 2 mg given IV push every 3 hours PRN. J.S.'s blood pressure has been a bit labile, and he complains of dizziness when getting out of bed. He states this passes after several minutes, but he must sit very still until it does. He verbalizes fears of falling.

The PMH for this patient includes:

- **Diabetes type I.** Currently he is receiving sliding-scale insulin coverage, and his blood sugars via fingerstick have been running around 200.
- **COPD.** J.S. uses no oxygen at home but has been requiring 2–3 L via nasal cannula while hospitalized. His breath sounds are diminished posteriorly bilat- erally, but there are no rales or other adventitious breath sounds auscultated. The chest x-ray taken earlier shows no pneumonia or CHF. According to the medical record, his COPD stemmed from past work as a welder. He states he becomes moderately to severely short of breath (SOB) with activity and has not been able to make it to see his doctor in a while: "I haven't taken any medicines for that in a long time."
- **Hypertension.** J.S. takes lisinopril 10 mg daily for this. He has not checked his blood pressure at home but relies on his physician to check it in the office.

The social history for this patient indicates that he lives alone in a multistoried residence. He states that he has a great deal of difficulty "looking after it" and has been considering selling it soon. He says, "I wouldn't mind moving into one of those senior apartments where they help you do everything. Then maybe I would remember to take my medicines and get to see the doctor regularly. My wife is gone and my children don't seem to want to be bothered with what I need." He does not drive. He denies use of tobacco, alcohol, or illicit drugs—now or ever. He tells you his budget has been limited by Medicare cutbacks, and this makes it difficult for him to eat properly: "Many times I can't afford the sugar testing supplies and just eat the best I can. I haven't checked my blood sugar in a long time."

You can see that this patient has many complex, collaborative needs. Let's create a concept map demonstrating organization and prioritization of his care using the nursing process (see **Figure 8-32**).

Our concept map for J.S. stems from the admission diagnosis as well as all of the many other complex problems discovered. Because the assessment portion of the nursing process centers around patient problem identification, formulating the problem list is the launching point for your subsequent nursing actions. The *assessment* is an overall look at every piece of patient-related information—PMH, subjective and objective data, and col- laborative needs. Every problem identified impacts the plan of care, nursing actions, and

Figure 8-32 Example #2: Organization and prioritization within the nursing process.

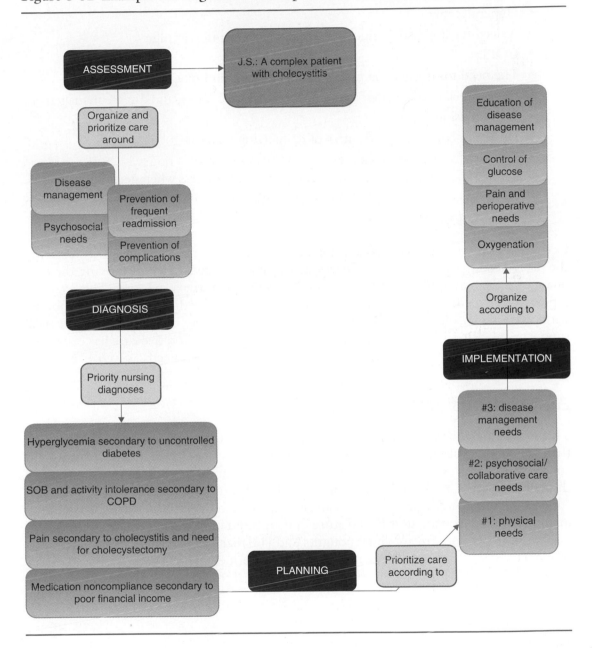

outcomes. While J.S.'s main problem or concern is the RUQ pain and need for surgery, the related problem list includes:

- Need for morphine for pain control
- Complaints of dizziness and postural hypotension
- Increased fall risk
- Labile blood pressure
- Verbalized fears of falling

- Diabetes type I
- Hyperglycemia
- A need for fingerstick glucose readings and insulin coverage
- COPD
- The need for oxygen via nasal cannula to maintain oxygen saturation
- Educational needs related to medications, disease states, and disease management
- Hypertension
- Difficulty completing activities of daily living (ADLs)
- Inability to care for his home
- Lack of a support system
- Inadequate health maintenance/management
- Social isolation

Certain associations quickly become apparent and can be grouped together. Clustering the related concepts by making connections and associations aids in prioritizing the next phase of the nursing process. Organization is occurring at the same time. This example typifies most medical-surgical patients today. Coexistent medical diagnoses combined with psychosocial and educational needs take priority in nursing care. Family and financial support are lacking in many situations, and the need for collaborative care has expanded greatly. Holism is a necessary ingredient in meeting all patient needs as well.

Associations and Connections

This section details the associations and connections you should be making as you plan the care for this patient. It may help to create categories under which the problems and concerns fall. This is another type of associating you can use. Another way to think of this entire process, meaning formulating the plan of care using the nursing process and concept mapping, is as a process of visualization. Whenever you think through a plan, no matter the stage, you are getting a picture in your mind of how to proceed. The concept map and the plan of care are your thoughts and visualizations on paper. Another way to think of concept mapping and the nursing process is as mental processing tools and extensions of thought processes—the results of your critical thinking and decision making.

Association Categories

Physical Problems/Concerns

Cholecystitis	Pain
	Need for pain medication
	Morphine-associated hypotension & dizziness
	Increased fall risk
	Labile blood pressure
	Orthostatic hypotension
	Need for surgical intervention

Disease-Related Problems/Concerns

COPD	Need for oxygen
	Dyspnea
	Altered oxygen saturation
	Need for COPD management
Diabetes type I	Hyperglycemia
	Need for insulin coverage
	Need for fingerstick glucose monitoring
Hypertension	Need for blood pressure monitoring
	Risk for not receiving medications because of current hypotension

Psychosocial/Collaborative Problems/Concerns

Physical activity intolerance	Inability to drive
	Inability to access health care
	Altered ability to complete ADLs
	Inadequate health maintenance
	Inability to live independently
Lack of a support system	**Social isolation**
	Need for altered living environment
	Need for social service/case management services

Educational Needs/Concerns

In-patient	Pain management
	Surgical procedure: pre-, intra-, & postoperative phases/management
	Blood pressure management
	Fall risk prevention
	Actions taken to address fears
	Diabetes management
	Disease processes
	Oxygen therapy
	Medications
	Physical activity planning/limitations
	Collaborator roles & responsibilities

(Continues)

Educational Needs/Concerns (Continued)

In-patient	Pain management
Out-patient/follow up	Importance of health maintenance
	Medication use, management, affordability
	Disease management—support groups
	Post-surgical care
	Pain management
	Complication & symptom management

Once you have this information, it is much simpler to make even more connections and associations. Many of the categories blend and overlap so that our actions must mirror this process. All of this now leads to formation of nursing diagnoses and use of differential diagnoses that will lead to actual nursing actions. Nursing diagnoses themselves create associations with the patient problem list so that use and understanding of nursing knowledge is reinforced.

You have no doubt realized that some problems stem from medical needs and necessitate physician management and collaboration. These problems may not seem to fit into nursing diagnosis categories. They are truly collaborative problems. Although they might not fit the nursing diagnosis template, they require nursing actions provided for in the plan of care. They will have links to NANDA-approved nursing diagnoses. The *diagnosis* phase is simply a continuation of the assessment phase where identification of the patients' problems plays a key role.

You now know that *planning* involves using concept mapping to address or plot out how all problems will be addressed through specific nursing actions. This is a goal-setting phase where short-term, acute care needs are addressed. In addition, long-term goals can be set to address post-acute care needs. You always need to consider and include the entire healthcare continuum because this is also an integral part of collaborative and holistic care. In the case of J.S., short-term goals managed through the application of nursing actions would include:

1. **Control pain.** This includes all pain, and in this case that includes preoperative and postoperative pain.

2. **Preoperative preparation.** Patient education is completed in collaboration with the physician and anesthesiologist. Educational needs must be nursing action based as well as medical-treatment based.

3. **Maintaining adequate oxygenation.** A history of untreated COPD indicates higher surgical risk and possible complications. Planning and goal setting need to include anticipation of complications.

4. **Maintain diabetic control with insulin coverage.** This includes setting goals for anticipating hyperglycemia and monitoring the patient for hyperglycemia but also hypoglycemia.

5. **Decreasing fall risk.** This is currently associated with use of morphine for pain control and may continue into the postoperative period. Any significant blood loss leading to hypovolemia during surgery would exacerbate this.

6. **Anticipating hypertension.** J.S. has labile blood pressure readings and is not exhibiting hypertension. Nevertheless, you must anticipate the possibility of hypertension if blood pressure medications are held or severe pain leads to higher readings.

7. **Assisting the patient with activity management.** These goals are based on the patient's difficulties carrying out ADLs due to shortness of breath. Additionally, the patient's pain and postoperative status will impact this.

8. **Prevention of complications.** In addition to complications from existing diseases and surgery, you will need to prevent bed rest complications for J.S.

9. **Addressing psychosocial needs.** J.S. has multiple collaborative care needs in this area.

You may be able to think of additional goals and planning objectives for nursing care of this patient. Remember to research all resources at your disposal.

Implementation

Implementation is the phase in which nursing actions are put into practice or applied. After discussing this in some detail, we can create concept maps demonstrating nursing actions. To provide effective care standards, you need to create thorough and complete nursing actions. Each problem must be identified and addressed so that nursing actions exist for all of them. In addition, nursing actions must follow up and follow through on problems. This means that a single nursing action is not enough. Most problems require multiple or multiple-step nursing actions. Ongoing repeat assessments and monitoring are required for many types of patient problems. Questions to ask yourself during this phase can include:

1. Can this problem be solved easily with only one nursing action?
   - What about the problem necessitates more than one nursing action?
   - How must these nursing actions be carried out?
   - What collaborative component exists with the problem or concern?

Obviously, there are many more that must be determined for each unique patient situation. All of the problems for J.S. will require multiple nursing actions. His chronic disease states have the potential for causing a status change and must have ongoing monitoring. The patient's age and baseline health status make the likelihood of complications and/or altered responses greater, which also intensifies care along with the type and number of focused assessments required.

Now, let's create small concept maps that isolate this patient's needs. The first two examples (see **Figures 8-33** and **8-34**) demonstrate how problems and the nursing actions used to address them overlap. In the first example, one of the main factors to address and control is the patient's pain. That goal will not be totally effective, however, unless you also address the patient's symptomatic hypotension. Critical thinking is clearly demonstrated when this is made part of the concept map. Advocacy and anticipation, as well as collaborative actions, are also clearly demonstrated. A concept map for an actual patient will contain factual information and data, actual or anticipated nursing actions,

Figure 8-33 Example #1.

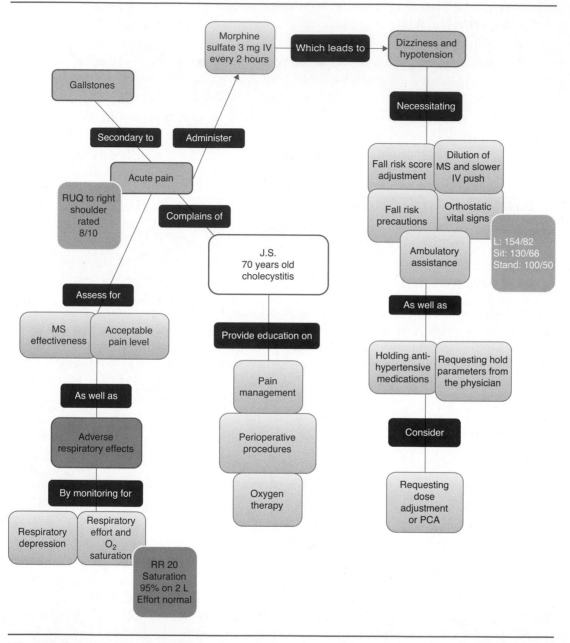

MS = Morphine, PCA = patient controlled analgesia

and follow up necessary to completely assess and evaluate any problem. You can also include alternate but acceptable actions to take, such as administering the morphine sulfate. Options to dilute a medication to be administered via IV push can be found in accepted nursing resources and are sometimes mandated as part of a unit or facility protocol. In the case of J.S., rapid or undiluted administration of the morphine may exacerbate symptoms and lead to complications.

The second concept map would become part of the entire concept map for this patient. What has been created is a small part of what would need to be included if you

Figure 8-34 Example #2.

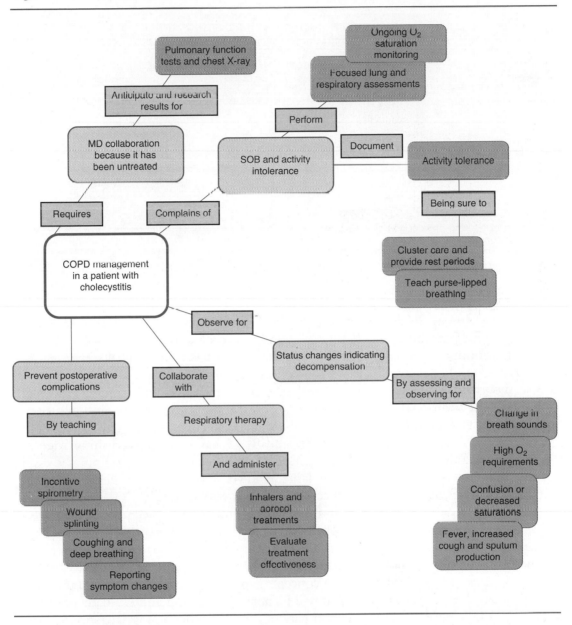

were to address every problem or concern. Although concept map assignments such as this can become quite large, they are most effective at reinforcing theory, stimulating and demonstrating critical thinking, and allowing for reflection and self-evaluation.

Please keep in mind that your own concept map for a patient such as this would be uniform in color and no doubt a bit more symmetrical. Many student concept maps I have seen cluster categories of like information together in sections. See **Figure 8-35**. This accomplishes several things. First, it allows you to organize your thoughts. From that point, you can then prioritize. This method also allows for some room to include all necessary information. It also makes use of white space in a way that aids in interpretation

Figure 8-35 **Common student concept map template.**

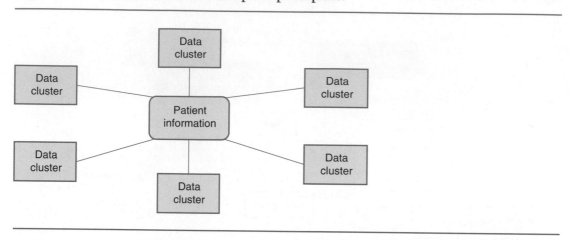

of the concept map. Each student's approach is individualized and slightly different, depending on what learning style is present and how problems are processed.

In this common example, each problem the patient has would have its own section. Clustered around that would be related concepts, nursing actions, and outcomes. Of course, descriptive phrases and all necessary concept map components would be included, along with any additional lines linking associations. If this example is helpful, please feel free to use it. However, be sure to use it only if it is congruent with your learning style.

The two examples in **Figures 8-36** and **8-37** have pulled everything together and have also considered legalities and ethics. You can see that when you put the entire concept map together it would be quite large. And yet, it contains all necessary information and effectively demonstrates concept mapping theory through critical thinking and relationship analysis. Lines, color, and descriptive phrases have been utilized in a way that allows for easy interpretation of the concept map—establishing connections and links. Each concept map tells a part of the story about who this patient is. Problems are emphasized, nursing actions are detailed, and all phases of the nursing process are built in. Once you have a mental picture of the concept map's subject and the care you provided, it becomes a great reflection tool. You will be able to reflect on and evaluate all of your skills as you have applied them to direct patient care. Whether you isolate specific skills, such as how you communicated, or consider the overall actions taken, you are applying critical thinking and reinforcing theory for meaningful learning.

Evaluation

The last phase to cover is evaluation. Evaluation has many purposes, as I am sure you are aware now. The main purpose of this phase is a focus on patient outcomes. Not addressing this phase would be akin to providing nursing care and then never looking at how effective or complete that care really was. From this phase evolves nursing actions

Figure 8-36 Example #3: Diabetes.

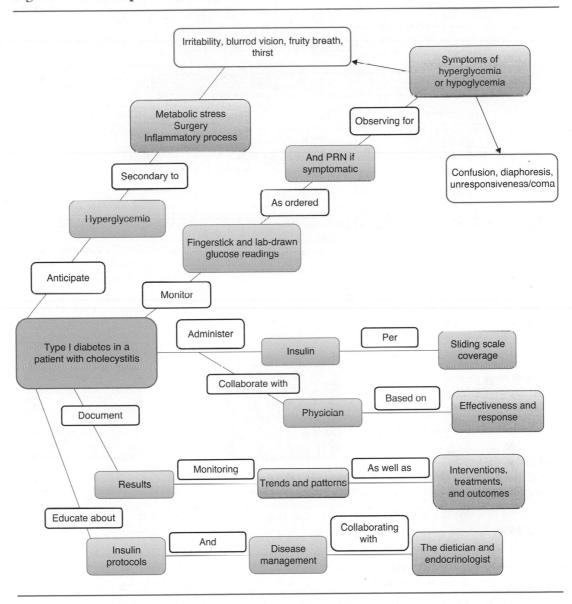

that are repeated or ongoing. Nursing care outcomes stem from specific nursing actions and are studied within nursing research in relation to:

- Readmission rates
- Patient satisfaction
- Complication rates
- Implementation of evidence-based practice
- Maintenance of care standards
- Infection rates

Figure 8-37 Example #4.

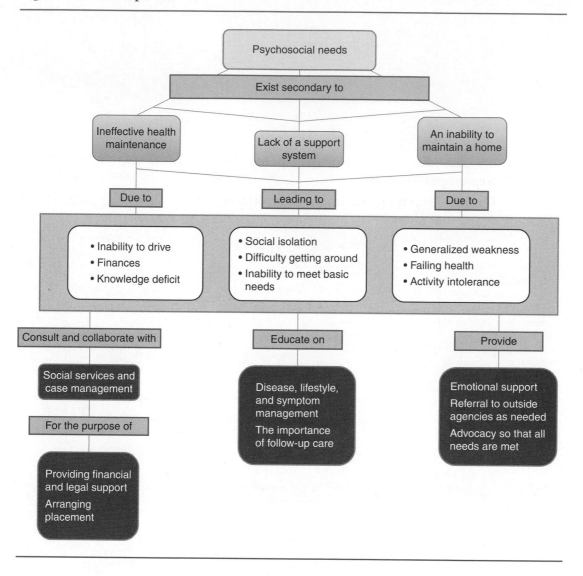

At that point you would reassess the problem or concern and begin following the steps of the nursing process all over again. The plan of care is a constantly changing and ever-evolving plan based on the patient's needs in response to the treatment plan.

If you look back over the problem list for J.S., you would see the following outcomes. Nursing actions may be repeated or continuous, depending on initial outcomes:

- **Cholecystitis**
  1. The patient would proceed through surgery without complications.
  2. J.S.'s pain would be controlled without further dizziness or other adverse reactions.
  3. The pain rating would be an acceptable one to the patient.

4. There would be no occurrence of COPD exacerbation.

5. The patient would be able to perform incentive spirometry and cough and deep breathe effectively.

6. J.S. would demonstrate understanding of splinting.

7. The patient's blood pressure would normalize to his baseline readings.

- **COPD**

  1. The patient's status would not change from baseline.

  2. Oxygen requirements would diminish over time, and J.S. would tolerate weaning to room air.

  3. Oxygen saturation readings and respiratory system base vital signs would remain at this patient's baseline.

  4. The chest x-rays would show no indication of atelectasis or pneumonia.

- **Diabetes**

  1. Blood sugars would be maintained at the patient's baseline.

  2. Only mild fluctuations would be seen with trended results.

  3. Only mild dosing adjustments would be needed to maintain glucose control.

  4. The patient would exhibit no signs of hypoglycemia or hyperglycemia.

And so the evaluation would continue for each problem. This is another reason why I say that all nursing-based actions and thought processes are related and every thing is connected. The assessment and planning phases look at actual and potential problems, alike. Anticipation becomes a key player in identifying and predicting trouble spots toward which your actions are addressed. This is how complications are prevented. Each phase is blended and overlaps with the other. As the plan of care changes, the process repeats until complete resolution, or in any case the best resolutions that can be attained.

Some questions to ask during this phase of care include:

- Has the main problem been identified and addressed?
- Has the healthcare team identified all problems and concerns?
- How has the plan of care changed over time and what caused that change?
- What new problems or areas of concern have surfaced?
- Have all collaborative and holistic concerns been addressed?

Evaluation is also used as a barometer of nursing skills. Applying knowledge through the use of evidence-based practice, critical thinking, and other nursing care standards strongly and directly affects patient outcomes. In this way outcomes reflect care effectiveness. This is where reflection comes in. So many things can influence status and outcomes. Critical thinking is used to continuously review the plan to ensure that all patient needs are identified and addressed. Practice reflection can be used for specific nursing units and an entire facility just as it can for individual care providers.

Summary

You have chosen a noble profession and want to be successful. This chapter has explored additional ways for you to be successful by using concept mapping in all phases of your nursing education. True academic success is always a combination of active and passive learning. The companion piece to teaching is an eagerness to learn and explore, making learning an active experience. This is especially true in light of so many individualized learning and mental processing styles. You need to actively pursue those learning strategies that give meaning to each and every piece of information you need to be successful and competent. Nursing education blends critical thinking with hands-on skills, both of which are necessary in attaining competencies and providing an adequate standard of care. You need to continuously strive for the highest standard attainable.

Using concept mapping for success in studying is an opportunity for you to tailor your learning to your needs. You will be able to clearly see connections and links that will make what you learn "stick." Comprehending theory or skills in this way internalizes knowledge, allowing you to draw on it and reapply it to many other varied situations and circumstances. This type of learning is invaluable to you.

Critical Thinking Questions and Activities

1. Kylie is studying the hematologic system, specifically iron-deficiency anemia. She is having trouble making associations between the symptoms and what is happening pathophysiologically. How can she use concept mapping to enhance her learning?

2. Initiate a discussion regarding proactive learning and its components.

3. Describe what is meant by RECQ and its use and rationale in note taking.

4. Share ideas about what study methods have been successful for you and how you might need to adjust them based on what you have learned from this chapter.

Case Studies

Directions: Read through each case study and answer the questions using the chapter material provided.

1. Ellen wants to try to use a concept map blank copy to take notes during class. Help her to create a template she can easily use. (To use a Concept Map Creator, see the Student Companion Website at http://go.jblearning.com/schmehl.)

2. Review the theory associated with a hip fracture. Create study notes using RECQ, and then answer the following questions:

   a. How is this knowledge applied during an assessment for a suspected fracture?

   b. How does that compare to how it is applied for an actual, confirmed fracture?

   c. What rationales exist between the pathophysiology and your nursing actions?

   d. How does the theory apply to anticipating complications?

    e. What nursing actions accompany this anticipation?

    f. If you still have questions, what resources will you use to answer them?

3. You have admitted a 30-year-old patient with Down syndrome. She lives at home with her parents. Her admitting diagnosis is community-acquired pneumonia. She has been pleasant and cooperative but her mother, who is present, states that the patient has a tendency to act out at times and has difficulty processing information. She normally needs to repeat things multiple times and demonstrate something while explaining it.

    One of her orders is for a Foley catheter placement. The physician has also ordered a chest x-ray.

    a. What patient-related factors need to be considered prior to carrying out both orders?

    b. Outline your approach for educating this patient regarding her care, tests, and procedures.

    c. How would the approach be different for a patient without Down symdrome?

    d. How is it similar?

    e. What equipment-related factors need to be considered?

    f. Identify the collaborative needs this patient has.

    g. Verbalize communication techniques you will need to employ when approaching this patient.

    h. How will all of these considerations affect time management?

4. You are caring for, T.M., a 68-year-old male patient admitted with a ruptured appendix and peritonitis. He has undergone a successful appendectomy and is now 3 days postop. He has been progressing well using morphine for pain—4 mg every 4 hours as needed. T.M. has been receiving the morphine regularly to maintain an acceptable pain level of 4 (on a scale of 1–10) since surgery. This morning during the assessment, T.M. states his "belly doesn't feel right." A focused abdominal assessment reveals a slightly distended lower abdomen with hypoactive bowel sounds in all four quadrants. He states he has not passed any flatus since surgery and feels too full to eat.

    a. What additional information is necessary to fully evaluate the patient's complaint?

    b. What are some differential diagnoses for his complaints?

    c. What are at least three nursing diagnoses you can create for this patient?

    d. What are some nursing actions needed in response to this complaint and status change?

    e. What nursing actions can be anticipated based on this change?

    f. How do both organization and prioritization play a role in your nursing actions?

5. Using Case Study 4, create a problem list for this patient. Create a main list of all problems and then additional lists as needed to identify all relationships.

    a. What connections and links did you establish?

    b. How will you follow up on and evaluate all of your nursing actions related to T.M.'s complaints?

For a full suite of assignments and additional learning activities, use the access code located in the front of your book to visit this exclusive website: http://go.jblearning.com/schmehl. If you do not have an access code you can obtain one at the site.

WWW   For a full suite of assignments and additional learning activities, use the access code located in the front of your book to visit this exclusive website: **http://go.jblearning.com/schmehl**. If you do not have an access code, you can obtain one at the site.

References

Jennings, B. M., Scalzi, C. C., Rodgers, J. D., & Keane, A. (2007). Differentiating nursing leadership and management competencies. *Nursing Outlook, 55*(4), 169–175.

Smith, E. L., Cronenwett, L., & Sherwood, G. (2007). Current assessments of quality and safety education in nursing. *Nursing Outlook, 55*(3), 132–137.

Walsh, T., Jairath, N., Paterson, M. A., & Grandjean, C. (2010). Quality and safety education for nurses clinical evaluation tool. *Journal of Nursing Education, 49*(9), 517–522.

Wilgis, M., & McConnell, J. (2008). Concept mapping: An educational strategy to improve graduate nurses' critical thinking skills during a hospital orientation program. *The Journal of Continuing Education in Nursing, 39*(3), 119–126.

Glossary

Academic performance competencies: course and program competencies to be demonstrated, accomplished, and achieved through written assignments and examinations

Active problems: problems contributing to the current plan of care and that threaten homeostasis

Advanced concept map setup: an extension of basic concept map setup where shape and color differentiation are utilized to refine the map for translation and readability

Brain processing: the brain's ability to accept, categorize, create associations, process, and give meaning and understanding to knowledge input

Clinical performance competencies: course and program competencies to be demonstrated, accomplished, and achieved through patient care in the clinical setting

Computer-generated concept map composition: concept maps composed via use of a computer

Concept map: a diagrammatic teaching and learning tool demonstrating relationship analysis between a main concept and its related concepts; it promotes critical thinking skills

Concept map clarity: the ability to interpret and follow the path of a concept map

Concept map formatting: physical layout of concept map construction to demonstrate critical thinking and relationship analysis

Concept map key: a coded guide to color and shape included on the map to aid in interpretation

Concept map symmetry: balance of the map contents for more organized visual interpretation and appearance

Concept map uniformity: use of one style throughout a concept map for clarity and interpretative ease

Critical thinking: an in-depth thought process utilizing multiple information resources to question, make associations, and analyze data to form conclusions and consider actions and outcomes

Descriptive phrases: phrases used within a concept map to explain interrelationships between and among concepts as well as to denote an action between concepts

Focus-based nursing concept map: concept map composition concentrated on a specific patient care concept

Free-form method of concept map composition: creative concept map composition via sketching or drawing and the use of nonconfigured concept map components

Hand-drawn concept map composition: concept maps composed via use of pencil and paper

History of present illness (HPI): the circumstances surrounding the patient's hospital admission; the symptomatology and events leading the patient to seek medical care

Inactive problems: problems not related or contributing to the current plan of care

Learning continuum: the process of learning that begins with attaining simple knowledge and continues to comprehension and ultimately application

Learning domains: categories of learning skills, behaviors, and outcomes a student must master within the continuum of learning, from simple to complex, comprising the cognitive, affective, and psychomotor spheres

Learning styles: methods through which one is able to effectively comprehend theory for meaningful learning from input related to aural, verbal, written, or visual information

Living concept maps: Concept maps demonstrating multiple, complex interrelationships and actions for in-depth, complex application related to analysis

Main concept: the focal point of a concept map from which all ideas and relationships stem

Nursing-based concept maps: concept maps containing information based on applying nursing knowledge through analysis of skills and nursing care–related actions

Nursing performance competencies: goals set to be accomplished and achieved satisfactorily for successful course and program completion

Objective data: patient information the nurse obtains from patient assessments, behaviors, nonverbal cues

Open copy templates: blank, pre-formatted concept maps adapted to a student's preferences based on learning style and mental processing

Past medical history (PMH): the patient's inclusive past medical history

Past surgical history (PSH): the patient's inclusive past surgical history

Patient problems: a listing of patient concerns contributing to the plan of care as derived from subjective, objective, and related diagnostic data

Practice reflection: the continuous and ongoing action of evaluating nursing knowledge and its application to refine and expand

Primary related concepts: data, information, and ideas that have direct interdependent relationships with the main concept

Process-based nursing concept map: concept map composition concentrated on core processes affecting nursing standards, planning of care, and patient care outcomes

Purpose-based nursing concept map: concept map composition emphasizing components of concept mapping theory as they relate to nursing actions, reasoning, and judgment

Realism: utilization of life-like situations and content in learning

Related concept: any data, information, or idea that has a relationship with the main concept

Related diagnostic data: patient information utilized in formulating nursing diagnoses and planning care, originating from laboratory results, diagnostic testing, procedure outcomes, and treatment responses

Relationship analysis: the process of comparing and contrasting concepts to make associations; interpreting similarities and differences between and among concepts which allows for comprehensive learning

Secondary related concepts: data, information, and ideas that have indirect but interdependent relationships with the main concept

Software-based concept map generator: software designed specifically for concept map composition

Static concept maps: concept maps demonstrating simple interrelationships and concepts for simple application related to knowledge and comprehension

Structured method of concept map composition: creative concept map composition via computer generation and the use of preconfigured concept map components

Subjective data: patient-related information obtained directly from patient statements

Symmetrical concept map formatting: balanced symmetry within a concept map for visual appeal and interpretation

Theory Rationale (related to nursing theory): a statement explaining causation of a disease, symptom, or treatment

Theory to practice application: the action of establishing a knowledge base and enabling utilization of that knowledge to enact practice decisions; providing rationales for decision making in practice

Uniformity (as it applies to concept maps): selective use of shapes and colors with the advanced setup of a concept map

White space: unfilled spaces within pages, lines of text, and words or drawings that aid in separating words, drawings, and ideas

Afterword

As you have found, I am as dedicated to the use of concept mapping in nursing education as I am to the profession itself. I am very excited to present you with this book and would love to know more about your thoughts on this topic, as well as how you have used it and benefitted from that use. I would enjoy hearing from students as well as educators. I think it is essential to network whenever possible and to learn all we can from each other. Please feel free to contact me.

—Pat Schmehl
pksbsn@aol.com

Index